EVERYDAY EATS

EVERY EATS

100 SIMPLE AND HEALTHY RECIPES FOR REAL LIFE

wm
WILLIAM MORROW
An Imprint of HarperCollins*Publishers*

DAY

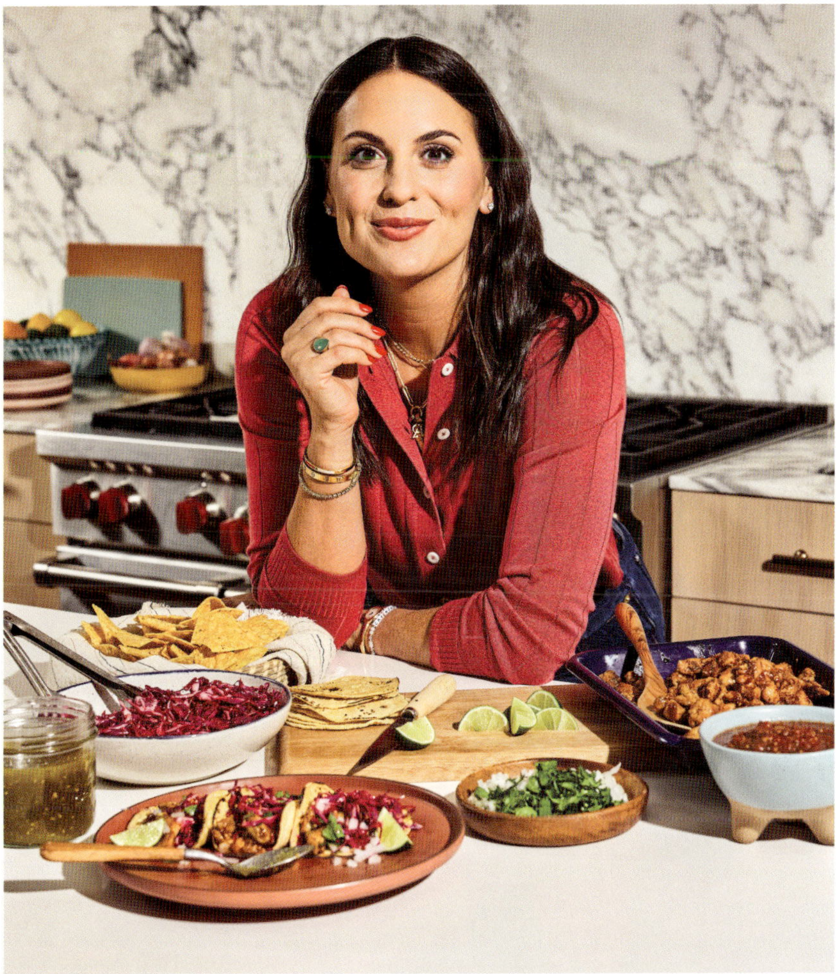

ALEX SNODGRASS

PHOTOGRAPHY BY EVA KOLENKO

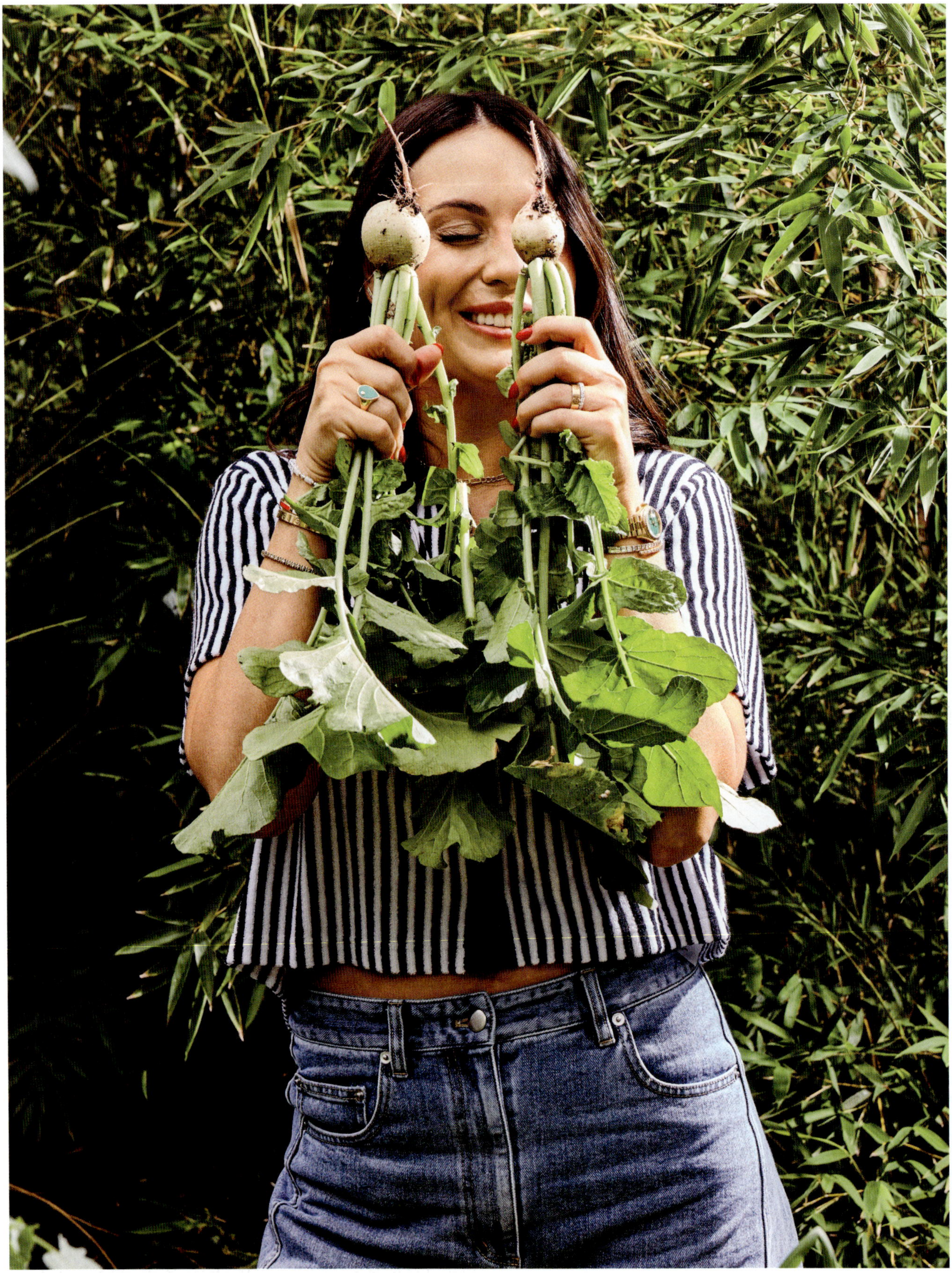

TO MY PARENTS

SOME OF MY FONDEST MEMORIES ARE THOSE MADE AROUND OUR FAMILY TABLE. THANK YOU FOR SHOWING ME THE JOY OF GATHERING THE ONES I LOVE, THE VALUE OF A HOME-COOKED MEAL, AND THE BEAUTY IN EVERYDAY MOMENTS.

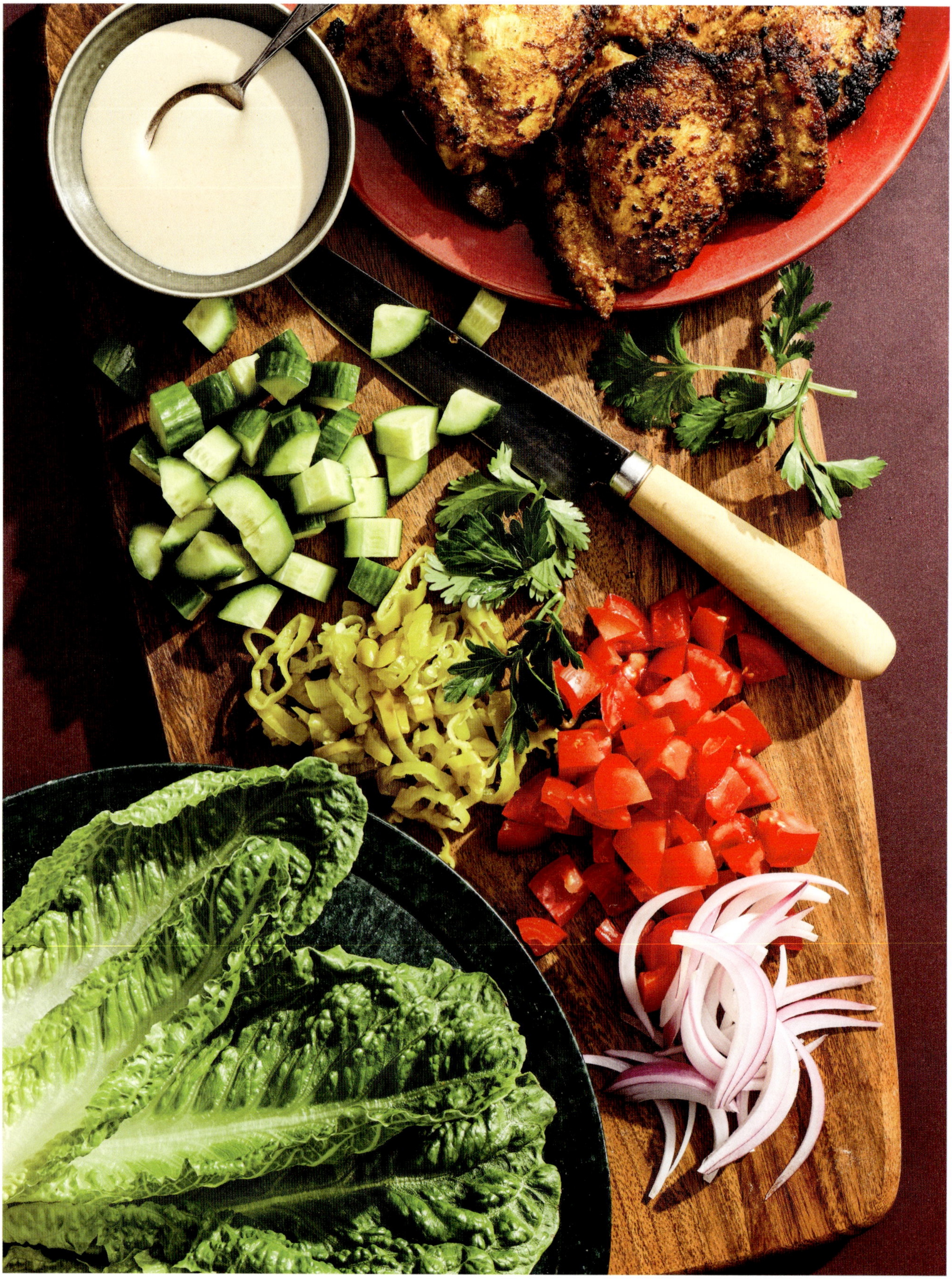

CONTENTS

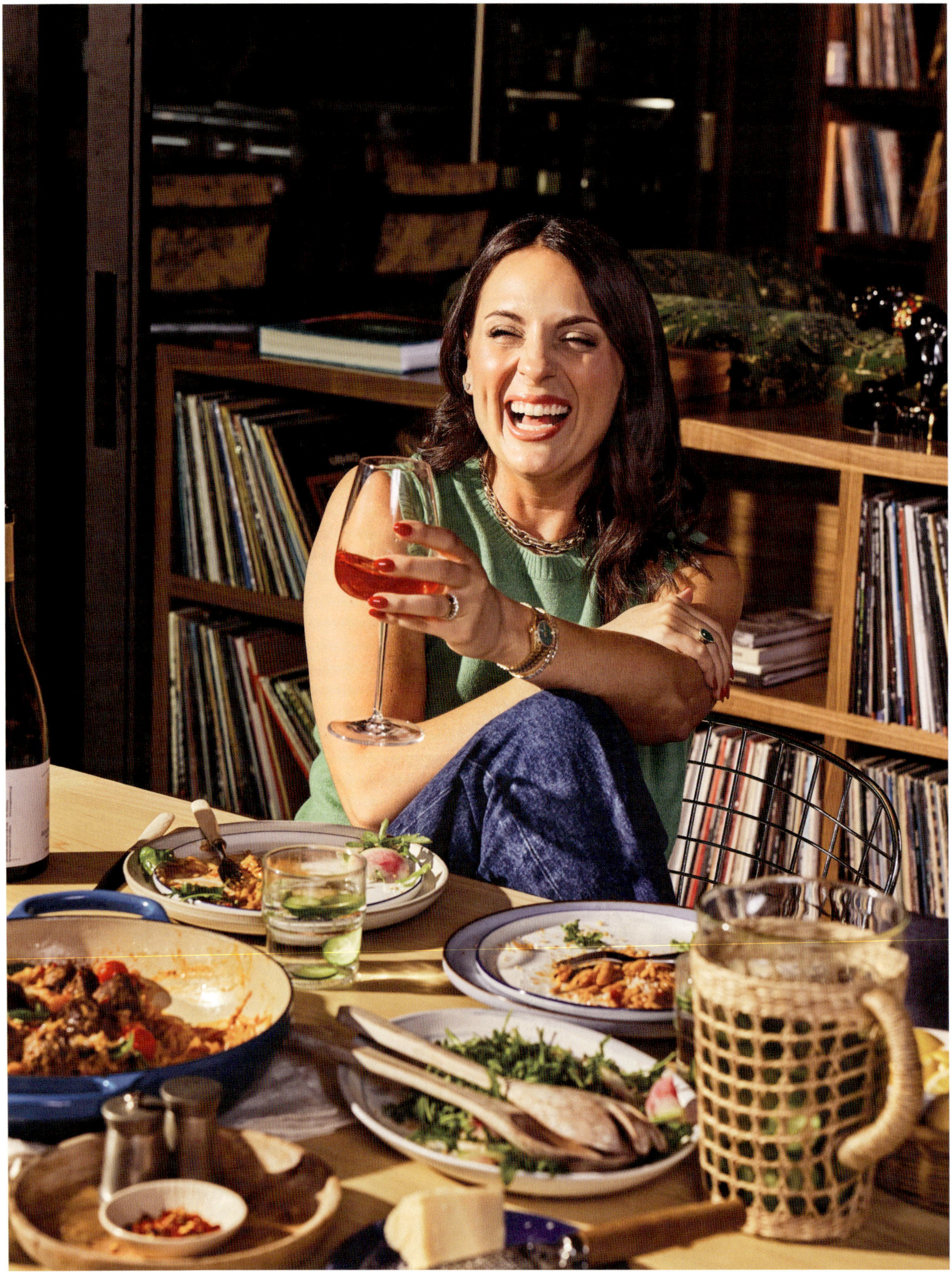

When people ask me why I love cooking and how this whole crazy journey got started, it always brings me right back to my childhood. I've mentioned it in my other books, but it's worth saying again: My favorite memories are in the kitchen with my mom and grandmother, or squeezed around the table with my siblings, laughing and eating.

Since writing my first cookbook, I can hardly believe how everything has unfolded. The gratitude I feel when someone tells me my recipes have changed the way they cook makes my heart absolutely burst. Writing these books has become the pride and joy of my business—and every single day, I'm grateful I get to keep doing it.

Meanwhile, I blink, and my kids are growing up right before my eyes. So when it came time to dream up book number four, I'll admit: The ideas in my mind began to run a little wild. I felt like it was time to do something . . . different.

And while this book is a little different, I've stuck to my roots. My goal? To inspire you. To make cooking feel doable, joyful, and worth gathering around your table for. This is a book for the everyday. The mornings that start fast, the lunches you actually look forward to, and the dinners that are there for you when life is full. Maybe it's the Slow Cooker or Pressure Cooker BBQ Beef Lettuce Wraps (page 169) after soccer practice, or maybe it's my 20-Minute Wonton Soup (page 80) after a long day. Whatever your day looks like, these recipes are here to carry you through.

FIND JOY IN THE EVERYDAY

When I was growing up in a small town, dining out wasn't really an option without a bit of a drive. My mom, who worked full-time (and still does!), always managed to get dinner on the table. Sure, she had her "famous" lasagna, but most nights she kept things super simple and weeknight-friendly—ground beef tacos and Hamburger Helper were on regular rotation. It wasn't anything extravagant, but it brought us to the table and fed us, and no one complained. I always remind myself of this fact. It's easy to get caught up in making meals feel impressive or picture-perfect, but some of the best family dinners are the simplest ones. The real magic is just in showing up and feeding the people you love.

I'm in a season of motherhood where the more elaborate recipes are reserved for Sundays or special occasions. Between running my business and keeping up with my two kids—now thirteen and ten—life feels busier than ever, with school events, after-school activities, and all the social commitments. For the first time in a long time, I'm leaning harder on pantry staples and becoming more efficient by sticking with quick and easy meals. But for me, quick and easy never means boring. My versions of simple meals still leave me feeling excited and satisfied in the kitchen. More importantly, they get us around the dinner table. That part matters most. Even in the chaos, carving out those moments to pause, connect, and enjoy a meal together brings a kind of satisfaction that goes well beyond what's on the plate.

This book wasn't just created with my current season of life in mind—it was shaped by your feedback, too. You asked for even simpler, faster recipes for busy weeknights, and I'm here to deliver. When I was developing this book, I focused on streamlined techniques like skillet dinners and sheet pan wonders, and I kept ingredient lists as short as possible—without ever compromising on flavor.

More than ever I found myself asking: What can I cook with what I already have? If there was half a can of chipotles in adobo or a spoonful of red curry paste in the fridge, I challenged myself to use it up in a fresh, creative way. I leaned into pantry staples, aiming to make the most of what was on hand and keeping things practical, resourceful, and still full of flavor.

Whether you're a confident home cook who needs some easy-breezy dinner ideas for the middle of a crazy week or you're just starting to find your groove in the kitchen, this book was made with you in mind. Each recipe is designed to guide you in the kitchen without overwhelming you and, most importantly, to actually fit into your real life.

Because let's be honest: With all the hustle and bustle, it's way too easy to lose sight of the magic in the everyday. Cherish dinnertime. Reconnect. Share a laugh. Put your phone down! I am constantly reminding myself of these very lessons that we can all easily forget. I believe the ritual of dinnertime is an art we can't just let die. It's the glue that connects us to each other—to our families, our friends, our people, ourselves.

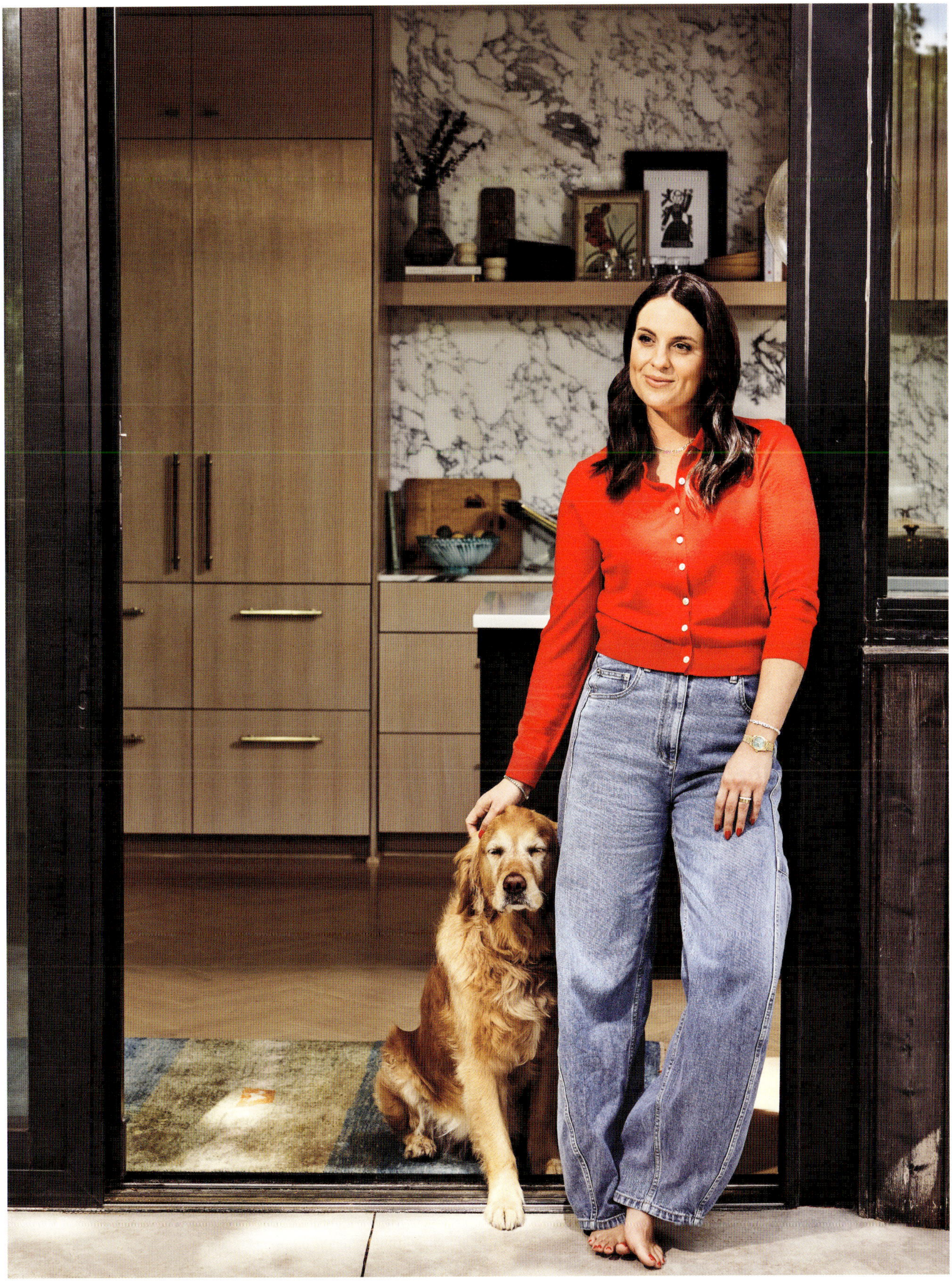

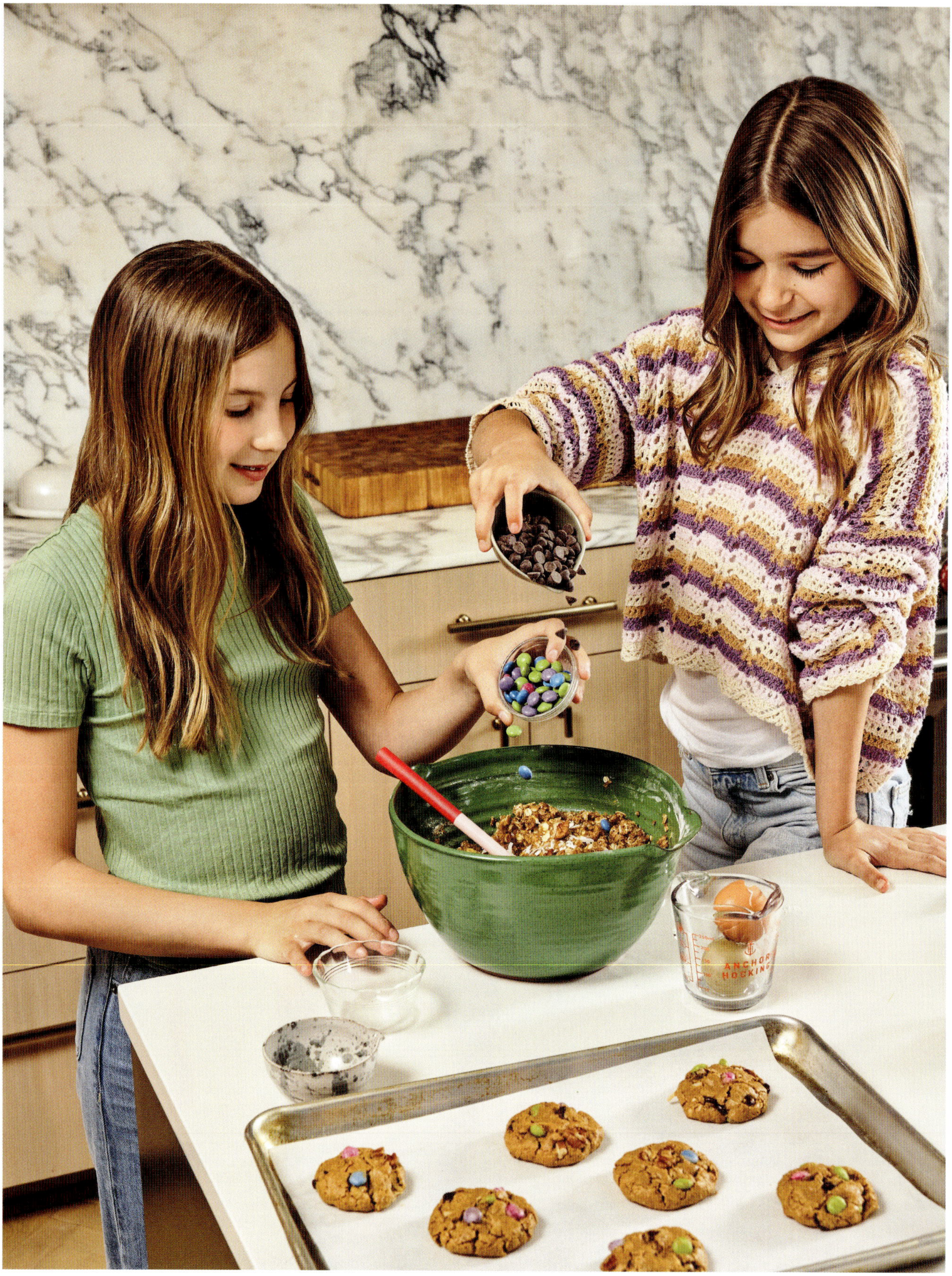
ANCHOR HOCKING

This book is here to help you romanticize your everyday just a little more—with recipes designed for less thinking, fewer dishes, fewer ingredients, and way less stress so you can slam a stunning meal like Skillet French Onion Chicken with Mushrooms (page 145) down on the table and watch your people dive in. Trust me: That moment is pure magic.

And hey (plot twist!)—this time I even added a breakfast chapter! Cue the confetti! With easy, make-ahead breakfasts you can prep on a Sunday, you'll start your day with a wholesome meal while making the week feel a little less hectic.

Now, while this isn't a full-blown meal-prep book, if you appreciate a little plan-ahead magic or just want something nourishing and ready to grab, I've labeled options throughout that are great for meal prep. From nourishing breakfasts to protein-packed grab-and-go items like my Classic Tuna Salad (page 62) and more, there are a variety of recipes that can set you up for success during the week.

This book is designed to guide you through your everyday. Wake up and reheat two Bacon Gruyère Egg Cups (page 23) before walking out the door. Pop open that Italian Deli Chicken Salad (page 46) at your desk and bask in the joy of knowing you already prepped lunch on Sunday. And after a full day, come home and make the One-Pot Chicken Marsala Orzo (page 113) for dinner. It's all doable. It gives you space to be intentional about how you're fueling your body in a way that's both realistic and creative.

Bottom line, this book isn't just about the food—it's about creating a little space in the everyday chaos. It's about sitting down, looking around the table at the people you love, and feeling grateful that you made the time for one another. Because dinner doesn't have to be fancy to matter. It doesn't have to be complicated to be memorable. It just has to happen. And if I can help you make it happen a little more often and with a little more ease, a little more laughter, and a whole lot of flavor, then I'll consider this book a job well done.

Thank you for picking up this book. I hope it brings a little extra joy to your everyday.

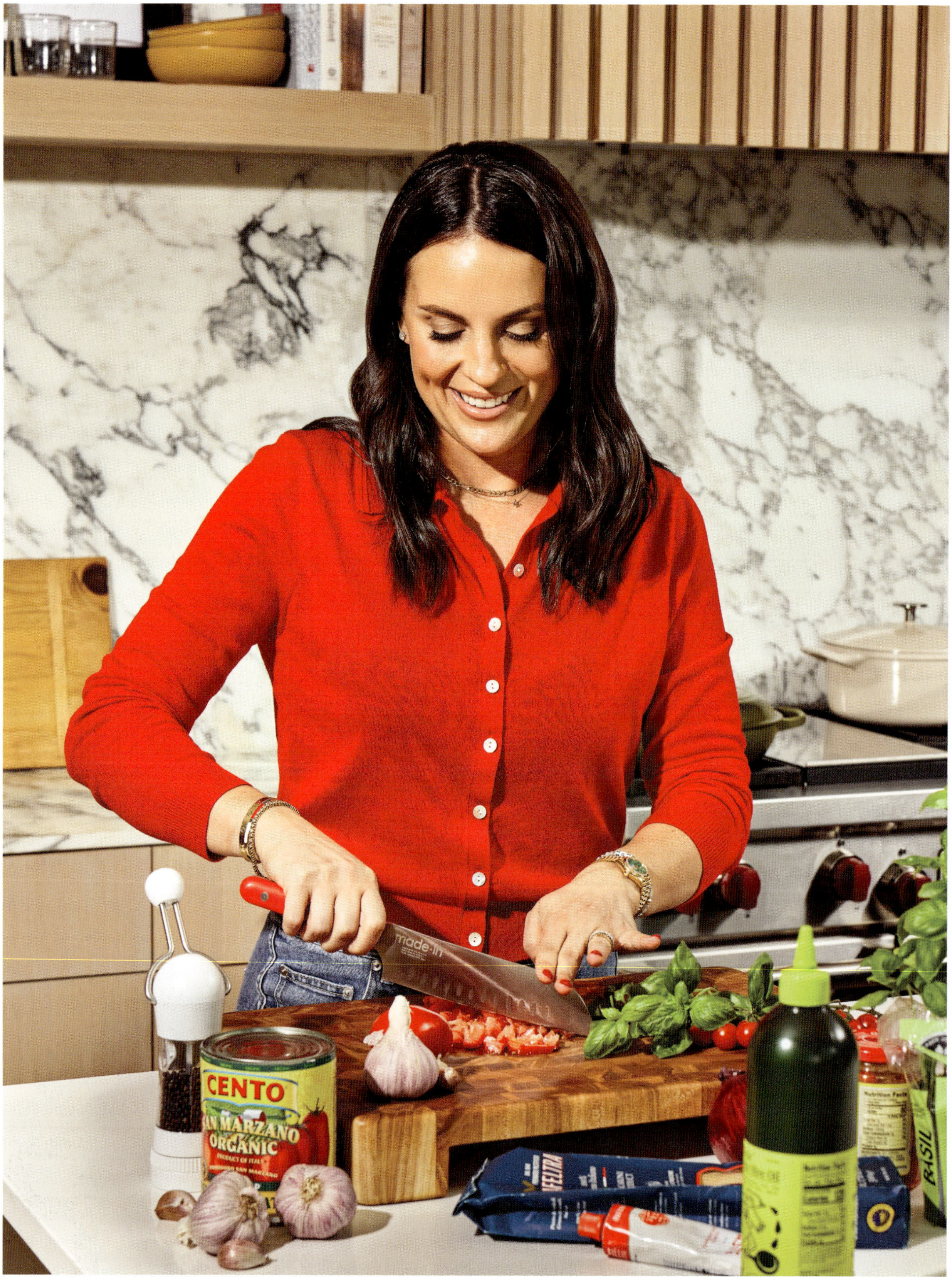
made in
CENTO
ORGANIC
BASIL

MY 5 TIPS FOR A SUCCESSFUL WEEK

On Sundays, I love to take a little time to set myself up for a smoother, more successful week. Here are my best tips to help you stay on top of meals for the week ahead.

1. FRIDGE CHECK AND INVENTORY

First things first, take stock of your fridge. Toss anything that's gone bad and give the shelves a quick wipe down; it only takes five minutes and will keep things from getting out of hand. Then take inventory of what you already have and plan around those ingredients.

Have half a head of cabbage? Make my Shortcut Chicken Pozole Verde (page 94) or Skillet Unstuffed Cabbage Rolls (page 200). An open jar of red curry paste? Add my Chicken Khao Soi–Inspired Soup (page 87) or Thai Red Curry Shrimp Noodles (page 110) to the menu. As you flip through this book, look out for my notes on leftover ingredients—they're there to make your planning even easier!

2. MENU PLANNING

Speaking of planning, I use a weekly meal planner to map out our dinners. On Sunday mornings, I sit down with a cup of coffee and look at what the week holds. I jot down what I'm making for dinner each night and prop it up like a little menu in my kitchen to keep me on track. It also saves me from answering the ever-present question "What's for dinner?" from my family. For busy days, like an event or a track meet, I'll plug in a super-quick stir-fry, like my Honey-Orange Pork and Snap Pea Stir-Fry (page 170) or a slow cooker recipe, like my Slow Cooker or Pressure Cooker Chicken, Lime, and Avocado Soup (page 91), so dinner doesn't add to the chaos.

SUNDAY SETUP

3. LIGHT MEAL PREP

I'm not a big-batch cook, but I do like to prep a few things to take pressure off during the week. Breakfasts are big for me, so I love having items like my Freezer-Friendly Mediterranean Breakfast Sandwiches (page 32) ready to go. I also like to have one nutrient-dense lunch option prepped, like a soup or a hearty salad, so I can grab and go. I have marked the recipes in this book that are great for making ahead so that you can easily find them!

4. MISE EN PLACE

In addition to planning the weekly menu, I use Sundays to take care of a few key tasks to lighten the load for the days ahead. One of the most impactful things I do is a bit of mise en place—a French culinary term that means "everything in its place."

This might include chopping vegetables, marinating proteins, washing herbs, or preparing sauces in advance. These small, simple steps help create a smoother flow during busy weeknights when time is limited and energy is low. A little organization up front truly makes home cooking feel more manageable and even more enjoyable.

5. MAKE IT WORK FOR YOU

Here's your permission slip: It's totally okay to write DINNER OUT on your weekly menu. Your time and energy matter . . . preserve them! One of the biggest mistakes I see people make is overcommitting and burning out. If you're new to cooking, start small. Aim for two or three home-cooked meals a week. That's plenty. Once you're in a groove, you can build from there. This is about loving your time in the kitchen, not dreading it.

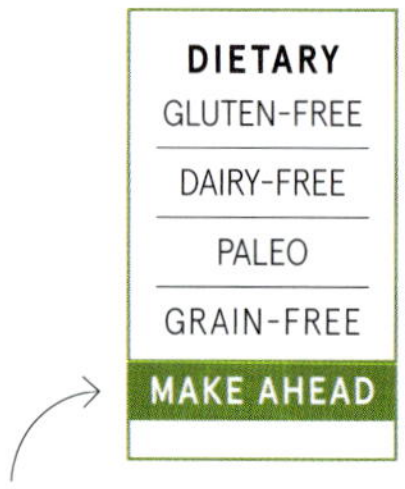

Need meals you can prep in advance? Look for this icon on recipes that are make-ahead approved!

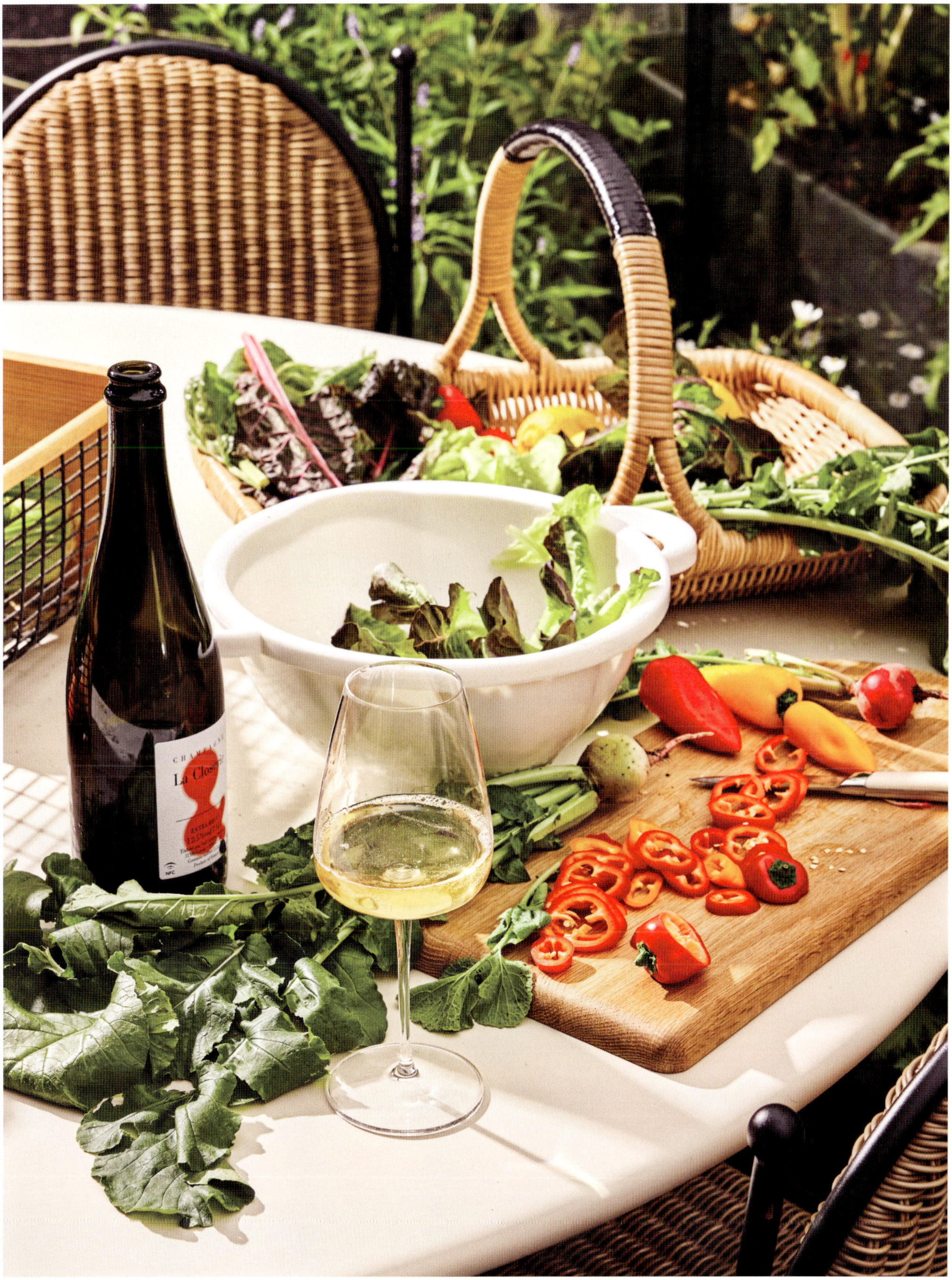

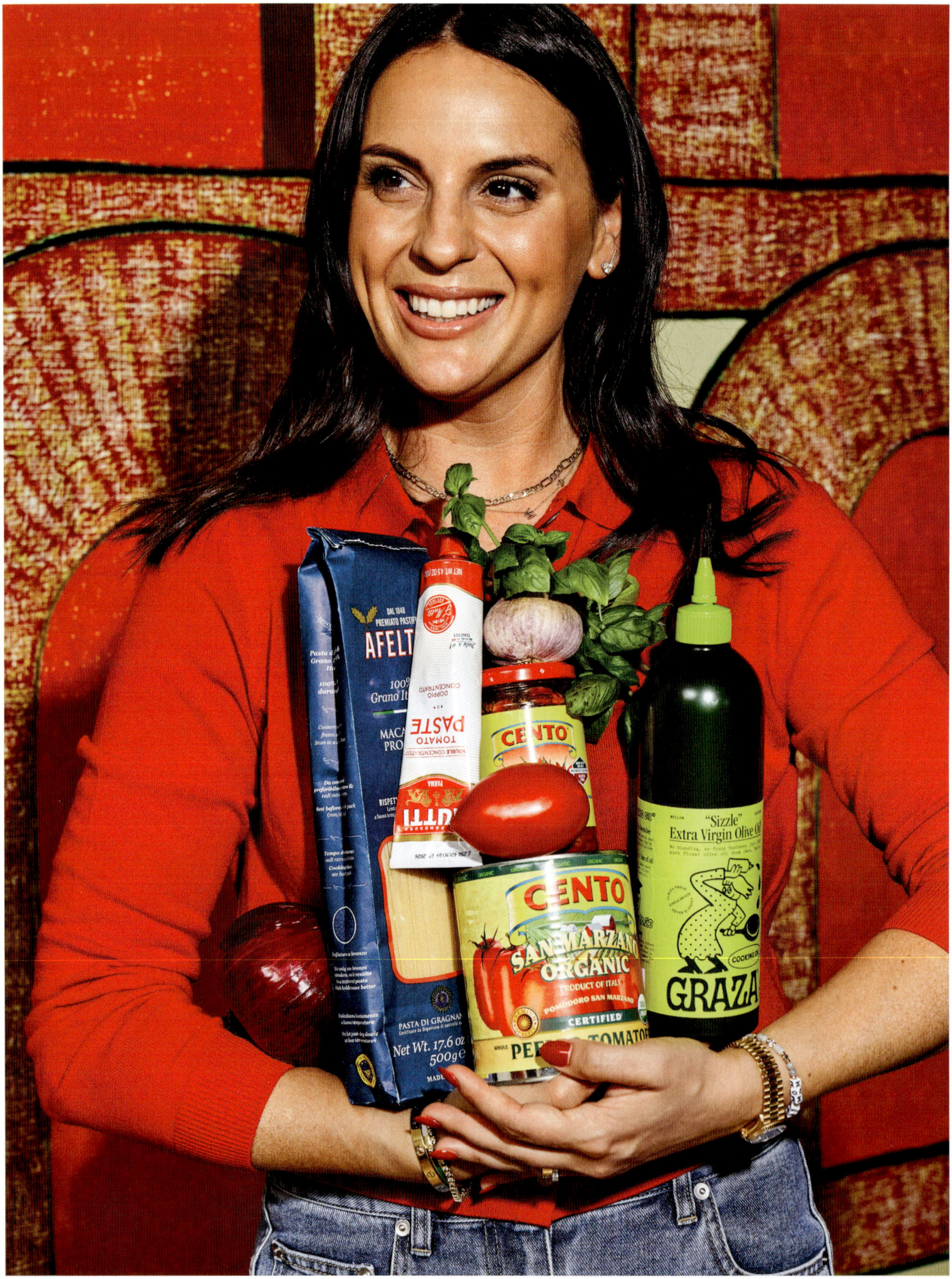
CENTO
SAN MARZANO
ORGANIC
PRODUCT OF ITALY
CERTIFIED
"Sizzle"
Extra Virgin Olive Oil
GRAZA
PASTA DI GRAGNANO
Net Wt. 17.6 oz
500g

STOCK THE PANTRY

As you cook your way through this book, you'll notice that a well-stocked pantry is your best friend. Having these staples on hand makes weeknight dinners so much easier because you won't be running to the store for every little ingredient, and you can pull together something delicious at a moment's notice. Once you've built up your pantry, you'll find your grocery runs are lighter, your stress levels are lower, and you'll feel a whole lot more confident whipping up dinner with what you've got. Think of this list as the building blocks for flavorful, fuss-free cooking.

BEANS AND LEGUMES

- Black-eyed peas
- Brown lentils
- Cannellini beans
- Chickpeas

CONDIMENTS, SAUCES, AND PASTES

- Avocado oil mayonnaise
- Barbecue sauce
- Buffalo sauce
- Chili crisp or chili oil
- Chipotle chiles in adobo
- Chopped Calabrian peppers
- Coconut aminos
- Enchilada sauce (red and green)
- Fish sauce
- Gochujang
- Green curry paste
- Mild diced green chiles
- Mild harissa paste
- Miso paste
- Mustard (Dijon, yellow, whole-grain Dijon)
- Salsa verde
- Sriracha
- Tamari
- Thai red curry paste

DRIED SPICES AND HERBS

- Allspice
- Bay leaves
- Black peppercorns
- Cayenne pepper
- Chili powder
- Chipotle powder
- Curry powder
- Dried oregano
- Dried rosemary
- Dried thyme
- Garam masala
- Garlic powder
- Ground coriander
- Ground cumin
- Ground ginger
- Herbes de Provence
- Italian seasoning
- Kosher salt
- Mustard powder
- Paprika
- Red pepper flakes
- Saffron threads
- Smoked paprika
- Turmeric

EXTRACTS

- Pure almond extract
- Pure vanilla extract

FLOURS AND STARCHES

- Almond flour
- Arrowroot flour
- Baking powder
- Baking soda
- Cassava flour
- Gluten-free panko breadcrumbs
- Tapioca flour

GRAINS AND PASTA

- Barley
- Farro
- Israeli or pearl couscous
- Pasta (spaghetti, linguine, fusilli, orzo, rigatoni, bowtie)
- Quinoa
- Rice (basmati, brown)
- Rice noodles

NUTS AND SEEDS

- Black sesame seeds
- Cashews
- Peanuts
- Pistachios
- Walnuts
- White sesame seeds

OILS

- Avocado oil
- Extra-virgin olive oil
- Liquid coconut oil
- Toasted sesame oil

PICKLES AND OLIVES

- Capers
- Castelvetrano olives
- Kalamata olives
- Peperoncini
- Pickled jalapeños

SWEETENERS

- Coconut sugar
- Honey
- Pure maple syrup

TINNED FISH

- Albacore or skipjack tuna
- Anchovy paste

TOMATO PRODUCTS

- Crushed tomatoes
- Diced tomatoes
- Fire-roasted diced tomatoes
- Sun-dried tomatoes (packed in oil)
- Tomato paste
- Whole peeled tomatoes

VINEGARS

- Apple cider vinegar
- Balsamic vinegar
- Red wine vinegar
- Rice vinegar
- White wine vinegar

OTHER PANTRY ESSENTIALS

- Low-sodium beef broth
- Low-sodium chicken broth
- Unsweetened full-fat coconut milk

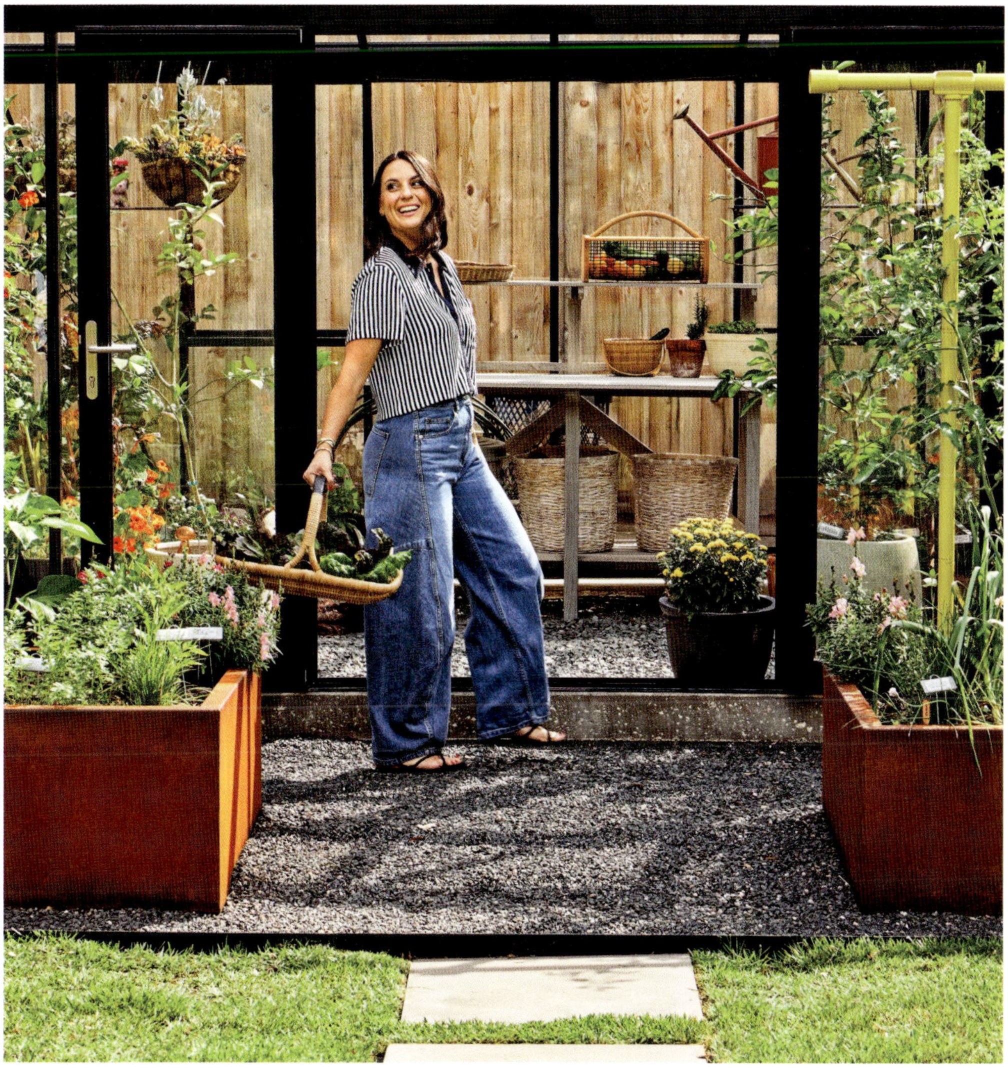

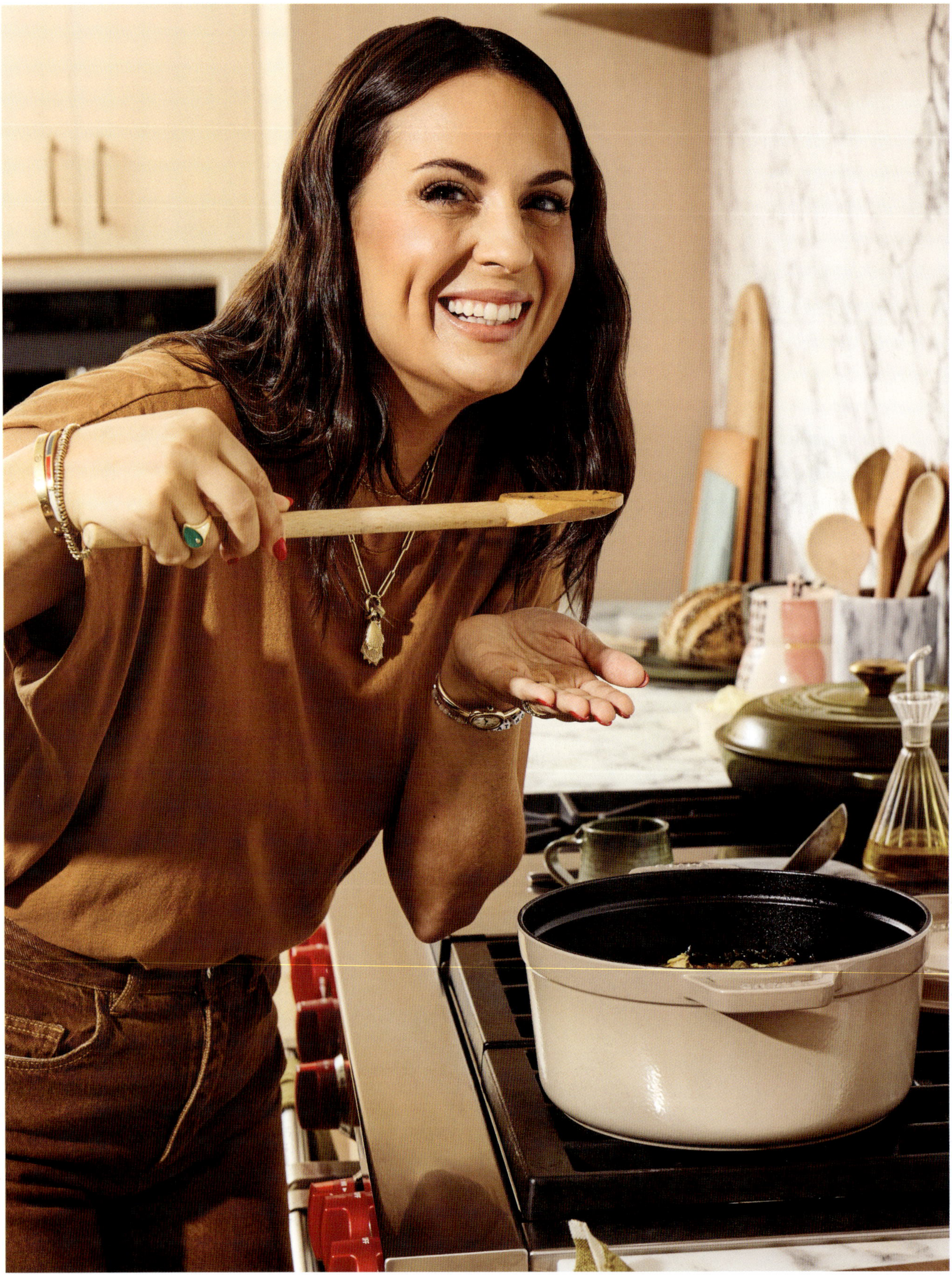

Cooking is so much easier (and more fun!) when you've got the right tools at your fingertips. This isn't about having every gadget under the sun; it's about a handful of essentials that really make a difference in the kitchen. These are the pots, pans, and small tools I rely on every day to keep meals stress-free and delicious. A few are true investments, others are simple basics, but together they'll set you up for success no matter what you're cooking.

BRAISER: When it comes to skillet dinners, my 3.5-quart braiser is one of my most-used pans. The wide base, tall sides, and fitted top are perfect for braising saucy dishes, shallow-frying, or building a one-pan meal complete with a grain and protein. It's oven-safe, versatile, and beautiful enough to take from the stovetop to the table. It's an investment piece, but an absolutely timeless one.

CAST-IRON SKILLET: Talk about versatile. A cast-iron skillet can sear steaks, bake cornbread, roast chicken, or even make a Skillet Peach Crumble (page 230). It holds heat wonderfully and lasts forever with proper care—a well-seasoned skillet only gets better with age. Think of it as an heirloom in the making.

TOOLS OF THE TRADE

COLANDERS: Simple but essential, colanders make draining pasta, washing produce, and rinsing beans a whole lot easier. I like to keep both a large colander and a small mesh strainer around—they cover just about every draining or rinsing task you'll come across.

CUTTING BOARDS: A reliable, sturdy cutting board is one of the most-used items in any kitchen. I like to keep a few on hand in various sizes and materials as they are being used in constant rotation for everyday chopping, prepping, and more.

DIGITAL SCALE: I'm not the kind of baker who carefully measures every gram of flour—I'm not that sophisticated. But I do love having a digital scale around. It's great for portioning proteins (like cutting a fish into even fillets), weighing grains, or measuring out ingredients when you really need precision. It's small, inexpensive, and one of those tools you'll be glad to have on hand.

DUTCH OVEN: A 5-quart Dutch oven is the workhorse of my kitchen. It's ideal for soups, stews, roasts, and bread baking, and it retains heat well. The 5-quart size is big enough for most family meals without being bulky, making it a sweet spot for everyday cooking.

FOOD PROCESSOR: This is a wonderfully versatile tool to have in the kitchen. It helps to quickly create sauces, dips, and dressings, but it's also fantastic for pulsing nuts, oats, or flours into a coarse, crumbly texture for desserts like my Cowboy Cookies (page 241) or Baklava-Inspired Energy Bites (page 233). You can also use it to shred or slice veggies in seconds!

HIGH-SPEED BLENDER: For silky smoothies, soups, or nut-based sauces, a good blender is worth every penny. I love a large-batch, high-speed blender because it can handle anything you throw at it. For smaller quantities or quick sauces, I reach for my bullet blender, as it's compact and easy to clean.

IMMERSION BLENDER: This is forever a top-notch kitchen must-have. From quickly blending soups right in the pot to making creamy dressings and sauces without dragging out a big appliance, an immersion blender is all about convenience. It's one of those tools you don't realize you need until you have one and can't imagine life without it.

INSTANT-READ THERMOMETER: While not an essential, this tool is a game changer if you ever second-guess whether something is cooked through. An instant-read thermometer takes all the guesswork out of cooking—no more poking or cutting into meat to "check." With quick, accurate readings every time, it gives you confidence and ensures perfectly cooked results.

TEMPERATURES FOR COOKING PROTEINS

POULTRY: 165°F
FISH: 135–145°F (depending on the type of fish and desired doneness)
LAMB: 125–130°F for medium-rare (cook longer for medium and above)
PORK: 145°F (followed by a 3-minute rest; it will rise slightly in temp)
BEEF: 125–130°F for medium-rare; 135–145°F for medium

KNIVES: A sharp chef's knife is the most essential tool in any kitchen. You truly don't need a huge set—just a reliable chef's knife, a serrated knife, and a small paring knife will cover almost all your needs. Keep them sharp, and cooking becomes safer, faster, and much more enjoyable.

LOAF PANS: For recipes like my Morning Glory Loaf (page 35), a sturdy loaf pan is handy to have around. I recommend keeping at least two so you can bake a double batch when you need to. Look for heavy-duty pans that bake evenly and won't warp over time.

MIXING BOWLS: A good set of mixing bowls is essential. I like a stackable assortment of glass or metal bowls in small, medium, and large sizes so I'm covered whether I'm whisking a quick dressing, tossing a salad, or mixing up cookie dough. They nest neatly for storage, and having the right size on hand always makes prep easier.

NONSTICK SKILLETS AND PANS: I recommend keeping at least one large nonstick pan in your kitchen for those foods that just love to cling, like eggs, pancakes, or even a quick stir-fry. They make cooking (and cleanup) so much easier. And if you're newer to the kitchen and feel most comfortable cooking everything in nonstick instead of stainless steel, go for it! Whatever makes you feel confident in the kitchen is the right choice.

RICE COOKER: As a busy mom with rice as an everyday staple in our house, I love having a rice cooker around. It takes all the guesswork out and delivers perfectly fluffy rice every single time. I also appreciate that I can focus on the main course while the rice cooker does the work. Many models handle other grains like quinoa or farro, and most will keep rice warm until you're ready to eat. It may not be essential for everyone, but if you cook rice often, it's a huge convenience.

SHEET PANS: Sheet pans are the unsung heroes of the kitchen. From roasting vegetables to baking cookies or building easy one-pan dinners, they get used constantly. I recommend keeping a couple of half sheet pans (the most common size at 18 × 13 inches) and at least one quarter sheet pan (9½ × 13 inches). The quarter sheet pans aren't just for baking—they're perfect during prep mode for dredging chicken, holding prepped ingredients, and more. Look for heavy-duty uncoated aluminum. They bake evenly and hold up well over time.

SILICONE MUFFIN PAN: If you're tired of muffins sticking, this pan will change your life. Muffins and recipes like my Bacon Gruyère Egg Cups (page 23) pop right out without fuss, and cleanup is a breeze. I still love a classic metal muffin tin, but the silicone version is lightweight, flexible, and a nice addition to your bakeware lineup.

SLOW COOKER OR PRESSURE COOKER: Both of these appliances are about hands-off cooking. A slow cooker is wonderful for soups, stews, and braises you want to set in the morning and come home to at night—it's a tried-and-true classic for low and slow cooking. The pressure cooker can yield similar results as the slow cooker in a much quicker way—plus you can even sauté in it. Which one you choose really depends on your style. For me, the slow cooker is the reliable staple I reach for most, while the pressure cooker is a versatile option if you're more of a gadget person and want your finished meal faster.

STAINLESS STEEL SKILLETS AND PANS: These are true workhorses. Stainless steel skillets give you a great sear and transition seamlessly from stovetop to oven. They're not nonstick, but with a little practice, you'll find they cook more evenly and last a lifetime.

STAND MIXER OR HAND MIXER: Both of these have their place in the kitchen, and your best option will depend on your space and how often you bake. A stand mixer is a kitchen powerhouse for kneading dough, whipping meringues, or mixing big batches of cake batter. Plus, it frees up your hands while it does the work. A hand mixer, on the other hand, is lightweight, affordable, and perfect for quick batters, whipped cream, or smaller jobs. If you bake often, the stand mixer is worth the investment; if not, a trusty hand mixer will cover your bases.

TWEEZER TONGS: Think of these as an extension of your hands. They give you the precision to flip delicate scallops, grab pasta from boiling water, or plate food with finesse. Once you start using them, you'll wonder how you ever managed with just big clunky tongs. Every time I use these on Instagram or TikTok I get asked what they are and where to find them!

SMALLER TOOLS

- Bench scraper
- Box grater
- Can opener
- Citrus juicer or reamer
- Fish spatula
- Garlic press (or garlic rocker)
- Kitchen shears
- Ladle
- Large tongs
- Measuring cups
- Measuring spoons
- Microplane
- Pastry brush
- Peeler (Y-peeler or swivel)
- Rolling pin
- Silicone spatulas
- Slotted spoon
- Small offset spatula
- Spider strainer
- Whisks
- Wooden spoons

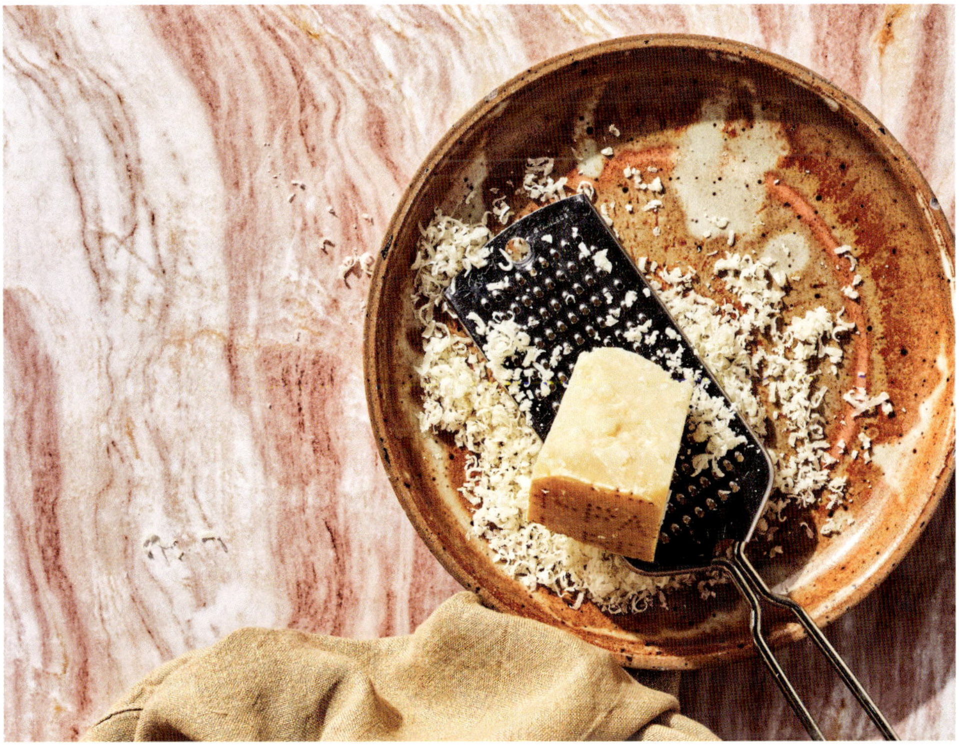

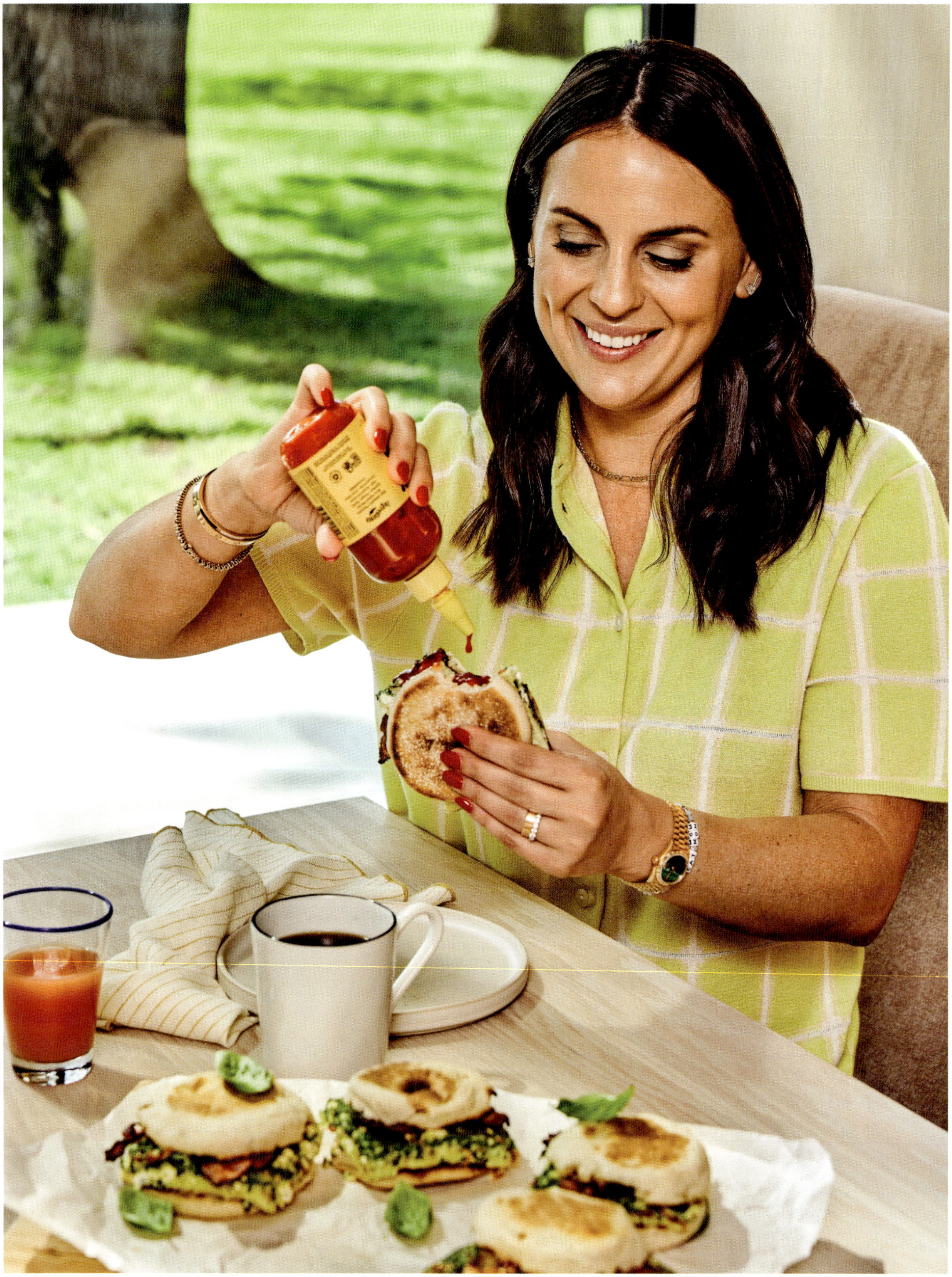

MAKE-AHEAD BREAKFASTS

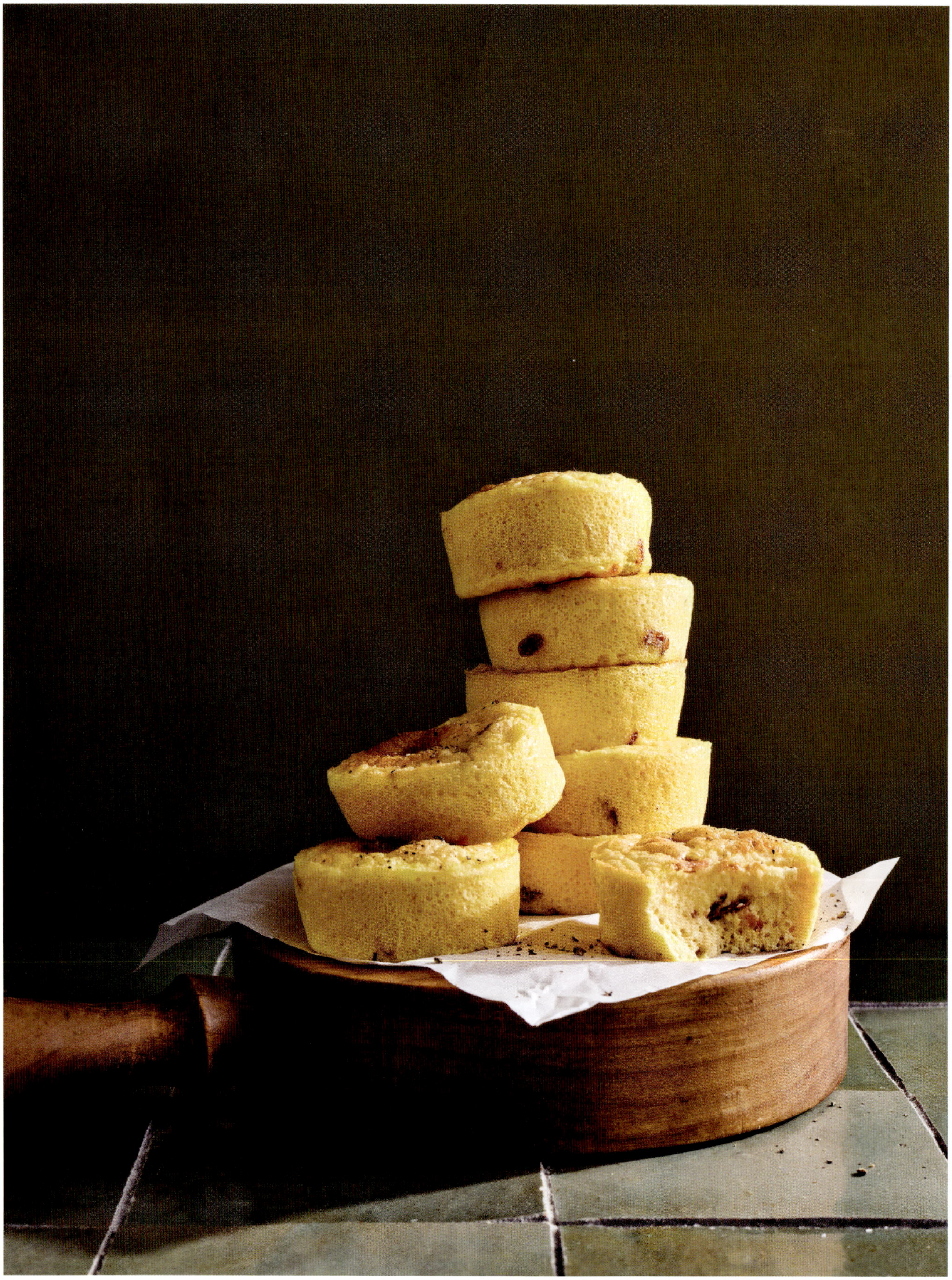

BACON GRUYÈRE EGG CUPS

MAKES 12 CUPS | **TOTAL TIME:** 30 MINUTES

DIETARY
GLUTEN-FREE
GRAIN-FREE
MAKE AHEAD

When I'm traveling, one of my go-to airport or road trip breakfasts is the Starbucks Bacon & Gruyère Egg Bites. Inspired by those flavors, I've crafted a homemade version that's perfect for busy mornings—a protein-packed, make-ahead delight. Simple to whip up and ideal for those on-the-go moments!

- Nonstick cooking spray
- 4 slices no-sugar-added bacon
- 10 large eggs
- ¾ cup whole-milk cottage cheese
- ¾ cup shredded Gruyère cheese
- 1 teaspoon kosher salt
- ½ teaspoon freshly ground black pepper
- ½ teaspoon garlic powder
- 1 teaspoon hot sauce

PREHEAT the oven to 375°F. Lightly grease a silicone 12-cup muffin pan with nonstick cooking spray. Place the silicone pan on a sheet pan. This will make it easier to transfer to the oven without spilling. (See note for muffin pan tips.)

LINE a plate with paper towels. In a large nonstick skillet, cook the bacon over medium heat until crisp, 3 to 4 minutes per side. Using tongs, transfer the bacon to the prepared plate.

ALLOW the bacon to cool enough to handle, then dice into very small pieces. Evenly divide the bacon among the prepared muffin cups.

IN a high-speed blender or food processor, combine the eggs, cottage cheese, Gruyère, salt, pepper, garlic powder, and hot sauce. Blend until smooth.

EVENLY distribute the egg mixture over the bacon bits until each muffin cup is about three-quarters of the way full.

TRANSFER to the oven and bake until the eggs have just set, taking care not to overcook them, about 15 minutes. The egg bites might puff up slightly, but they will deflate as they cool.

REMOVE from the oven and let cool in the pan for 5 minutes.

ONCE cool, carefully loosen the edges of each bite using a mini-silicone spatula or butter knife, then lift them out. Place leftover egg bites in an airtight container (in the fridge) for up to 3 days or in the freezer for up to 2 months. See note for reheating instructions.

FROM MY KITCHEN TO YOURS

MUFFIN PAN TIPS: I like to use a silicone muffin pan for this recipe to prevent the eggs from sticking. If you do not have a silicone muffin pan, you can use a classic metal muffin pan. Just be sure to spray the muffin cups generously with nonstick cooking spray.

REHEATING INSTRUCTIONS: If warming from the fridge, reheat in the microwave until just warm, about 60 seconds. If warming from frozen, defrost in the fridge overnight, then reheat using the microwave.

EASY BANANA NUT MUFFINS

MAKES 12 MUFFINS | **TOTAL TIME:** 35 MINUTES

DIETARY
- GLUTEN-FREE
- GRAIN-FREE
- DAIRY-FREE
- PALEO
- VEGETARIAN
- **MAKE AHEAD**

You know how some people turn their noses up at paleo treats? Well, these banana nut muffins are here to change minds! Seriously, they're some of the tastiest muffins out there. They're easy to make, packed with wholesome goodness, and downright delicious. In just thirty-five minutes, you'll have yourself a batch of these ready to enjoy with your morning coffee.

- 1 cup mashed overripe bananas (about 3 medium bananas)
- ½ cup pure maple syrup
- 2 large eggs
- ¼ cup liquid coconut oil (see note)
- 2 teaspoons pure vanilla extract
- 1½ teaspoons ground cinnamon
- ¼ teaspoon kosher salt
- 1½ cups almond flour
- 1 cup tapioca flour
- 2 teaspoons baking powder
- ½ teaspoon baking soda
- ¾ cup chopped walnuts, divided

PREHEAT the oven to 350°F. Line a 12-cup muffin pan with muffin liners.

IN a large bowl, combine the mashed banana, maple syrup, eggs, coconut oil, and vanilla extract. Whisk until smooth.

ADD the cinnamon, salt, almond flour, tapioca flour, baking powder, and baking soda. Stir until well combined and smooth. Fold in ½ cup of the chopped walnuts.

EVENLY distribute the batter among the muffin cups, filling each about three-quarters of the way full. Sprinkle the tops with the remaining ¼ cup chopped walnuts.

TRANSFER to the oven and bake until the muffins have set, 20 to 22 minutes, or until a toothpick inserted into the muffins comes out clean.

TO store, allow the muffins to cool completely, then keep in an airtight container at room temperature for 3 to 4 days.

FROM MY KITCHEN TO YOURS

FOR COCONUT OIL: I prefer using liquid coconut oil, which I find in the baking aisle of my local grocery store, but if you cannot find it, you can melt solid coconut oil and let it cool before using. Alternatively, use avocado oil.

MAKE IT CHOCOLATE CHIP: Swap the walnuts for mini dairy-free chocolate chips if you want banana chocolate chip muffins.

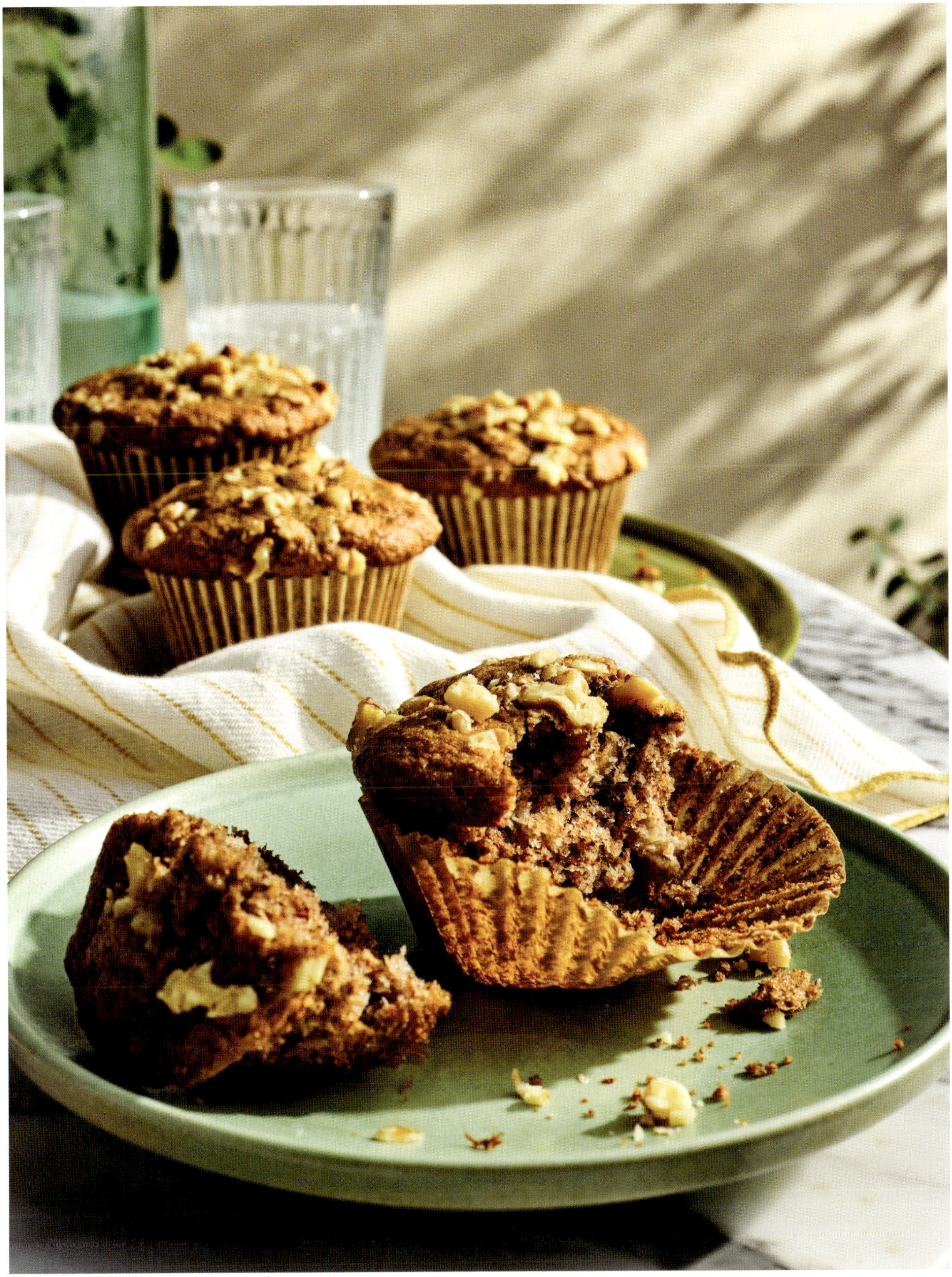

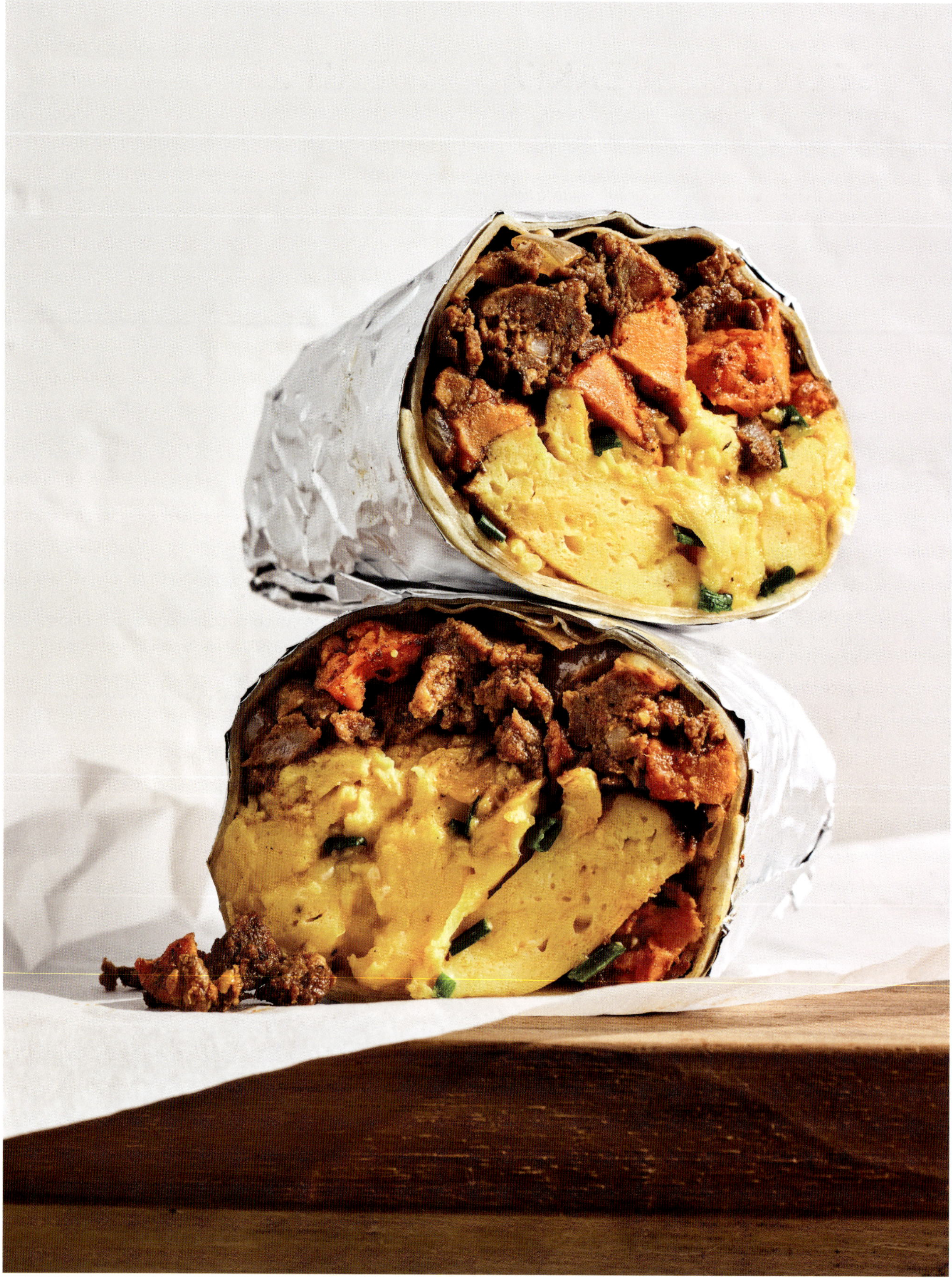

DELIVERY BREAKFAST BURRITOS

MAKES 6 BURRITOS | **TOTAL TIME:** 1 HOUR 10 MINUTES

DIETARY

GLUTEN-FREE (IF MODIFIED)

GRAIN-FREE (IF MODIFIED)

DAIRY-FREE (IF MODIFIED)

MAKE AHEAD

Whether you're meal-prepping for the week or have a loved one in need of some freezer meals, these burritos will be a hit. Tender sweet potatoes are folded into warm tortillas alongside soft-scrambled eggs and spicy chorizo to make the perfect, handheld comfort food.

FOR THE POTATOES

3 medium sweet potatoes, peeled and cut into ½-inch dice (about 6 cups)

4 teaspoons taco seasoning

½ teaspoon kosher salt

2 tablespoons avocado oil

FOR THE CHORIZO AND EGGS

1 tablespoon avocado oil

1 cup finely diced yellow onion (about ½ medium onion)

1 teaspoon taco seasoning

1 pound fresh Mexican chorizo sausage (see note, page 181)

10 large eggs

¼ cup whole milk (omit for dairy-free)

½ teaspoon kosher salt

¼ teaspoon freshly ground black pepper

⅓ cup shredded sharp cheddar cheese (omit for dairy-free)

2 tablespoons chopped fresh chives

FOR ASSEMBLY AND SERVING

6 large flour tortillas (sub grain-free tortillas for gluten-free and grain-free)

Your favorite salsa

POSITION a rack in the center of the oven and preheat the oven to 425°F. Line a sheet pan with parchment paper.

MAKE THE SWEET POTATOES: Toss together the sweet potatoes, taco seasoning, salt, and oil on the prepared sheet pan to combine. Spread the potatoes into an even layer and transfer to the oven. Bake until the potatoes are tender and browned, 22 to 25 minutes, tossing halfway through the cook time. Remove from the oven and allow to cool slightly before assembling.

PREPARE THE CHORIZO AND EGGS: While the sweet potatoes roast, in a large nonstick skillet, heat the oil over medium-high heat. Add the onion and taco seasoning and sauté until the onion slightly softens, about 2 minutes.

ADD the chorizo and spread it into an even layer. Cook, undisturbed, until the chorizo is deeply browned on one side, 4 to 5 minutes. Stir, breaking up the meat with a spatula, and continue to cook until the chorizo is fully cooked and deeply browned on all sides, about 4 more minutes. Using a slotted spoon, transfer the chorizo to a plate. Turn off the heat. You will cook the eggs in the fat that remains in the skillet.

IN a large bowl, whisk together the eggs, milk (if using), salt, and pepper. Turn the heat under the skillet to medium-low. Add the eggs and cook, undisturbed, for 30 seconds. Using a rubber spatula, slowly push the eggs to the middle of the pan. Repeat this process, stirring intermittently and cooking slowly, until the eggs are glossy and very soft scrambled, about 8 minutes. When the eggs are about 80 percent cooked, add the cheese (if using). Stir to combine and cook for 1 more minute, just to melt the cheese. Remove from the heat and gently stir in the chives.

ASSEMBLE THE BURRITOS: If the tortillas feel stiff, microwave them in 15-second increments until warm and pliable. Place the tortillas on a flat surface. In the middle of each tortilla, place ⅓ cup of the chorizo, ⅓ cup of the roasted sweet potatoes, and a heaping scoop of scrambled eggs. Fold over the ends of the tortilla and roll tightly. Repeat with the remaining tortillas. Serve warm with salsa, if desired.

continued

TO store, allow the burritos to cool completely. Wrap each one with parchment paper and then tightly in foil, then place them in a gallon zip-top bag. It's essential they are not warm when you wrap them because they will get soggy, especially if stored in the freezer. Store in the fridge for up to 4 days or in the freezer for up to 2 months. See note for reheating instructions.

FROM MY KITCHEN TO YOURS

FRIDGE REHEATING METHOD: If reheating from the fridge, remove the foil and parchment paper and place on a plate and microwave for 30 seconds. In a small skillet, heat ½ tablespoon butter or avocado oil over medium heat. Set the burrito in the pan seam side down and cook until golden brown, about 2 minutes.

FREEZER REHEATING METHOD: If cooking from frozen, remove the foil and parchment paper, wrap the burrito in a paper towel, and microwave it in 30-second increments until warmed through, 2 to 3 minutes total. In a small skillet, heat ½ tablespoon of butter or avocado oil over medium heat. Set the burrito in the pan seam side down and cook until golden brown, about 2 minutes.

EASY CRANBERRY AND ORANGE DROP SCONES

MAKES 16 SCONES | **TOTAL TIME:** 1 HOUR

DIETARY
GLUTEN-FREE
GRAIN-FREE
VEGETARIAN
DAIRY-FREE (IF MODIFIED)
MAKE AHEAD

Treat yourself to these delightfully easy drop scones! These tender and fluffy scones are a breeze to make using the "drop scone" method and are bursting with fruity goodness for a perfect breakfast bite or afternoon treat. These gluten-free and grain-free scones are light and oh so tasty.

FOR THE SCONES

- ½ cup coconut sugar
- Grated zest of 1 orange (about 1 tablespoon)
- 3 cups almond flour
- 1½ cups tapioca flour
- ½ teaspoon kosher salt
- 1 tablespoon baking powder
- ¼ teaspoon baking soda
- 1 stick frozen unsalted butter (sub vegan butter for dairy-free)
- ⅓ cup unsweetened full-fat coconut milk or buttermilk
- 2 tablespoons honey
- 1 large egg
- ½ teaspoon pure almond extract
- ¾ cup unsweetened dried cranberries

FOR THE ORANGE GLAZE (OPTIONAL)

- ¾ cup powdered sugar
- ¼ teaspoon kosher salt
- 1 to 2 tablespoons freshly squeezed orange juice

MAKE THE SCONES: In a large bowl, combine the coconut sugar and orange zest, using your fingers to massage the zest into the sugar until fragrant. Add the almond flour, tapioca flour, salt, baking powder, and baking soda and whisk to combine, making sure there are no clumps.

USING the large grates on a box grater, grate the frozen butter. Add it to the flour mixture. Using a pastry cutter or clean fingers, gently work in the butter so it is evenly incorporated and there are small bits of butter suspended throughout the dry ingredients. Set aside.

IN a medium bowl, whisk together the coconut milk, honey, egg, and almond extract until well combined and frothy.

USING a wooden spoon, make a well in the center of the flour mixture and pour the wet ingredients into the well. Mix until just combined. Add the dried cranberries and, using clean hands, fold them into the mixture just until they are well incorporated and the dough is formed into a cohesive ball. Transfer into the fridge to chill while you preheat the oven.

POSITION a rack in the center of the oven and preheat the oven to 350°F. Line a large sheet pan with parchment paper.

WHEN the oven is ready, remove the dough from the fridge. Using a large cookie or ice cream scoop, drop 2-inch round balls of the scone dough onto the prepared sheet pan. They do not need to be perfectly round, but ensure they are spaced at least 2 inches apart. With two clean fingers, gently flatten the tops of the scones so that they are about 1 inch thick.

TRANSFER to the oven and bake until the tops are golden brown, about 17 minutes.

REMOVE the pan from the oven and allow the scones to cool slightly, then transfer the scones to a wire rack to cool completely.

MAKE THE ORANGE GLAZE (IF USING): In a medium bowl, whisk together the powdered sugar, salt, and 1 tablespoon of the orange juice until smooth. If it

continued

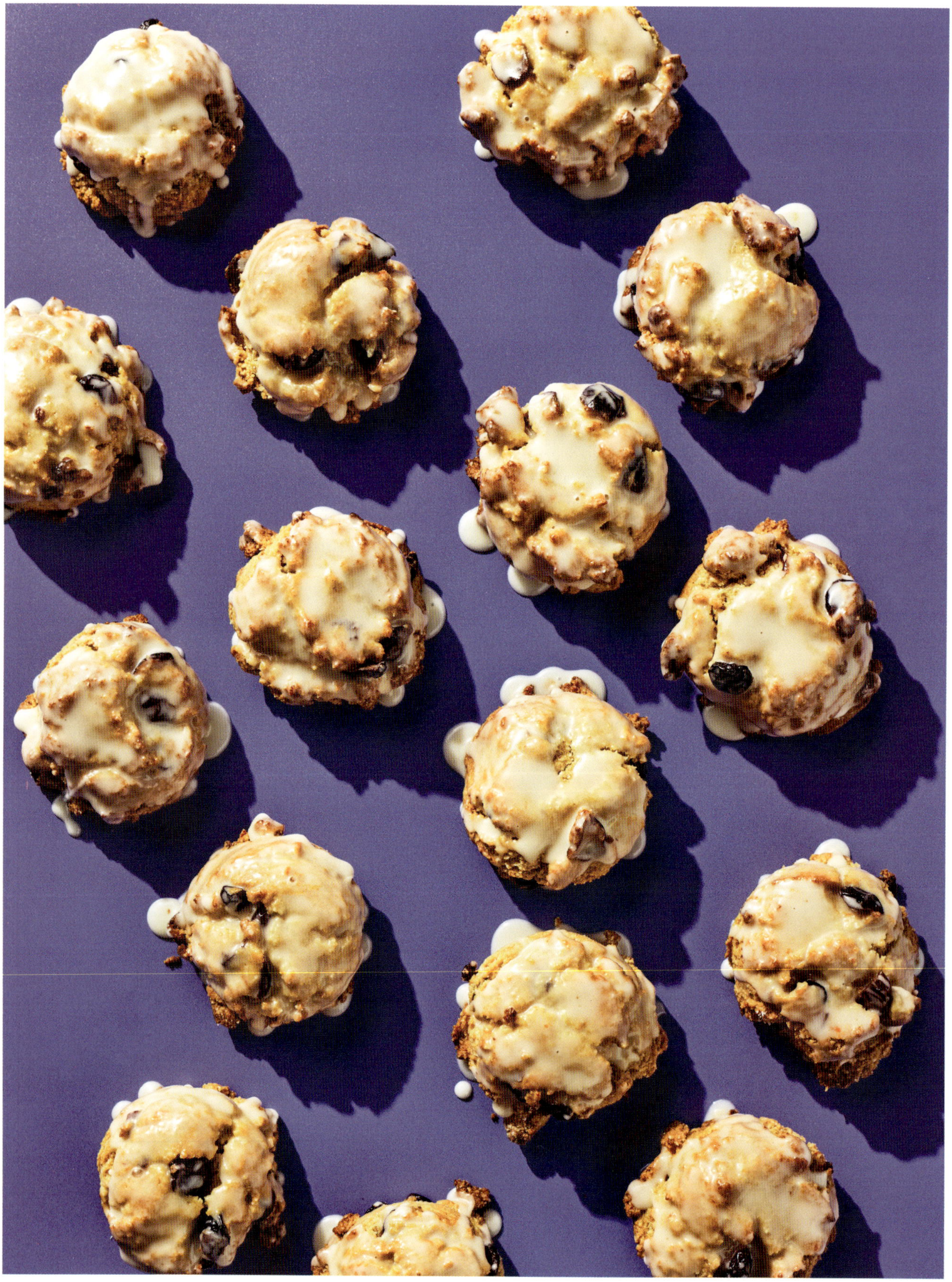

seems dry, add a bit more orange juice and whisk until smooth. Drizzle the glaze over the cooled scones.

TO store, allow the scones to cool completely, then keep in an airtight container at room temperature for up to 4 days.

FROM MY KITCHEN TO YOURS

FREEZER TIPS: Since this recipe yields quite a few scones, I always freeze half of the dough for later! After placing the drop scones on the sheet pan and gently pressing the tops to shape them, pop the whole tray in the freezer until the scones are fully frozen. Transfer the frozen scones to an airtight container or freezer-safe zip-top bag and store for up to 3 months. No need to thaw before baking—simply preheat the oven as instructed and add 2 to 3 extra minutes to the bake time. Top the cooled scones with the orange glaze, if using.

OTHER FLAVOR IDEAS: My kids love when I skip the orange zest, replace the almond extract with vanilla extract, and use chocolate chips in place of the dried cranberries. These are also great with lemon and blueberry! Swap the orange zest for lemon zest, use vanilla extract instead of almond extract, and add ½ cup freeze-dried blueberries plus ½ cup fresh blueberries in place of the dried cranberries.

FREEZER-FRIENDLY MEDITERRANEAN BREAKFAST SANDWICHES

MAKES 8 SANDWICHES | **TOTAL TIME:** 1 HOUR

DIETARY
GLUTEN-FREE (IF MODIFIED)
MAKE AHEAD

These freezer-friendly breakfast sandwiches are a lifesaver for busy mornings! Packed with protein-rich eggs, crispy no-sugar-added bacon, and Mediterranean-inspired flavors like sun-dried tomatoes, basil, and feta, they're both nourishing and delicious. Baking the eggs makes assembly a breeze, and the English muffins hold up beautifully in the freezer. Just heat one for a quick, satisfying breakfast that tastes fresh and flavorful—no stress required!

8 slices no-sugar-added bacon
Avocado oil spray
8 large eggs
⅓ cup whole-milk plain Greek yogurt
2 garlic cloves, minced
⅓ cup finely chopped fresh basil leaves
1 teaspoon kosher salt
½ teaspoon freshly ground black pepper
⅓ cup roughly chopped oil-packed sun-dried tomatoes, drained
2 cups finely chopped baby spinach
½ cup crumbled feta cheese
8 English muffins (sub gluten-free English muffins for gluten-free)
Hot sauce, optional for serving

LEFTOVER sun-dried tomatoes? Try my Marry Me White Bean Soup (page 76) or Creamy Sun-Dried Tomato Basil Chicken (page 153).

POSITION a rack in the center of the oven and preheat the oven to 325°F. Line a plate with paper towels and set aside. Line a large sheet pan with parchment paper.

COOK THE BACON: Arrange the bacon in a single layer on the prepared sheet pan, ensuring the slices do not overlap. Bake until the bacon is just crisp, about 20 minutes. Transfer to the prepared plate. Set aside.

GENEROUSLY spray a 9 × 13-inch quarter sheet pan or baking dish with avocado oil spray. Set aside.

IN a large bowl, combine the eggs, yogurt, garlic, basil, salt, and pepper. Whisk until very well combined and slightly frothy. Add the sun-dried tomatoes, spinach, and feta and mix once more until well combined.

POUR the mixture into the prepared sheet pan and spread it out evenly. Transfer to the middle rack of the preheated oven and bake until the eggs are fully cooked and set, 22 to 25 minutes. Remove the egg bake from the oven and let cool completely.

CUT the cooled egg bake into 8 even squares. Slice the English muffins in half. Place 1 egg square on the bottom half of each muffin. Break each bacon strip in half and place both halves on top of the egg. Top with the other muffin half. Continue with the rest of the sandwiches.

WRAP each sandwich tightly in parchment paper or foil and store in the fridge for up to 3 days, or place them in a large freezer-safe zip-top bag and freeze for up to 1 month.

TO reheat, unwrap from the parchment or foil and place on a microwave-safe dish. Microwave for 60 to 90 seconds from the fridge, or 90 to 120 seconds from frozen. Serve with hot sauce, if desired.

FROM MY KITCHEN TO YOURS

If making these fresh for a crowd rather than prepping ahead, lightly spray the halved English muffins with avocado oil spray and arrange them on a sheet pan. Transfer to the preheated oven and toast for about 8 minutes, until lightly golden. Assemble as directed with the egg and bacon.

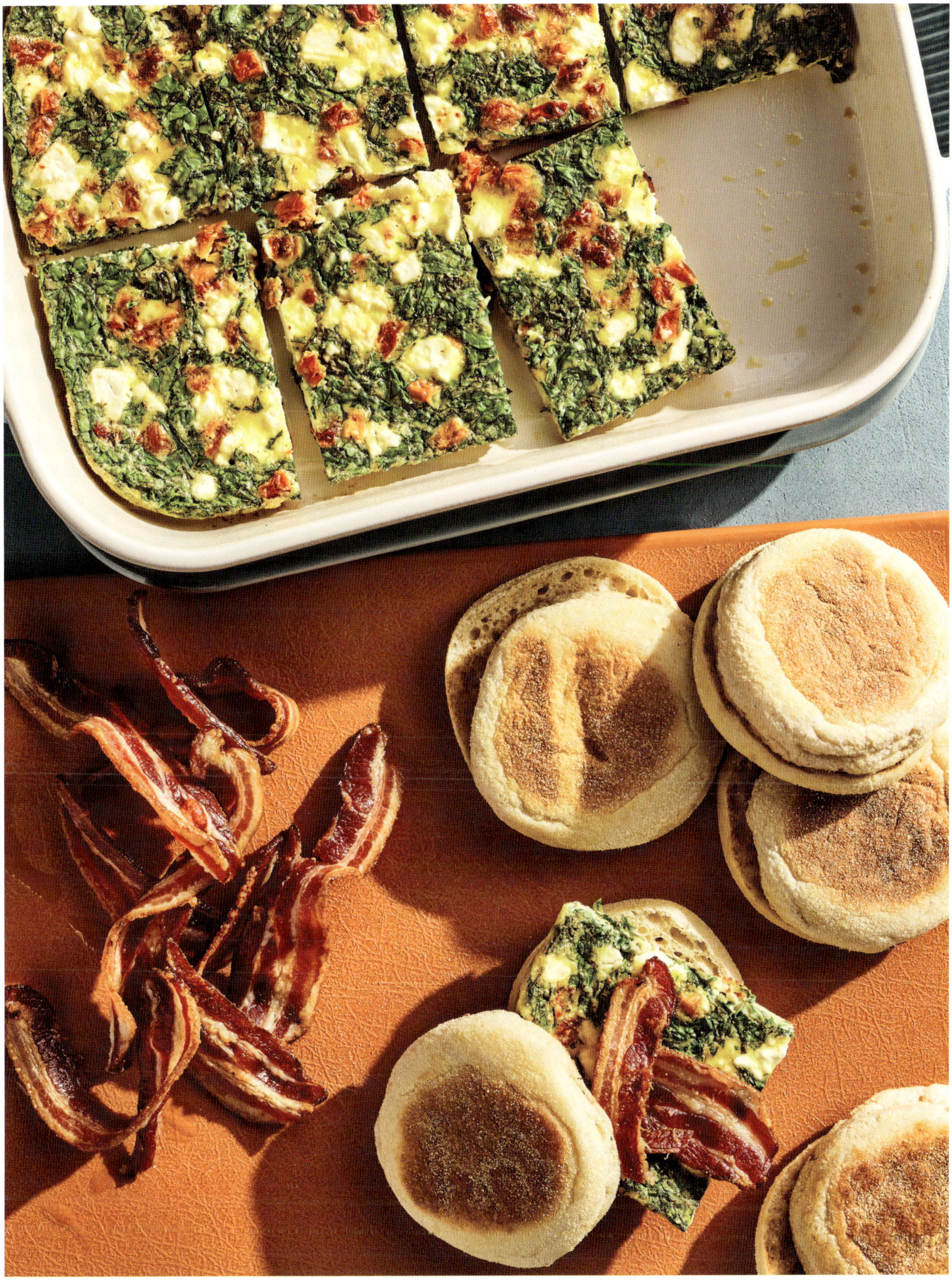

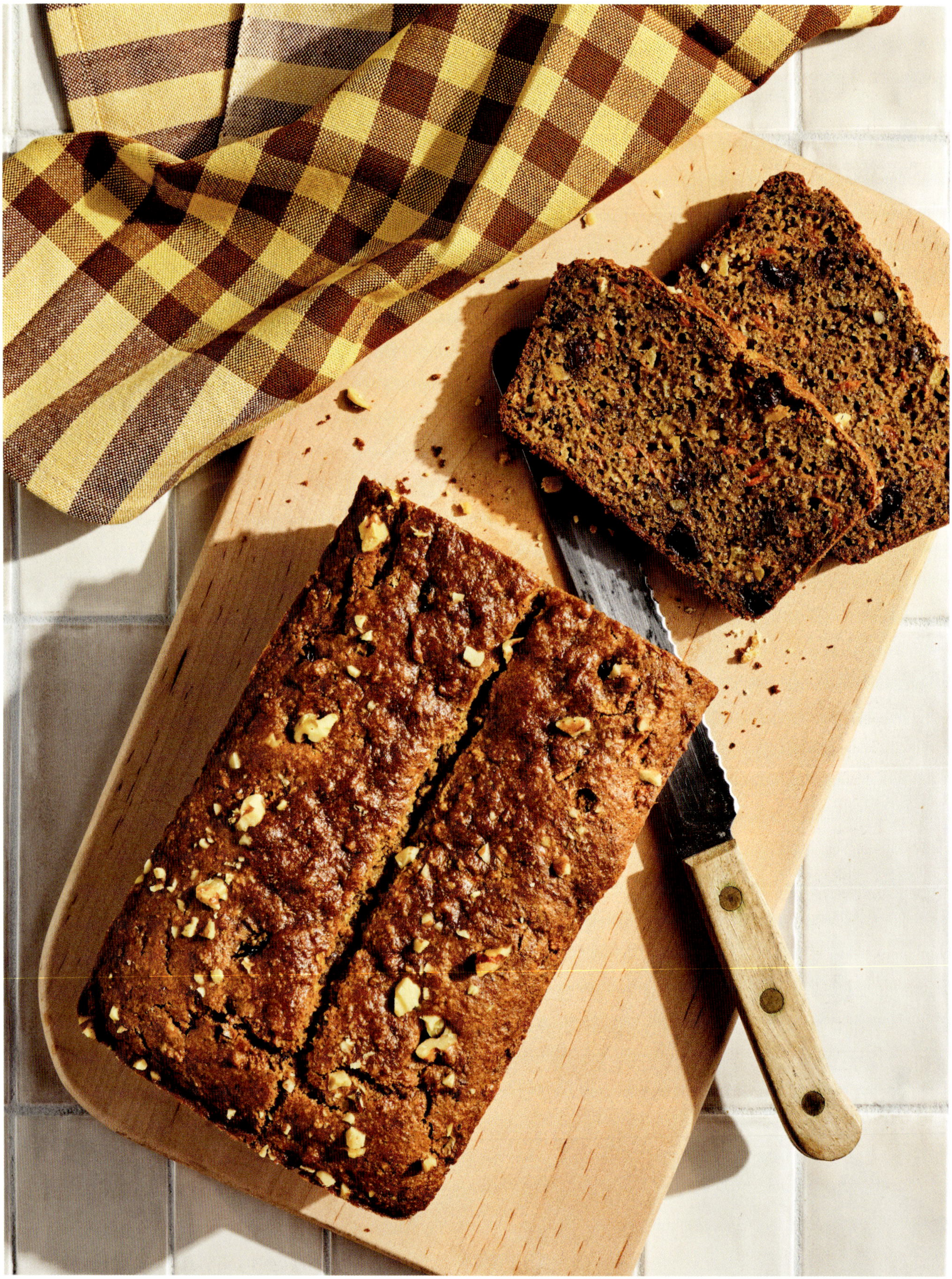

MORNING GLORY LOAF

MAKES ONE LOAF | **TOTAL TIME:** 1 HOUR 15 MINUTES

DIETARY

GLUTEN-FREE

GRAIN-FREE

DAIRY-FREE (IF MODIFIED)

PALEO (IF MODIFIED)

MAKE AHEAD

This grain-free breakfast loaf is packed with nutrients from flaxseed, carrots, apples, walnuts, and olive oil, making it as wholesome as it is delicious. Warming spices from the pumpkin pie spice add a cozy flavor, and a slice pairs perfectly with a cup of coffee or tea for a midmorning treat. Prefer muffins instead? This recipe works beautifully in muffin form too—I've included those instructions in the notes so you can choose your favorite!

Nonstick cooking spray

2 cups almond flour

1 cup tapioca flour

¼ cup flaxseed meal

1 teaspoon baking powder

½ teaspoon kosher salt

1 tablespoon pumpkin pie spice or 2 teaspoons ground cinnamon

3 large eggs, at room temperature

½ cup extra-virgin olive oil

⅓ cup whole-milk plain Greek yogurt (sub coconut milk yogurt for dairy-free and paleo)

Grated zest of ½ lemon

½ cup coconut sugar

¼ cup pure maple syrup

2 teaspoons pure vanilla extract

2 tablespoons freshly squeezed lemon juice (about 1 lemon)

1½ teaspoons baking soda

¼ cup raisins

½ cup peeled and small-diced Honeycrisp apple

½ cup chopped walnuts

1½ cups grated carrots (about 4 medium carrots; see note)

POSITION a rack in the center of the oven and preheat the oven to 350°F. Line a 9 × 5-inch loaf pan with a parchment paper sling and grease it generously with nonstick cooking spray. Set aside.

IN a medium bowl, whisk together the almond flour, tapioca flour, flaxseed meal, baking powder, salt, and pumpkin pie spice. Set aside.

IN a large bowl with a hand mixer or a stand mixer fitted with the whisk attachment, beat the eggs on medium-high speed until pale yellow and fluffy, 3 to 4 minutes. Add the oil, yogurt, lemon zest, coconut sugar, maple syrup, and vanilla extract. Mix on medium for 1 minute, until slightly thickened and smooth. Add the lemon juice and baking soda. Mix on low to combine, then set aside for 1 minute for the baking soda to activate.

ADD half of the dry ingredients into the wet mixture and mix on low until just combined. Scrape down the sides of the bowl and add the remaining dry ingredients. Mix until just combined. Using a rubber spatula, fold in the raisins, apples, walnuts, and carrots. Mix until evenly distributed throughout the batter.

POUR the batter into the prepared loaf pan and smooth out the top. Transfer to the oven and bake for 45 to 55 minutes, or until a cake tester inserted into the center comes out totally clean.

ALLOW the loaf to cool for at least 30 minutes then remove from the pan. Cut it into 1-inch slices to serve. Store leftovers in an airtight container at room temperature for up to 3 days or in the fridge for up to 1 week.

FROM MY KITCHEN TO YOURS

FOR THE CARROTS: Do not use preshredded carrots! They do not have the moisture needed for the loaf. After the carrots are washed and peeled, you can either hand-shred them or use a food processor with the shredding blade.

FOR MUFFINS: Set a rack in the center of the oven and preheat to 350°F. Line the cups of a muffin tin with paper liners or lightly grease them. Divide the batter evenly among the cups, filling each about three-quarters of the way full. Bake for 18 to 22 minutes, or until a toothpick inserted into the center comes out clean. Allow the muffins to cool in the pan for 5 minutes, then transfer them to a wire rack to cool completely.

PALEO PROTEIN WAFFLES

MAKES 12 WAFFLES | **TOTAL TIME:** 25 MINUTES

DIETARY
- GLUTEN-FREE
- GRAIN-FREE
- DAIRY-FREE
- PALEO
- VEGETARIAN
- **MAKE AHEAD**

These protein-filled waffles are light, fluffy, and just the thing when you want a feel-good breakfast with a little extra staying power. They're grain-free, dairy-free, and come together fast—perfect for busy mornings or lazy weekends. Add chocolate chips if you're feeling fancy, or just top with fresh berries and a good drizzle of maple syrup. Bonus: They freeze like a dream, so you'll always have a stack ready to go!

2 large eggs
1 cup unsweetened almond milk or milk of choice
2 teaspoons apple cider vinegar
¼ cup pure maple syrup
¼ cup avocado oil
1½ cups almond flour
1 cup tapioca flour
¼ cup vanilla protein or collagen powder
1 tablespoon baking powder
½ teaspoon ground cinnamon
Nonstick cooking spray

OPTIONAL

½ cup dairy-free chocolate chips
Fresh berries, for serving
Pure maple syrup, for serving

IN a medium bowl, whisk together the eggs, almond milk, vinegar, maple syrup, avocado oil, and ¼ cup water. Set aside.

MEANWHILE, in a separate large bowl, stir together the almond flour, tapioca flour, protein powder, baking powder, and cinnamon, breaking up any clumps until well combined.

ADD half of the wet mixture to the dry mixture and stir until well combined. Add the remaining wet mixture and continue stirring until there are no longer any clumps. Add the chocolate chips (if using) to the batter and stir to combine. Set aside to rest for a few minutes to allow the batter to thicken slightly.

WHILE the batter is resting, preheat the waffle iron to medium-low heat.

WHEN the waffle iron is hot, spray with nonstick cooking spray. Cook the waffles according to your waffle iron's manufacturer instructions. For my four-square waffle iron, I pour about 1¼ cups of the batter into the waffle iron and the waffles cook in 3 minutes.

USING a fork, carefully remove the waffles from the iron and set aside. Continue making the rest of the waffles. To serve, plate and top with fresh berries and drizzle with maple syrup, if desired.

FROM MY KITCHEN TO YOURS

FREEZER TIPS: To freeze, place the cooked waffles in a single layer on a sheet pan lined with parchment paper. Transfer the sheet pan to the freezer and freeze until the waffles are solid, about 2 hours. Transfer the frozen waffles to a freezer-safe zip-top bag or container for up to 3 months.

REHEATING TIPS: Warm the frozen waffles in a toaster until heated through and crispy. You can also reheat them in a 350°F oven for 5 to 7 minutes, until warmed through.

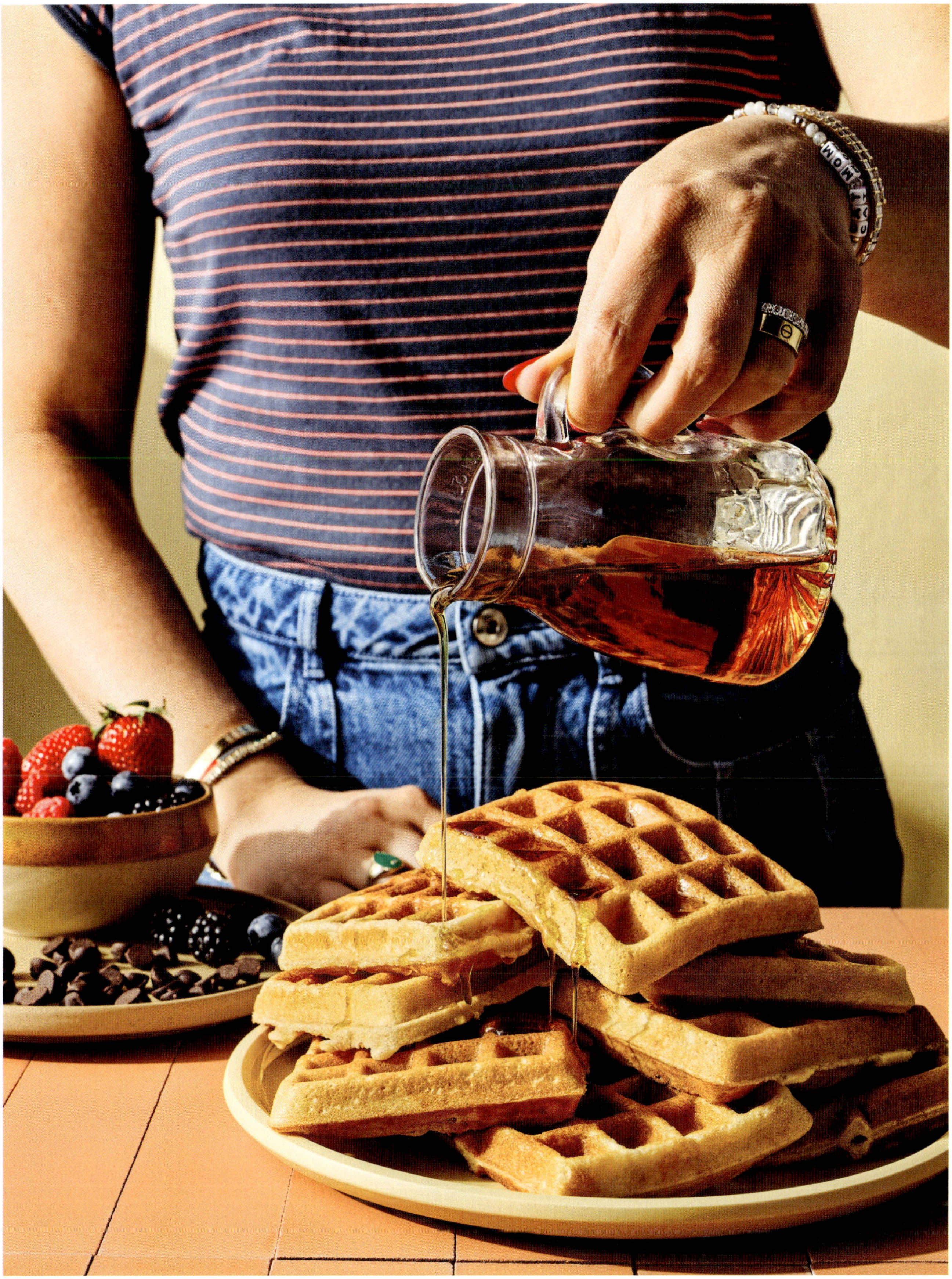

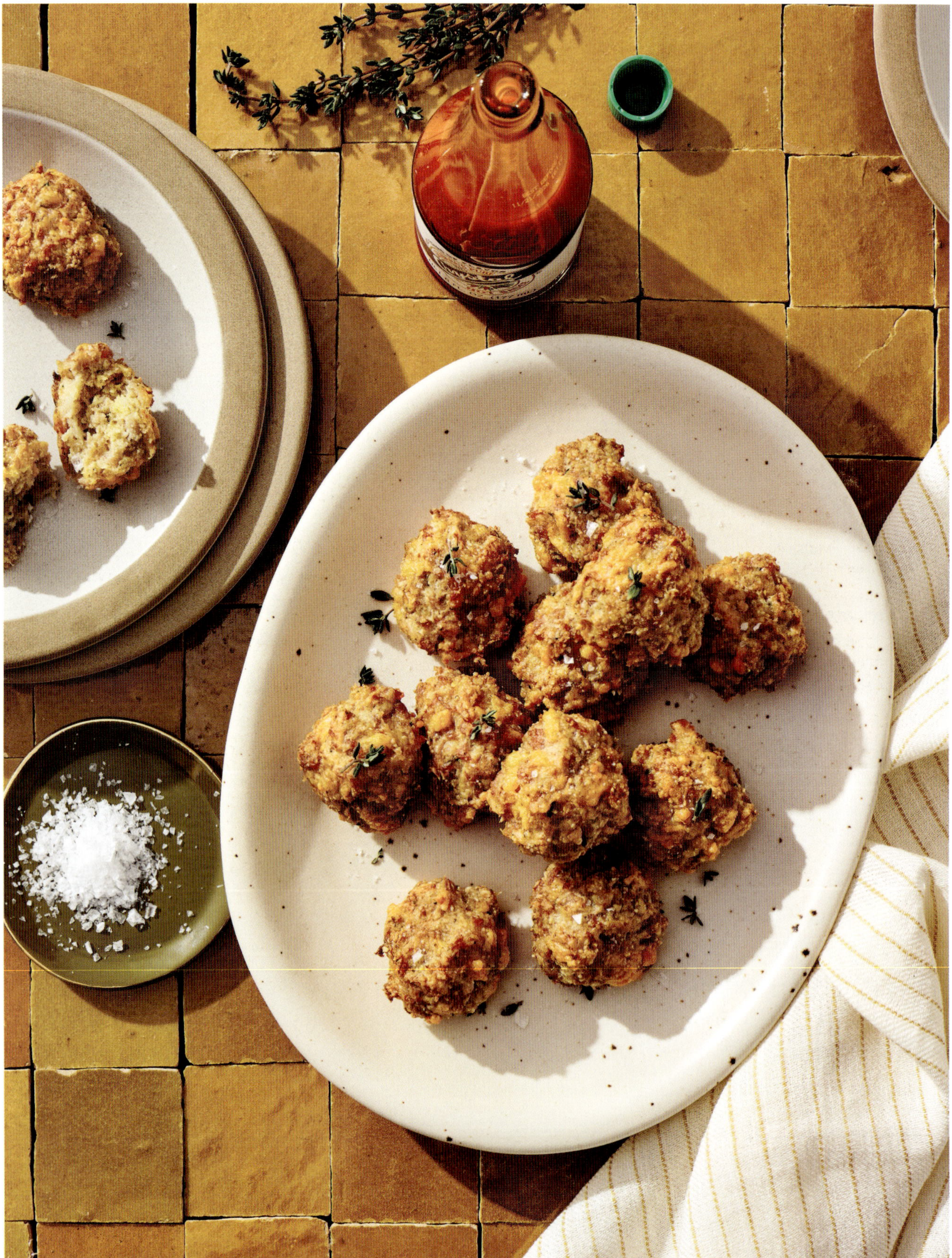

SAUSAGE AND CHEESE BALLS

MAKES 20 TO 24 BALLS | **TOTAL TIME:** 25 MINUTES

DIETARY
GLUTEN-FREE
GRAIN-FREE
MAKE AHEAD

Sausage balls—if you know, you know! Growing up, these childhood favorites were made with Bisquick, breakfast sausage, and cheese. Not only are these sausage balls irresistibly delicious, but they are made with more wholesome ingredients and are grain-free, too! The best part? They freeze well, making them perfect to have on hand for a quick breakfast or to serve when entertaining!

- 1 cup almond flour
- ½ cup tapioca flour
- 2 teaspoons baking powder
- ½ teaspoon baking soda
- 1 teaspoon kosher salt
- ½ teaspoon freshly ground black pepper
- 1 teaspoon roughly chopped fresh thyme leaves or ½ teaspoon dried
- 1 pound ground pork breakfast sausage
- 1 cup grated sharp cheddar cheese
- 2 large eggs, whisked

PREHEAT the oven to 400°F. Line a sheet pan with parchment paper and set aside.

IN a large bowl, combine the almond flour, tapioca flour, baking powder, baking soda, salt, pepper, and thyme. Stir to combine and break up any clumps.

ADD the sausage, cheese, and eggs. Using clean hands, break up the sausage into smaller pieces and work it into the flour mixture until well combined.

USING damp hands, roll the mixture into 1½-inch round meatballs and place them in an even layer on the prepared sheet pan.

TRANSFER to the oven and bake until the sausage is cooked through and the bites are golden brown, 15 to 18 minutes.

REMOVE from the oven and let cool slightly before serving.

TO store, let cool completely, then keep in an airtight container in the fridge for 4 to 5 days. To reheat, pop them in the microwave for 45 seconds to 1 minute.

FROM MY KITCHEN TO YOURS

FREEZER TIP: To freeze, form the sausage balls, but do not bake them. Arrange them on a sheet pan and freeze until solid. Transfer the frozen balls to an airtight container or freezer-safe zip-top bag. Store for up to 3 months. To bake, cook directly from frozen, adding just a few extra minutes to the baking time.

SHEET PAN BREAKFAST POTATOES WITH BACON AND EGGS

MAKES 6 SERVINGS | **TOTAL TIME:** 50 MINUTES

DIETARY
GLUTEN-FREE
GRAIN-FREE
DAIRY-FREE
PALEO
MAKE AHEAD

A hearty and wholesome way to start your morning, this sheet pan breakfast is the ultimate one-pan wonder. Crispy potatoes, caramelized veggies, and smoky bacon all roast together before eggs are added and baked to perfection. With simple ingredients and bold flavor, this is an easy, satisfying breakfast that also works beautifully for meal prep. Just portion it out and reheat throughout the week—because weekday mornings deserve something delicious, too.

1 pound yellow potatoes, unpeeled, cut into ½-inch cubes

½ cup small-diced white onion (about ½ small onion)

1 cup small-diced green bell pepper (about 1 small pepper)

1 cup small-diced red bell pepper (about 1 small pepper)

4 slices thick-cut no-sugar-added bacon, cut into small cubes

3 tablespoons avocado oil

1 teaspoon kosher salt

1 teaspoon freshly ground black pepper

1 teaspoon garlic powder

½ teaspoon smoked paprika

½ teaspoon dried thyme

¼ teaspoon cayenne pepper, optional

6 large eggs

1 tablespoon finely chopped fresh chives

1 tablespoon finely chopped fresh parsley

OPTIONAL FOR SERVING

Shredded sharp cheddar cheese (omit for dairy-free and paleo)

Sliced avocado

POSITION a rack at the top of the oven and preheat the oven to 425°F. Line a sheet pan with parchment paper.

PLACE the potatoes, onion, bell peppers, bacon, avocado oil, salt, black pepper, garlic powder, paprika, thyme, and cayenne (if using) on the prepared sheet pan. Toss until very well combined and the veggies are evenly coated. Spread into a single layer.

TRANSFER to the oven and bake until the potatoes are cooked through and crisp on the edges and the bacon is crisp, about 35 minutes, tossing halfway through the cook time.

REMOVE from the oven and create six wells in the potato hash to hold the eggs. Crack an egg into each well and carefully transfer back to the oven. Bake for 5 to 6 minutes, until the egg whites are just set and the yolks are slightly runny (for an over-easy egg).

REMOVE from the oven and garnish with fresh chives and parsley.

TO SERVE: Plate an egg with the potato hash around it. Serve with shredded cheese and sliced avocado, if desired.

FROM MY KITCHEN TO YOURS

STORAGE AND REHEATING: Allow the hash and eggs to cool completely, then transfer individual portions to airtight containers and refrigerate for up to 4 days. For the best texture, reheat in a 375°F oven or toaster oven for 8 to 10 minutes, until warmed through. You can also microwave these in 30-second intervals until hot, though the eggs and potatoes will be softer. If you don't love reheated eggs, you can skip baking them on the sheet pan! Just prep the hash portion and top with a freshly cooked egg each morning.

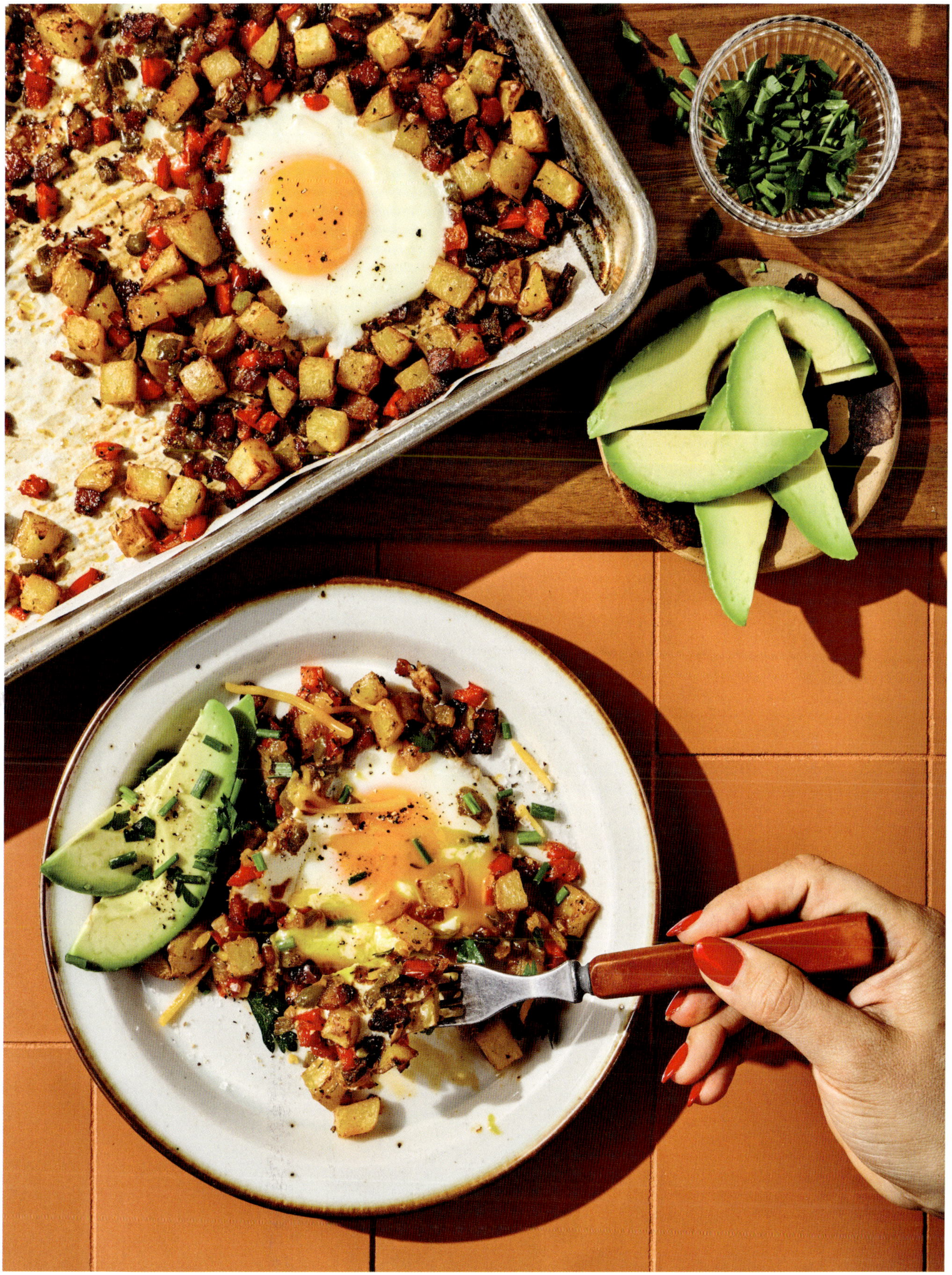

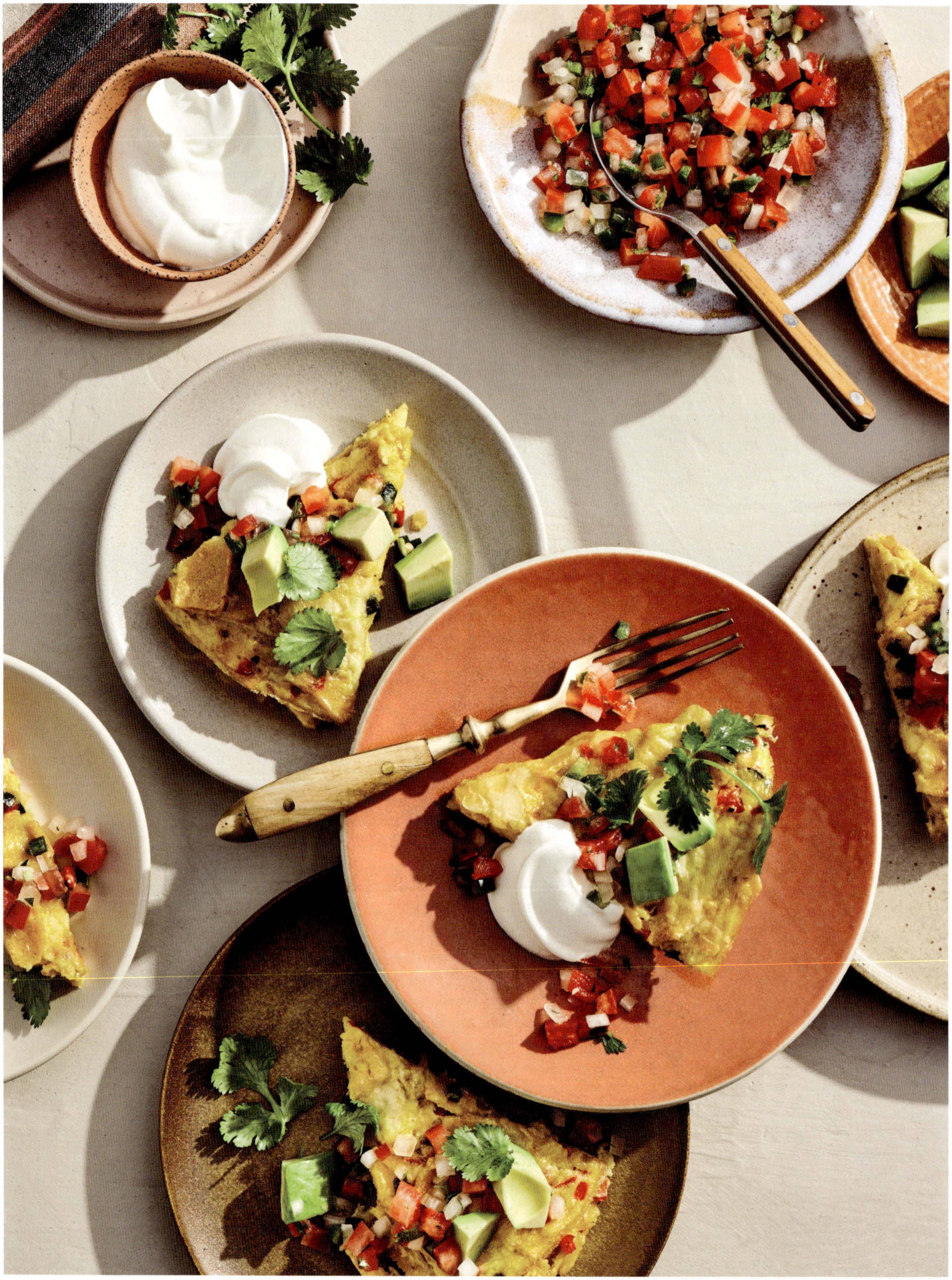

SKILLET MIGAS BREAKFAST FRITTATA

MAKES 8 SERVINGS | **TOTAL TIME:** 35 MINUTES

DIETARY

GLUTEN-FREE

DAIRY-FREE (IF MODIFIED)

MAKE AHEAD

Have leftover corn tortillas? Normally I'd whip up a classic migas for breakfast, but with this recipe I'm bringing those flavors to a convenient skillet meal that is ideal for reheating during the week. Sauté the veggies, pour in the eggs, and into the oven it goes! While the tortillas aren't crispy, they infuse the dish with a delightful corn essence. This one is a reheat favorite but also lovely when we have company and I want to impress my guests.

9 eggs

½ cup whole-milk (sub unsweetened full-fat coconut milk for dairy-free)

½ cup salsa verde

2 tablespoons avocado oil

½ cup small-diced poblano pepper (about 1 medium pepper)

¾ cup small-diced red bell pepper (about ½ medium pepper)

½ cup finely diced yellow onion (about ½ small onion)

2 garlic cloves, minced

1½ teaspoons kosher salt

½ teaspoon freshly ground black pepper

6 corn tortillas, cut into 1-inch pieces

½ cup shredded Monterey Jack cheese (omit for dairy-free)

OPTIONAL FOR SERVING

2 tablespoons fresh cilantro leaves

Pico de gallo

Diced avocado

Sour cream (omit for dairy-free)

POSITION a rack in the middle of the oven and preheat the oven to 375°F.

IN a large bowl, whisk together the eggs, milk, and salsa verde until very well combined. Set aside.

IN a large, deep oven-safe skillet, preferably cast iron, heat the oil over medium heat. Add the poblano pepper, bell pepper, onion, garlic, salt, and black pepper. Cook, stirring, until the veggies are tender, about 6 minutes.

ADD the corn tortillas to the skillet and toss until well combined. Remove from the heat and spread the veggie and corn tortilla mixture into an even layer. Pour the egg mixture into the skillet. Sprinkle the top with the cheese (if using) and transfer to the oven. Bake until the eggs have set and the cheese is golden, 18 to 20 minutes.

TO SERVE: If serving immediately, allow the frittata to cool for 5 minutes, then cut it into 8 slices and serve. Serve alone or top with the fresh cilantro, pico de gallo, diced avocado, and sour cream, if desired.

FROM MY KITCHEN TO YOURS

STORAGE TIP: Allow the frittata to cool completely, then cut it into 8 slices. Store in an airtight container and keep in the fridge for up to 4 days.

REHEATING TIPS: To reheat in the microwave, cover a slice of frittata with a damp paper towel and heat until warmed through, 1 to 2 minutes. To reheat in a skillet, place a slice of the frittata in a nonstick skillet over medium-low heat, cover, and heat until warm, 3 to 4 minutes, flipping halfway through.

LEFTOVER salsa verde? Try my Steak Street Taco Salad with Salsa Verde Vinaigrette (page 69).

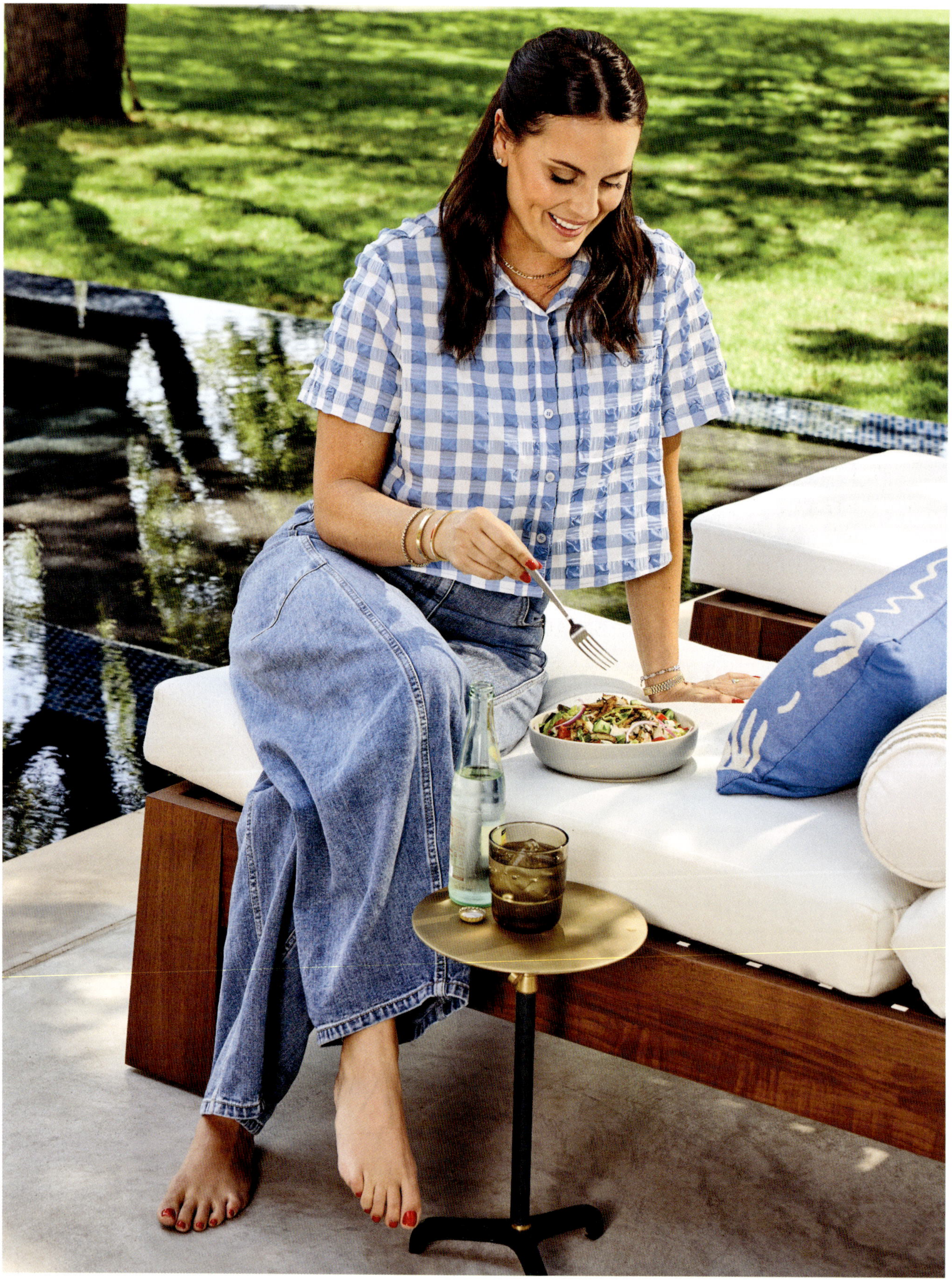

SALADS AND SUCH

ITALIAN DELI CHICKEN SALAD

MAKES 6 SERVINGS | **PREP TIME:** 15 MINUTES | **CHILL TIME:** 30 MINUTES

DIETARY
GLUTEN-FREE
GRAIN-FREE
DAIRY-FREE (IF MODIFIED)
PALEO (IF MODIFIED)
MAKE AHEAD

This Italian deli-inspired chicken salad comes together quickly, thanks to bold ingredients like kalamata olives, salami, and peperoncini. This is a versatile recipe designed to help you use those jars of pickled and briny ingredients you have on hand, or if your grocery store has an olive bar, it's a convenient one-stop shop for gathering the perfect amount of all the flavorful add-ins that make this dish irresistible.

¼ cup avocado oil mayo

¼ cup whole-milk plain Greek yogurt (sub avocado oil mayo for dairy-free and paleo)

3 garlic cloves, minced

2 tablespoons red wine vinegar

Grated zest of ½ lemon

2 tablespoons freshly squeezed lemon juice (about 1 lemon)

1 tablespoon brine from a peperoncini jar

½ teaspoon kosher salt

½ teaspoon freshly ground black pepper

1 teaspoon dried oregano

¼ cup grated parmesan cheese (omit for dairy-free and paleo)

4 cups small-diced cooked chicken (I use rotisserie)

½ cup small-diced Genoa salami (about 6 slices salami)

½ cup chopped peperoncini slices, drained

1 cup small-diced red bell pepper (about 1 small pepper)

½ cup small-diced celery (about 1 stalk)

½ cup small-diced shallot (about 1 large shallot)

½ cup chopped pitted kalamata olives

½ cup finely chopped fresh parsley leaves

OPTIONAL FOR SERVING

Greens of your choice

Gluten-free wrap of choice

Seedy brown rice crackers

IN a large bowl, whisk together the mayo, yogurt, garlic, vinegar, lemon zest, lemon juice, peperoncini brine, salt, black pepper, oregano, and parmesan (if using).

ADD the chicken, salami, chopped peperoncini, bell pepper, celery, shallot, olives, and parsley. Mix until coated in the sauce. Cover and refrigerate for at least 30 minutes to allow the flavors to meld.

TO SERVE: Serve over greens, in a wrap, or with seedy brown rice crackers, if desired.

STORE in an airtight container in the fridge for up to 5 days.

LEFTOVER sliced peperoncini? Try my Creamy Peperoncini Chicken (page 146).

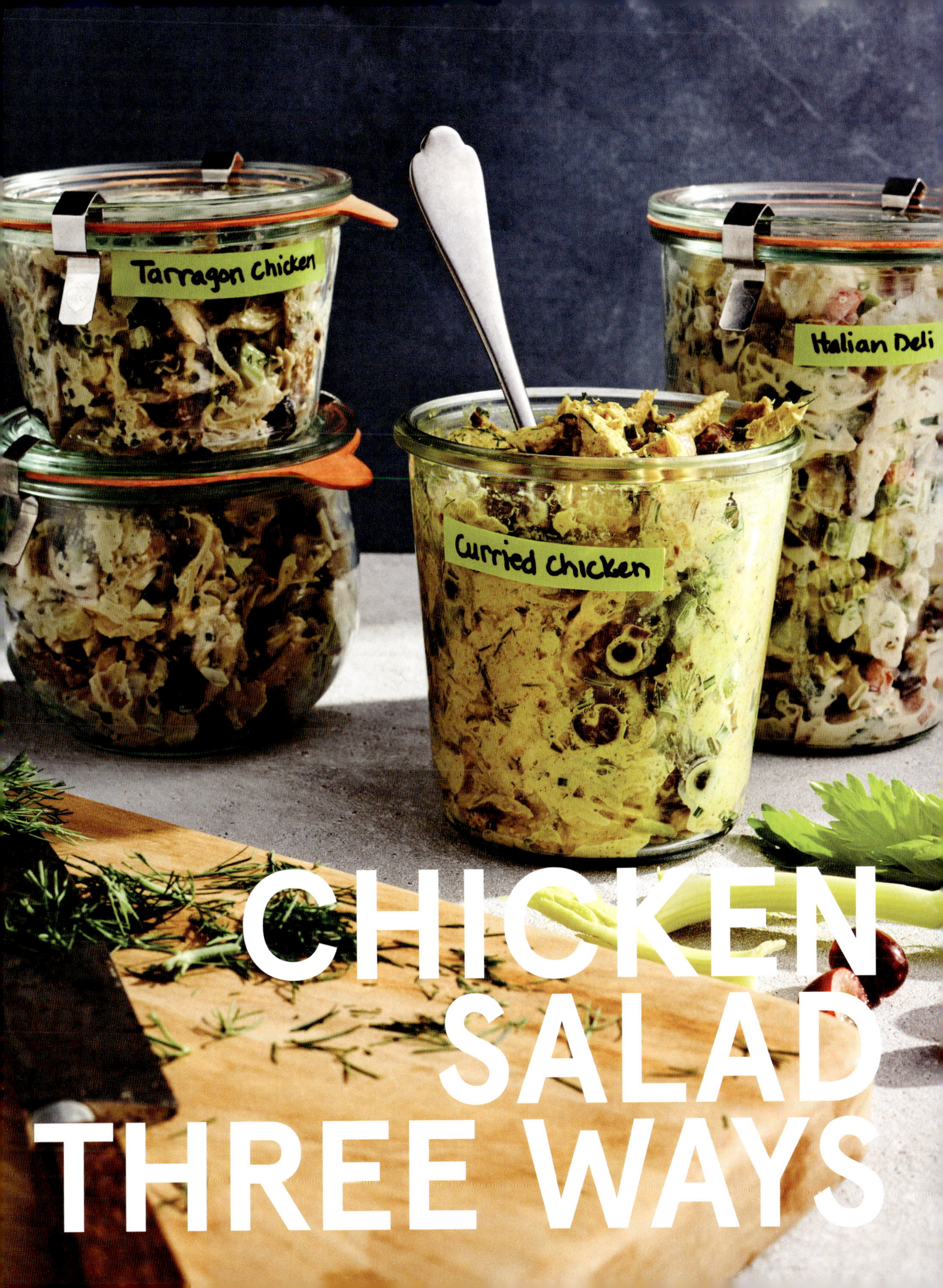

CHICKEN SALAD THREE WAYS

PERFECT CURRIED CHICKEN SALAD

MAKES 4 SERVINGS | **PREP TIME:** 15 MINUTES | **CHILL TIME:** 30 MINUTES

DIETARY

GLUTEN-FREE

GRAIN-FREE

DAIRY-FREE (IF MODIFIED)

PALEO (IF MODIFIED)

MAKE AHEAD

This quick and tasty curried chicken salad is perfect for any meal and great for meal prep. It's bursting with warm spices, bright herbs, and creamy yogurt-curry dressing that keeps you coming back for more. It's even better the next day as the flavors deepen; the kind of dish that instantly elevates your everyday lunch routine.

¼ cup whole-milk plain Greek yogurt (sub avocado oil mayo for dairy-free and paleo)

2 tablespoons avocado oil mayo

3 teaspoons curry powder

1 teaspoon garlic powder

½ teaspoon ground cumin

¼ teaspoon cayenne pepper, optional

1 teaspoon kosher salt, plus more to taste

½ teaspoon freshly ground black pepper

¼ cup freshly squeezed lemon juice (about 2 lemons)

4 cups shredded cooked chicken (I use rotisserie)

½ cup small-diced celery (about 1 stalk)

¼ cup finely diced red onion (about ¼ small onion)

¼ cup finely chopped fresh dill

¼ cup finely chopped fresh chives

¾ cup halved seedless red grapes

OPTIONAL FOR SERVING

Greens of your choice

Gluten-free wrap of choice

Seedy brown rice crackers

IN a large bowl, whisk together the yogurt, mayo, curry powder, garlic powder, cumin, cayenne (if using), salt, black pepper, and lemon juice until well combined.

ADD the chicken, celery, onion, dill, and chives. Mix until coated in the sauce.

GENTLY fold the grapes into the chicken salad. Cover and refrigerate for at least 30 minutes to allow the flavors to meld.

TO SERVE: Serve over greens, in a wrap, or with seedy brown rice crackers, if desired.

STORE in an airtight container in the fridge for up to 5 days.

TARRAGON CHICKEN SALAD

MAKES 4 SERVINGS | **PREP TIME:** 15 MINUTES | **CHILL TIME:** 30 MINUTES

DIETARY
GLUTEN-FREE
GRAIN-FREE
DAIRY-FREE
PALEO
MAKE AHEAD

Chicken salad is obviously a staple in my kitchen, and this tarragon version is my personal go-to when I am in the mood for a classic. The herb's delicate, aromatic flavor transforms a simple chicken salad into something truly special. It's perfect for lunches or light meals that you'll enjoy all week long.

¼ cup avocado oil mayo
1 teaspoon Dijon mustard
2 tablespoons freshly squeezed lemon juice (about 1 lemon)
½ teaspoon garlic powder
1 teaspoon kosher salt
½ teaspoon freshly ground black pepper
2 tablespoons finely chopped fresh tarragon leaves
4 cups shredded cooked chicken (I use rotisserie)
½ cup small-diced celery (about 1 stalk)
½ cup finely diced yellow onion (about ½ small onion)
½ cup unsweetened dried cranberries

OPTIONAL FOR SERVING
Greens of your choice
Gluten-free wrap of choice
Seedy brown rice crackers

IN a large bowl, stir together the mayo, mustard, lemon juice, garlic powder, salt, and pepper until well combined.

ADD the tarragon, chicken, celery, onion, and cranberries. Mix until coated in the sauce. Cover and refrigerate for at least 30 minutes to allow the flavors to meld.

TO SERVE: Serve over greens, in a wrap, or with seedy brown rice crackers, if desired.

STORE in an airtight container in the fridge for up to 5 days.

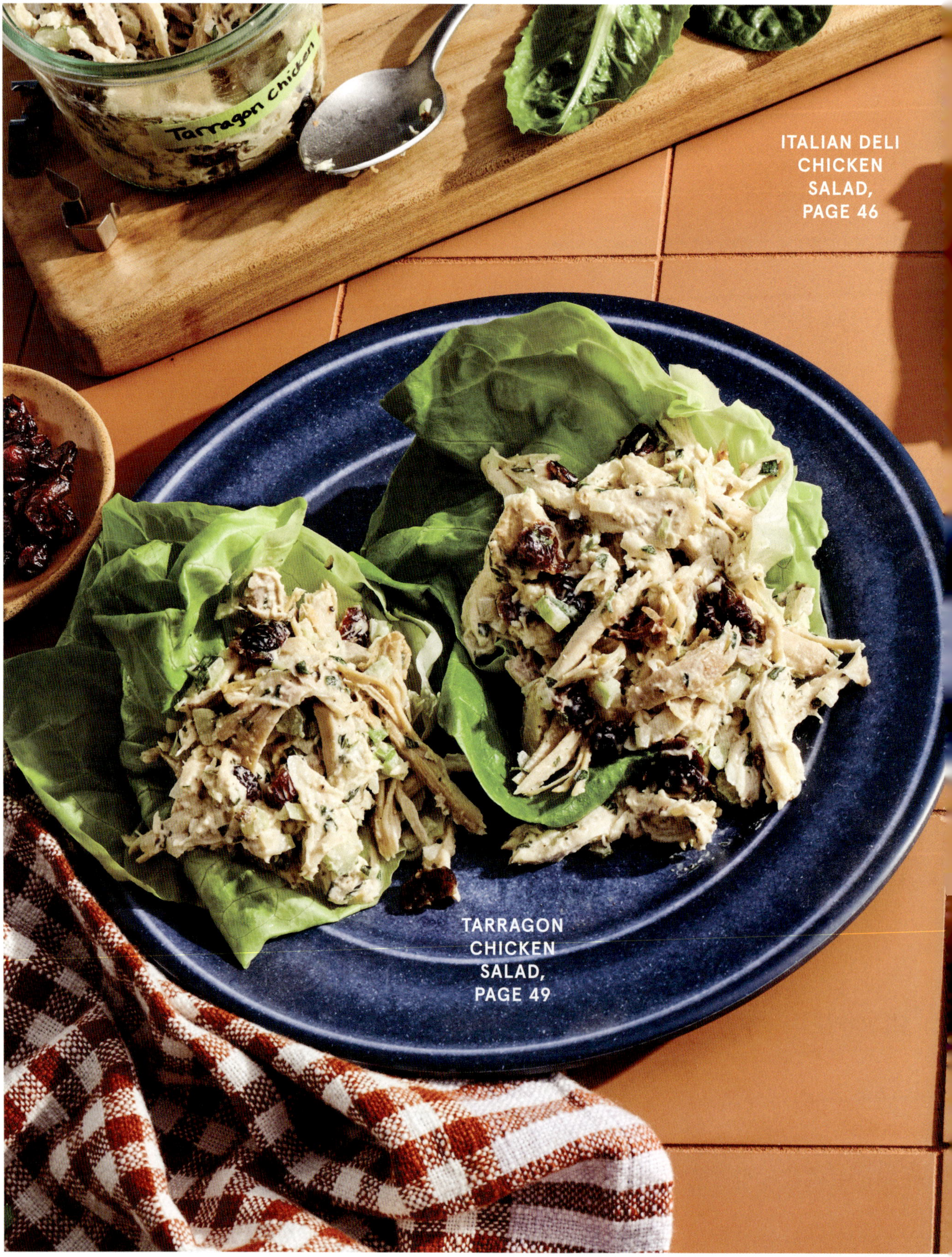

ITALIAN DELI CHICKEN SALAD, PAGE 46

TARRAGON CHICKEN SALAD, PAGE 49

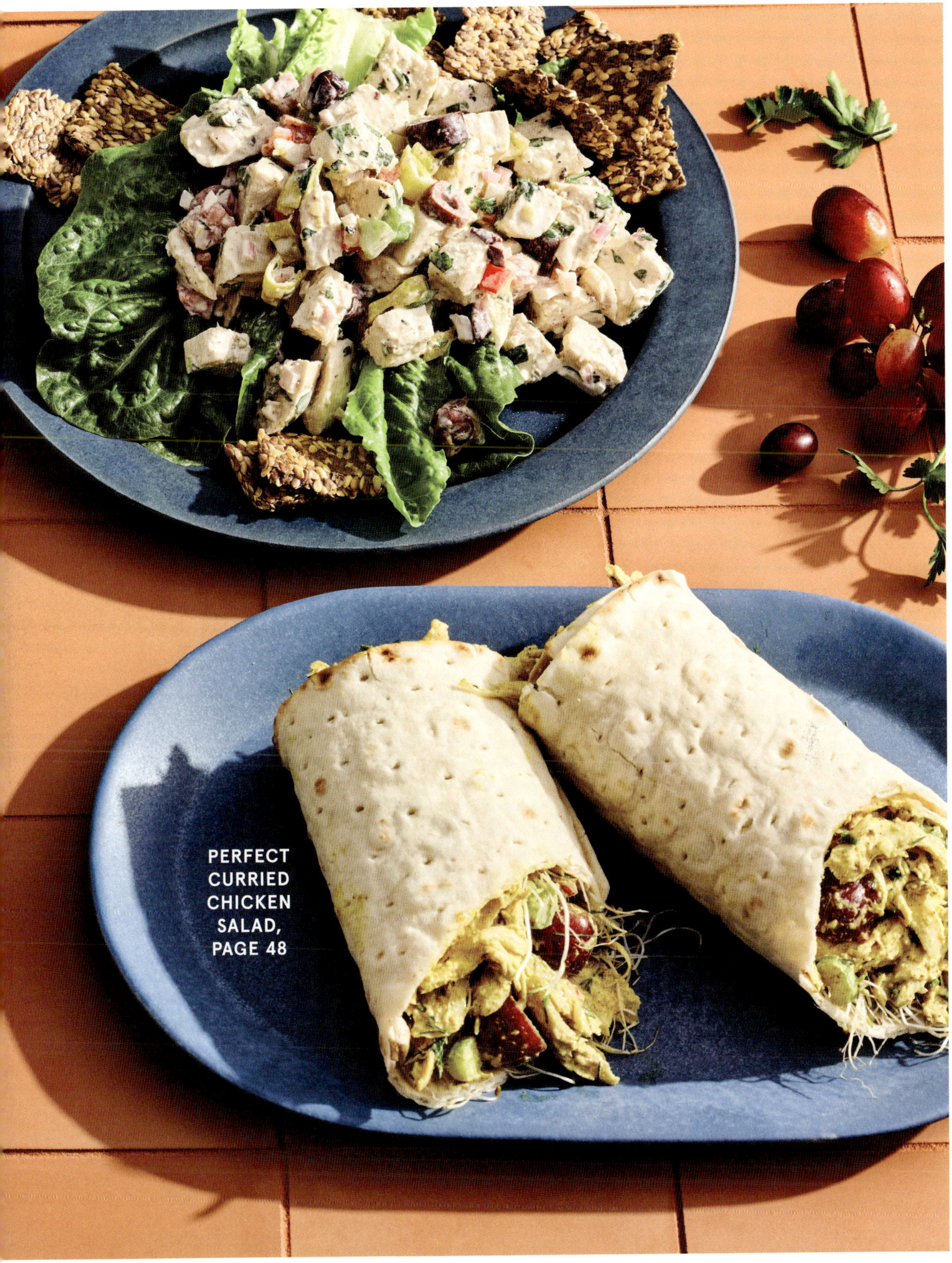

PERFECT CURRIED CHICKEN SALAD, PAGE 48

CHICKEN SHAWARMA SALAD

MAKES 6 SERVINGS | **MARINATING TIME:** 15 MINUTES TO 24 HOURS | **COOK TIME:** 35 MINUTES

DIETARY
GLUTEN-FREE
GRAIN-FREE
DAIRY-FREE
PALEO

This chicken shawarma salad is a dream come true. It's straightforward to make, but there's one key step that makes all the difference: marinating the chicken. While you can marinate it right before cooking and still have delicious results, for the best flavor and tenderness, I recommend marinating the chicken ahead of time—ideally in the morning or even the day before. When it's time to cook, simply sear the chicken on the stovetop or toss it on the grill, then pile it onto a vibrant, satisfying salad. For an extra-comforting meal, add a scoop of rice to the base and turn it into a hearty bowl.

FOR THE SHAWARMA-STYLE CHICKEN

- ¼ cup extra-virgin olive oil
- 2 teaspoons kosher salt
- ½ teaspoon freshly ground black pepper
- 3 teaspoons ground cumin
- 2 teaspoons smoked paprika
- 1 teaspoon ground coriander
- 1 teaspoon ground turmeric
- 1 teaspoon allspice
- ½ teaspoon cayenne pepper
- 4 garlic cloves, minced
- 2 tablespoons freshly squeezed lemon juice (about 1 lemon)
- 2 pounds boneless, skinless chicken thighs, trimmed of excess fat and patted dry

FOR THE TAHINI DRESSING

- ½ cup tahini
- 2 tablespoons freshly squeezed lemon juice (about 1 lemon)
- ½ teaspoon garlic powder
- ½ teaspoon kosher salt

PREPARE THE CHICKEN: In a large bowl, whisk together the oil, salt, black pepper, cumin, paprika, coriander, turmeric, allspice, cayenne, garlic, and lemon juice. Add the chicken thighs to the marinade and massage the mixture into the chicken, ensuring that each piece of chicken is well coated. Let marinate at room temperature for 15 minutes. Alternatively, you can cover and refrigerate for up to 24 hours for even more flavor.

MAKE THE TAHINI DRESSING: While the chicken is marinating, in a small bowl, whisk together the tahini, lemon juice, garlic powder, and salt. Tahini thickness can vary; if the dressing is too thick, add 2 to 4 tablespoons warm water until it reaches a Caesar dressing consistency. Set aside.

COOK THE CHICKEN: In a large skillet, preferably cast-iron, over medium-high heat, cook the chicken until golden brown on each side and fully cooked through, 4 to 5 minutes per side. Transfer to a cutting board and let rest for about 8 minutes, then slice into thin strips.

ASSEMBLE THE SALAD: Divide the lettuce, tomatoes, onion, cucumbers, and peperoncini among four bowls. Top with the sliced chicken and drizzle with the tahini dressing. Finish with a sprinkle of parsley and cilantro.

FROM MY KITCHEN TO YOURS

Alternatively, to grill the chicken, preheat a grill to medium-high heat and lightly oil the grates to prevent sticking. Place the marinated chicken thighs directly on the grill and cook for about 5 minutes per side, until the internal temperature reaches 165°F and the chicken is nicely charred. Remove the chicken from the grill and transfer to a cutting board. Let rest for about 8 minutes, then slice into thin strips.

FOR THE SALAD

6 cups thinly sliced romaine lettuce

1 cup medium-diced Roma tomatoes (about 2 medium Roma tomatoes)

½ cup halved and thinly sliced red onion (about ½ small onion)

1 cup medium-diced Persian (mini) cucumber (about 2 cucumbers)

½ cup sliced peperoncini, drained

2 tablespoons finely chopped fresh parsley leaves

2 tablespoons finely chopped fresh cilantro leaves

LEFTOVER tahini? Try my Harissa Salmon Bites with Sesame Cucumber Salad (page 214).

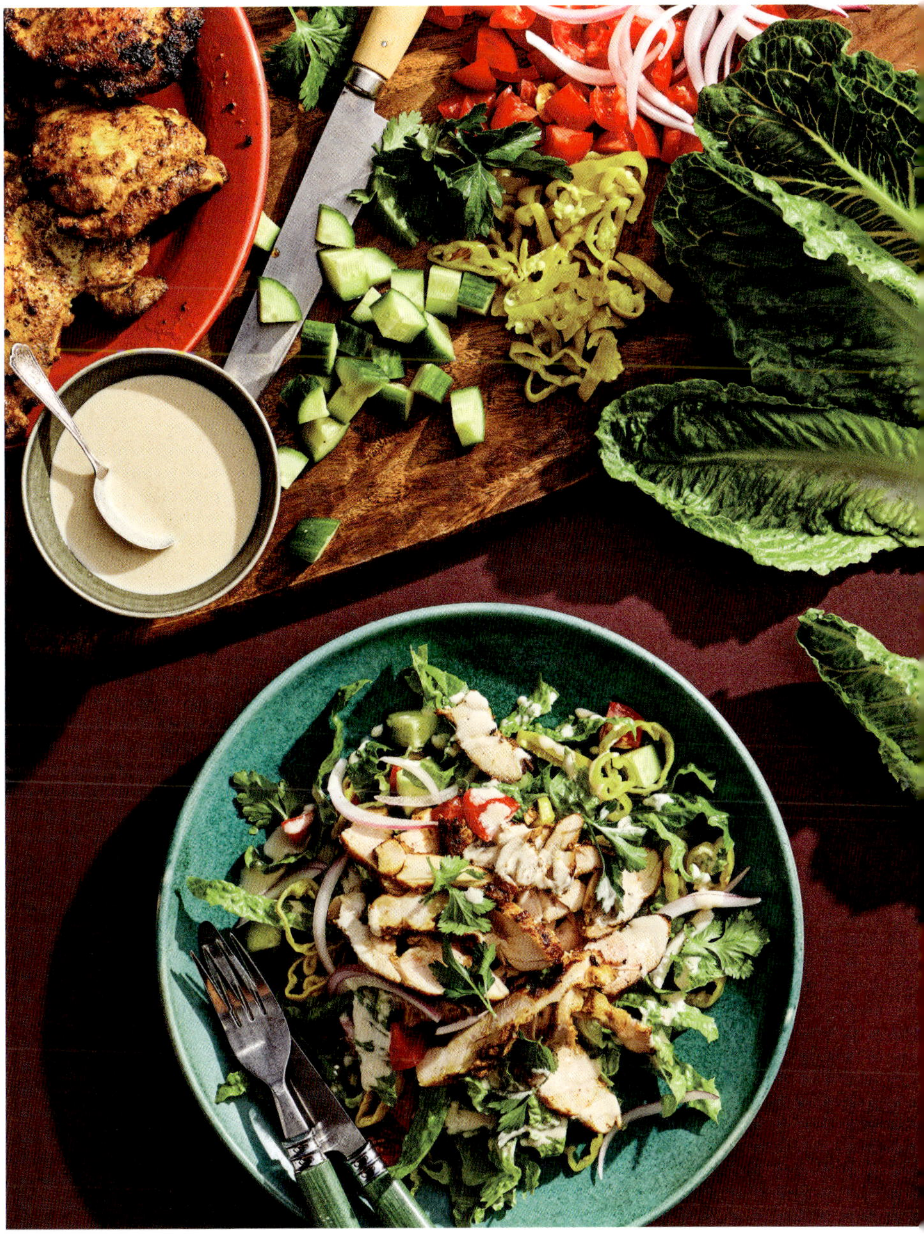

GOURMET DELI CHOP

MAKES 2 SERVINGS | **TOTAL TIME:** 20 MINUTES

DIETARY
GLUTEN-FREE
GRAIN-FREE
DAIRY-FREE (IF MODIFIED)

When you're craving a fresh, satisfying salad that comes together quickly, this recipe is for you. I love using deli meats and cheeses for a hearty chopped salad, and this simple truffle vinaigrette is a go-to in our home. Combined with crunchy potato chips for that irresistible finishing touch, this chopped salad brings big flavor with minimal effort!

FOR THE TRUFFLE VINAIGRETTE

2 tablespoons extra-virgin olive oil

2 teaspoons black truffle oil

3 tablespoons white wine vinegar

1 teaspoon Dijon mustard

½ teaspoon kosher salt

½ teaspoon freshly ground black pepper

2 garlic cloves, minced

1 large shallot, halved and thinly sliced (about ½ cup)

FOR THE SALAD

4 cups roughly chopped Little Gem lettuce or romaine hearts

2 cups roughly chopped romaine lettuce

2 Persian (mini) cucumbers, quartered lengthwise and sliced (about 2 cups)

¾ cup halved cherry tomatoes

⅓ cup sliced peperoncini peppers, drained

¼ cup roughly chopped fresh parsley leaves

¼ cup thinly sliced fresh chives

1 cup roughly chopped sliced deli ham

½ cup shredded Gruyère cheese (omit for dairy-free)

2 handfuls of gluten-free kettle-cooked potato chips

MAKE THE TRUFFLE VINAIGRETTE: In a small bowl, whisk together the olive oil, truffle oil, vinegar, mustard, salt, black pepper, and garlic. Add the shallot, stir, and set aside to allow the shallot to slightly soften and pickle while you prepare the salad.

ASSEMBLE THE SALAD: In a large bowl, combine the Little Gem lettuce, romaine, cucumbers, tomatoes, peperoncini, parsley, chives, ham, and cheese. Pour the dressing over the salad and toss until well combined.

TO serve, divide the salad between two bowls. Crumble the potato chips into smaller, bite-size pieces over each salad.

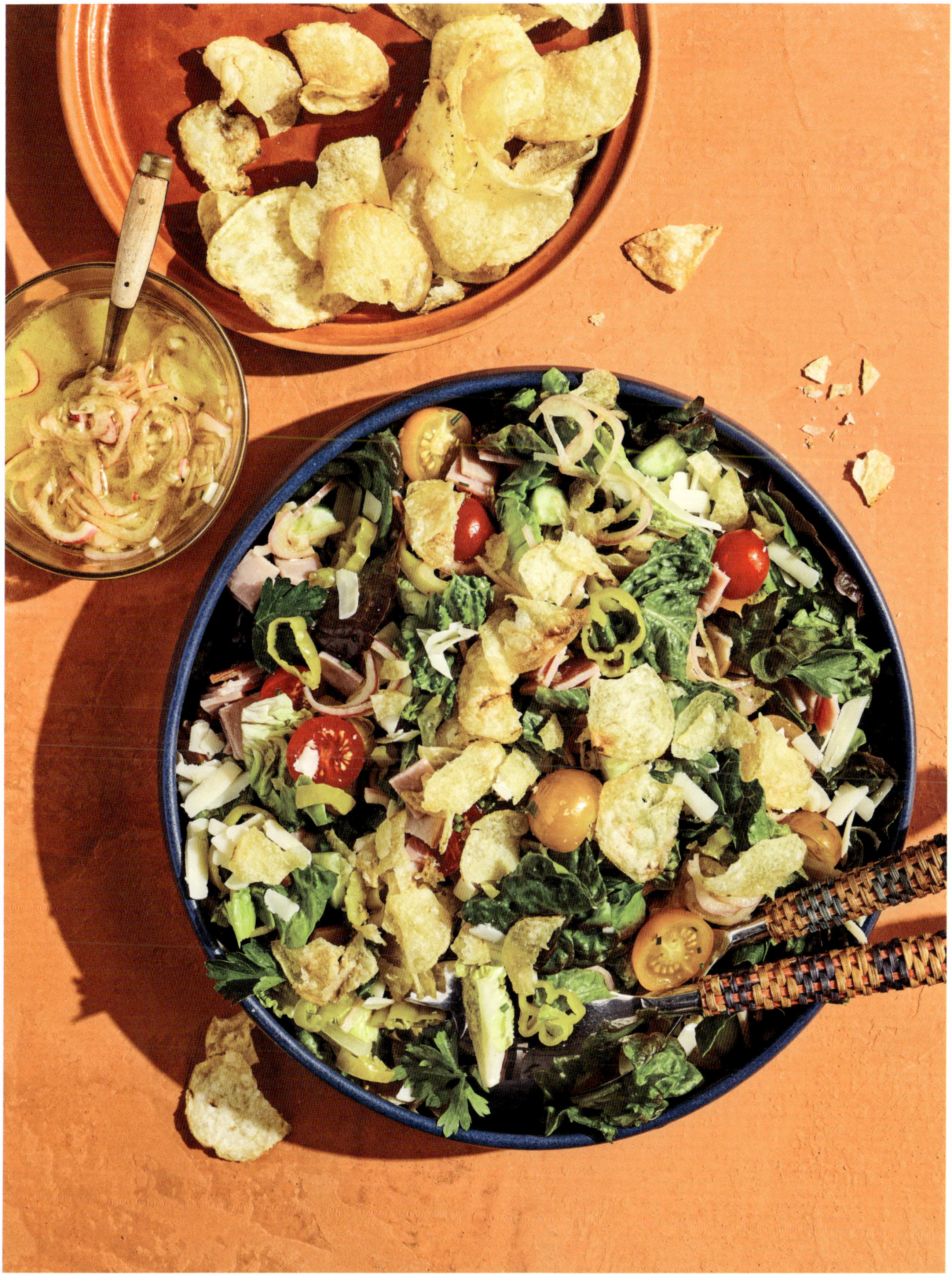

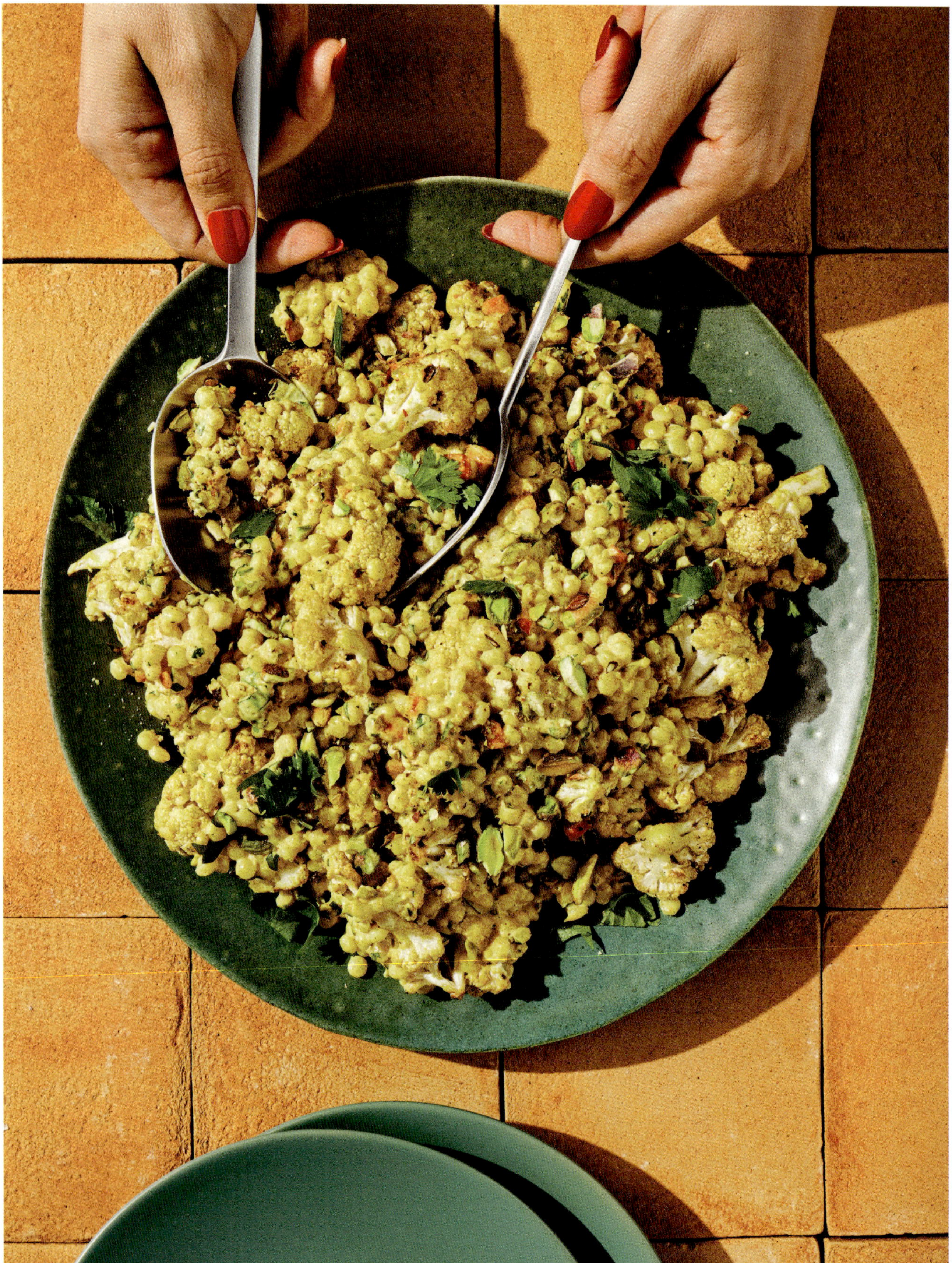

CURRIED COUSCOUS AND ROASTED CAULIFLOWER SALAD

MAKES 4 SERVINGS | **TOTAL TIME:** 40 MINUTES

DIETARY
VEGETARIAN
GLUTEN-FREE (IF MODIFIED)
MAKE AHEAD

This couscous salad takes inspiration from one of my favorite fast-casual lunch spots, Mendocino Farms. Filled with warm curry spices and roasted veggies, it's delicious served fresh but truly shines as a make-ahead option. The flavors deepen as they chill, making it an ideal meal-prep choice for lunch the next day!

4 cups small cauliflower florets (about 1 small head)

1 cup medium-diced carrot (about 1 large carrot)

2 tablespoons extra-virgin olive oil

Kosher salt

1 teaspoon freshly ground black pepper, divided

½ teaspoon ground cumin

½ cup whole-milk plain Greek yogurt

½ cup avocado oil mayo

2 teaspoons honey

2 garlic cloves, minced

½ teaspoon ground ginger

1 tablespoon curry powder

1 teaspoon ground turmeric

¼ teaspoon cayenne pepper

Grated zest of ½ lemon

2 tablespoons freshly squeezed lemon juice (about 1 lemon)

¼ cup finely chopped fresh cilantro leaves

1½ cups Israeli or pearl couscous (sub gluten-free orzo pasta for gluten-free)

½ cup chopped roasted pistachios

PREHEAT the oven to 400°F. Line a sheet pan with parchment paper.

PLACE the cauliflower and carrot on the prepared sheet pan and drizzle with the oil. Season with 1 teaspoon salt, ½ teaspoon of the black pepper, and the cumin. Toss until well coated. Roast until the veggies are fork-tender and the cauliflower is golden brown on the edges, about 20 minutes.

MEANWHILE, fill a medium saucepan with water and bring it to a boil.

WHILE waiting for the water to boil, in a large bowl, combine the yogurt, mayo, honey, garlic, ginger, curry powder, turmeric, cayenne, lemon zest, lemon juice, cilantro, ½ teaspoon salt, and the remaining ½ teaspoon black pepper. Whisk until well combined and set aside.

WHEN the water reaches a boil, add plenty of salt (I use 1 tablespoon) and the couscous. Cook the couscous according to package directions. Drain and rinse with cool water, then add to the bowl with the curry dressing. Toss until the couscous is well coated in the dressing.

WHEN the cauliflower and carrots are ready, add them to the bowl of couscous along with the roasted pistachios. Gently toss once more. Taste and add more salt, if desired.

SERVE this salad warm and eat it immediately or store in an airtight container and enjoy chilled. The salad keeps well in the fridge for up to 5 days.

SHEET PAN CHIMICHURRI SHRIMP AND CHICKPEA SALAD

MAKES 4 SERVINGS | **TOTAL TIME:** 30 MINUTES

DIETARY
GLUTEN-FREE
GRAIN-FREE
DAIRY-FREE

This sheet pan salad is a fantastic, healthy weeknight dinner that is fresh, flavorful, and quick to prepare. The chickpeas and shrimp are both roasted in the oven for minimal cleanup and topped with a vibrant, herbaceous chimichurri that pairs well with cool cucumber and avocado.

FOR THE CHIMICHURRI

1½ cups packed fresh cilantro leaves

1 cup packed fresh parsley leaves

2 garlic cloves, roughly chopped

¼ cup minced shallot (about 1 small shallot)

½ cup seeded and minced jalapeño (about 1 large jalapeño)

Grated zest of ½ lemon

2 tablespoons freshly squeezed lemon juice (about 1 lemon)

3 tablespoons red wine vinegar

½ teaspoon kosher salt

½ teaspoon freshly ground black pepper

⅓ cup extra-virgin olive oil

FOR THE SHRIMP AND CHICKPEAS

2 teaspoons ground coriander

2 teaspoons kosher salt

1 teaspoon paprika

POSITION a rack in the center of the oven and preheat the oven to 400°F. Line a large rimmed sheet pan with parchment paper and set aside.

MAKE THE CHIMICHURRI: In a blender or using an immersion blender in a wide-mouth jar, pulse the cilantro, parsley, garlic, shallot, jalapeño, lemon zest, lemon juice, vinegar, salt, black pepper, and oil until the mixture is combined but still slightly coarse. If you prefer a smoother consistency, continue to blend until smooth. Set aside.

PREPARE THE SHRIMP AND CHICKPEAS: In a small bowl, mix together the coriander, salt, paprika, garlic powder, black pepper, cumin, and pepper flakes (if using).

IN a medium bowl, combine half of the spice blend, 2 tablespoons of the oil, the shrimp, and the lemon juice. Toss until the shrimp are well coated, then set aside at room temperature. The shrimp will marinate slightly while the chickpeas roast.

PLACE the chickpeas on the prepared sheet pan. Add the remaining 2 tablespoons oil and the remaining half of the spice blend. Toss until the chickpeas are coated in the seasoning. Spread the chickpeas in an even layer, transfer to the oven, and roast for 15 minutes, until the chickpeas are just starting to crisp.

REMOVE from the oven and push the chickpeas to one side of the pan. Add the shrimp to the other side of the pan, spreading them into an even layer. Transfer

1 teaspoon garlic powder

½ teaspoon freshly ground black pepper, plus more for serving

½ teaspoon ground cumin

¼ teaspoon crushed red pepper flakes, optional

¼ cup extra-virgin olive oil, divided

1 pound peeled, deveined, and tail-off shrimp (31/40 count), patted dry

1 tablespoon freshly squeezed lemon juice (about ½ lemon)

One 14-ounce can chickpeas, drained, rinsed, and dried (see note)

FOR THE SALAD

4 cups roughly chopped butter lettuce

5 cups baby arugula

1 cup fresh cilantro leaves

2 cups halved lengthwise and thinly sliced Persian (mini) cucumbers (about 2 cucumbers)

1 large avocado, diced

back to the oven and roast for 8 to 10 minutes, until the chickpeas are golden and crisp and the shrimp are pink and cooked through. Remove from the oven and allow to cool slightly.

ASSEMBLE THE SALAD: In a large bowl, combine the butter lettuce, arugula, and cilantro. Add ¼ cup of the chimichurri and toss until well combined. Add the cucumbers and avocado and toss again. Distribute the salad among four bowls. Top each bowl with a scoop of chickpeas and shrimp. Drizzle with extra chimichurri and finish with extra freshly ground black pepper.

FROM MY KITCHEN TO YOURS

After draining and rinsing the chickpeas, dry them by placing them on a clean dish towel on a cutting board and topping them with another clean towel. Gently rub the top towel into the chickpeas. Drying them ensures they get extra crispy in the oven!

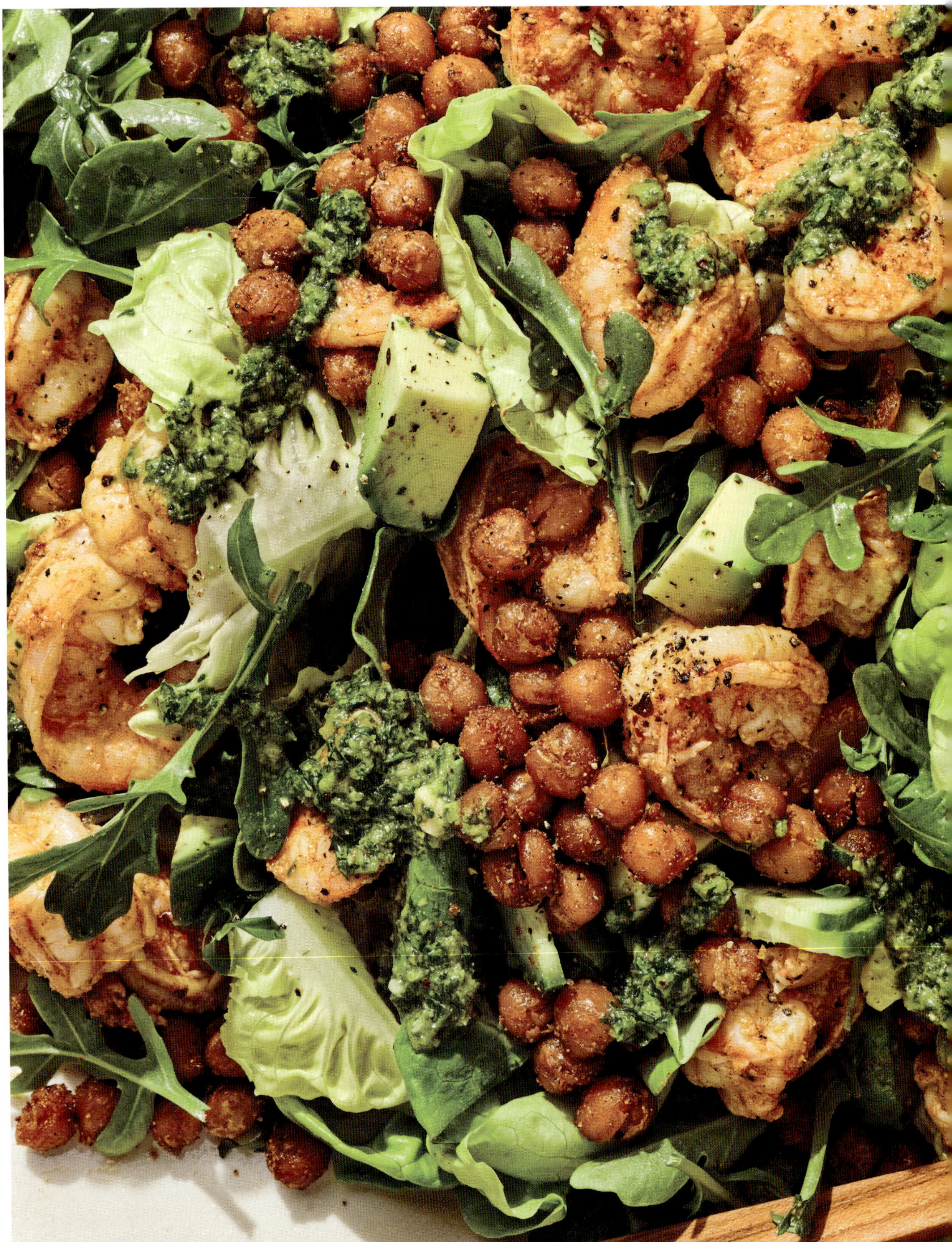

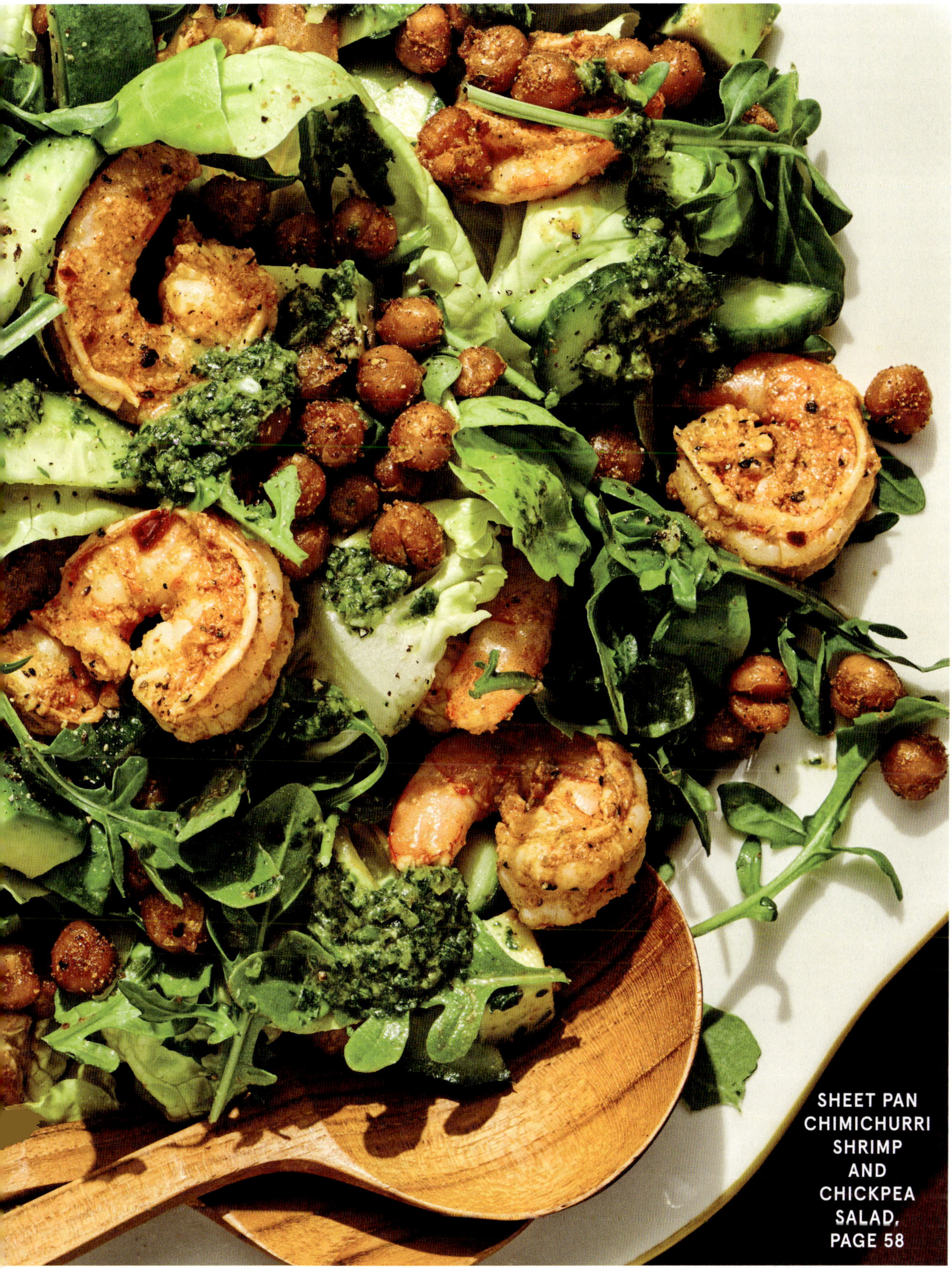

SHEET PAN CHIMICHURRI SHRIMP AND CHICKPEA SALAD, PAGE 58

CLASSIC TUNA SALAD

MAKES 2 SERVINGS | **COOK TIME:** 15 MINUTES | **CHILL TIME:** 1 HOUR

DIETARY
GLUTEN-FREE
GRAIN-FREE
DAIRY-FREE
PALEO
MAKE AHEAD

While chicken salad has its charm, tuna salad will always be my first choice for a quick and satisfying lunch. My mom instilled this love early on, and now it's a staple in my fridge—perfect for snacking or throwing together an easy meal. Depending on my mood, I'll serve it in crisp lettuce cups, piled onto crackers, or as a warm, cheesy tuna melt—topped with pickled jalapeños and Swiss cheese, of course! This tuna salad is versatile, comforting, and always hits the spot.

Two 4-ounce cans albacore or skipjack tuna, drained

½ cup finely diced celery (about 1 stalk)

¼ cup finely diced red onion (about ¼ small onion)

2 garlic cloves, minced

2 tablespoons finely chopped fresh dill

2 tablespoons avocado oil mayo

1 teaspoon Dijon mustard

1 tablespoon dill relish

1 tablespoon freshly squeezed lemon juice (about ½ lemon)

1 teaspoon coconut sugar

¼ teaspoon cayenne pepper, optional

Kosher salt and freshly ground black pepper, to taste

PLACE the drained tuna in a medium bowl and use a fork to break it up so there are no large chunks.

ADD the celery, onion, garlic, fresh dill, mayo, mustard, dill relish, lemon juice, coconut sugar, and cayenne (if using) and stir until very well combined. Season with salt and black pepper to taste.

TRANSFER to the fridge and let chill for at least 1 hour before serving. Serve as desired. This keeps well in the fridge for up to 4 days.

LEFTOVER dill relish? Try my Really Dilly Sheet Pan Salmon (page 207).

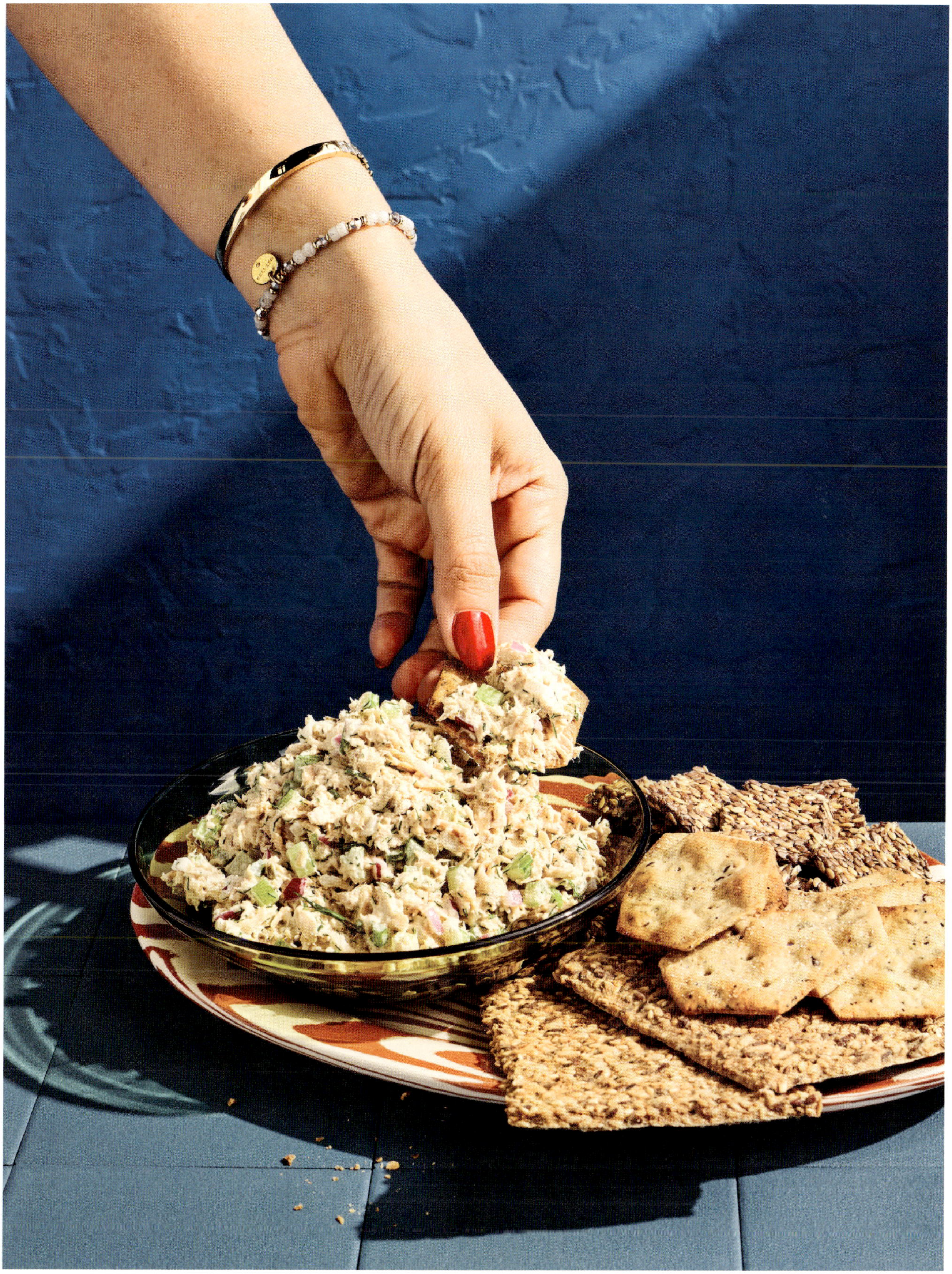

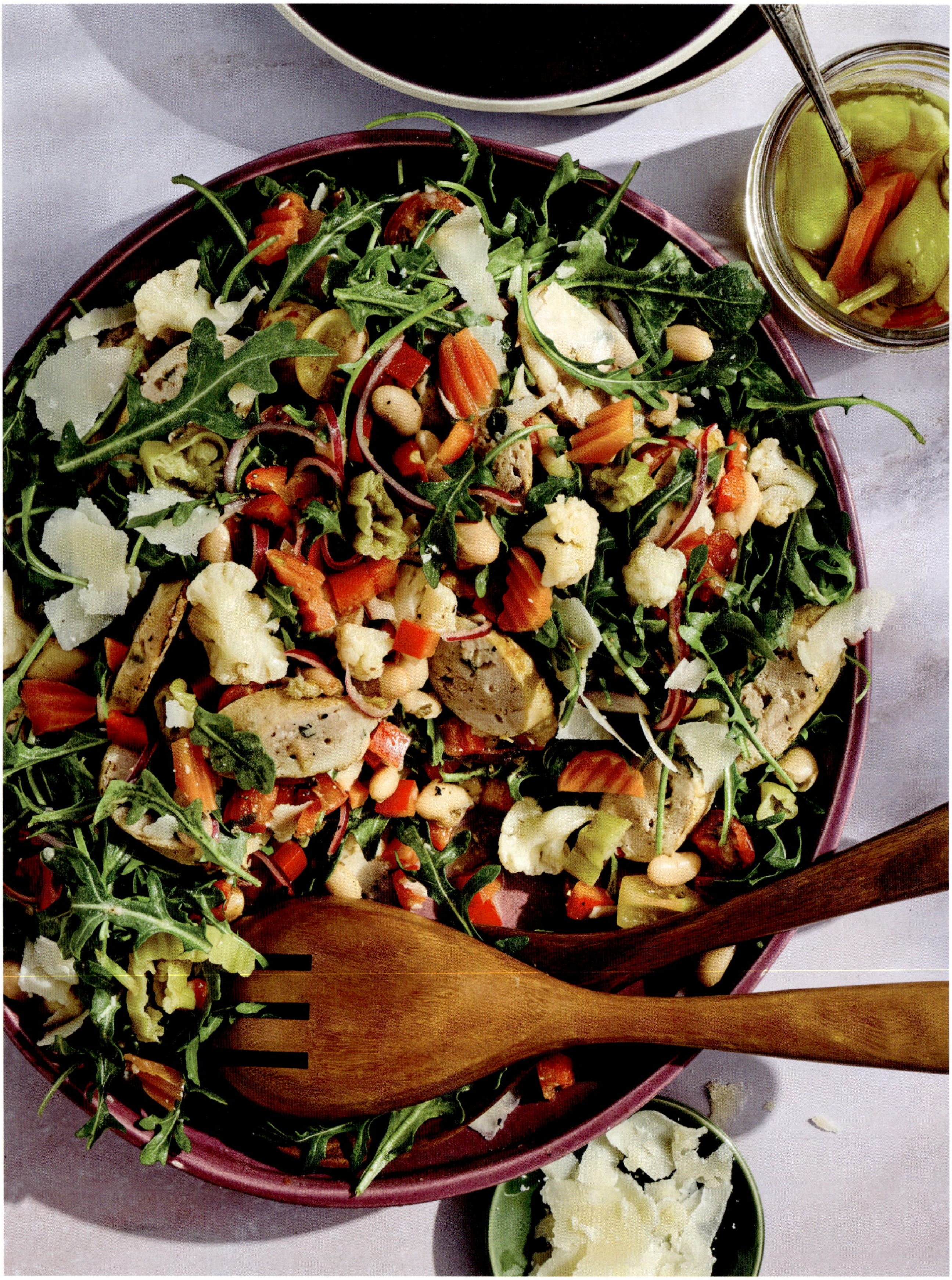

ITALIAN SAUSAGE AND GIARDINIERA GARDEN SALAD

MAKES 4 SERVINGS | **TOTAL TIME:** 35 MINUTES

DIETARY
GLUTEN-FREE
GRAIN-FREE
DAIRY-FREE (IF MODIFIED)

Get ready for a flavor-packed adventure with this hearty Italian-inspired salad! Two of my favorite ingredients, Italian sausage and giardiniera, make for an epic duo that brings a punch of flavor to every bite. The zesty mix of pickled veggies adds a crunchy kick, perfectly complementing the savory sausage and peppery arugula. This salad is hearty and refreshing, making it a delicious choice for any meal!

FOR THE DRESSING

2 tablespoons extra-virgin olive oil

2 tablespoons red wine vinegar

1 tablespoon freshly squeezed lemon juice (about ½ lemon)

1 teaspoon Dijon mustard

1 teaspoon dried oregano

½ teaspoon kosher salt

¼ teaspoon freshly ground black pepper, plus more for serving

FOR THE SALAD

One 15-ounce can cannellini beans, drained and rinsed

½ cup halved and thinly sliced red onion (about ½ small onion)

1 cup small-diced red bell pepper (about 1 small pepper)

1 cup halved cherry tomatoes

1 cup roughly chopped mild giardiniera, drained (see note)

1 tablespoon extra-virgin olive oil

4 hot or mild Italian chicken sausage links

5 cups baby arugula

¼ cup roughly chopped fresh parsley leaves

¼ cup shaved parmesan cheese (omit for dairy-free)

MAKE THE DRESSING: In a large bowl, whisk together the oil, vinegar, lemon juice, mustard, oregano, salt, and black pepper.

MAKE THE SALAD: Add the beans, onion, bell pepper, tomatoes, and giardiniera to the bowl with the dressing and toss until the salad ingredients are well combined and coated in the dressing. Allow the veggies to marinate while you cook the sausage.

IN a large skillet, heat the oil over medium heat. Add the sausage links in a single layer and cook until golden brown on each side, 2 to 3 minutes per side. Reduce the heat to medium-low and add ¼ cup water to the skillet. Cover and continue to cook, allowing the sausages to steam and fully cook through in the center, 3 to 5 more minutes.

TRANSFER the sausages to a cutting board. Let rest for 5 minutes, then thinly slice on the diagonal. Add to the bowl with the veggies and dressing.

ADD the arugula and parsley and gently toss until well combined. To serve, transfer to a platter and top with the shaved parmesan (if using) and extra freshly ground black pepper.

FROM MY KITCHEN TO YOURS

GIARDINIERA NOTE: Giardiniera is a traditional Italian pickled vegetable medley typically made with a colorful mix of peppers, carrots, and cauliflower. You can usually find it in jars in the condiment aisle, often near the pickles. For this salad, I recommend opting for the mild variety, as the hot flavor can pack a lot of heat.

STORAGE NOTE: This salad will keep in an airtight container in the fridge for up to 4 days. If prepping in advance, leave out the baby arugula and parsley until right before serving.

SPICY MISO CHICKEN SALAD

MAKES 4 SERVINGS | **TOTAL TIME:** 20 MINUTES

DIETARY
GLUTEN-FREE
DAIRY-FREE
MAKE AHEAD

This salad is essentially a deconstructed rendition of a chicken lettuce wrap, and while you can absolutely serve these in lettuce wraps, I like to chop up my greens and just eat with a fork to keep it simple! The ground chicken mixture is the real star of the show as the miso gives it a burst of umami and the sriracha adds a bit of a kick.

2 tablespoons avocado oil

½ cup small-diced shallot (about 1 large shallot)

2 garlic cloves, minced

1-inch piece fresh ginger, peeled and finely grated

½ teaspoon crushed red pepper flakes

1½ pounds ground chicken or turkey, preferably dark meat

1 teaspoon kosher salt

½ teaspoon freshly ground black pepper

4 green onions, thinly sliced on the diagonal, white and green parts kept separate

1 teaspoon toasted sesame oil

2 tablespoons gluten-free white miso paste (see note)

1 tablespoon sriracha, or more to taste

3 tablespoons coconut aminos

¼ cup roughly chopped fresh mint leaves, plus more for garnish

¼ cup roughly chopped fresh cilantro leaves, plus more for garnish

2 heads butter lettuce, roughly chopped

¼ cup roughly chopped unsalted dry-roasted peanuts

Lime wedges, for serving

LEFTOVER miso paste? Try my 20-Minute Wonton Soup (page 80).

IN a large skillet, heat the avocado oil over medium heat. Add the shallot, garlic, ginger, and pepper flakes. Cook, stirring, until tender, about 2 minutes.

ADD the ground chicken, salt, black pepper, and white part of the green onions. Cook, breaking up the meat with the edge of a spoon, until cooked through, 5 to 7 minutes.

ADD the sesame oil, miso paste, sriracha, and coconut aminos. Stir until well combined and smooth.

STIR in the mint, cilantro, and green parts of the green onions.

TO SERVE: Divide the lettuce among four bowls. Spoon the miso chicken mixture on top and garnish with additional mint and cilantro, the peanuts, and additional sriracha, if desired. Serve each bowl with a wedge of lime.

TO STORE: Store the leftover miso chicken in an airtight container in the fridge for up to 3 days, keeping the lettuce leaves and garnishes separate. Reheat the chicken in a skillet over medium heat until hot, or microwave in 1-minute increments, stirring between, until warmed through. Divide the miso chicken mixture over lettuce and garnish with mint, cilantro, peanuts, and additional sriracha, if desired. Serve with a wedge of lime.

FROM MY KITCHEN TO YOURS

Miso, a Japanese fermented paste, is made from various beans and/or grains that are both gluten-free and not gluten-free. To keep your miso dishes gluten-free, you'll need to look closely for a brand of miso paste that is gluten-free. I like Miso Master organic mellow white miso, which is labeled as certified gluten-free.

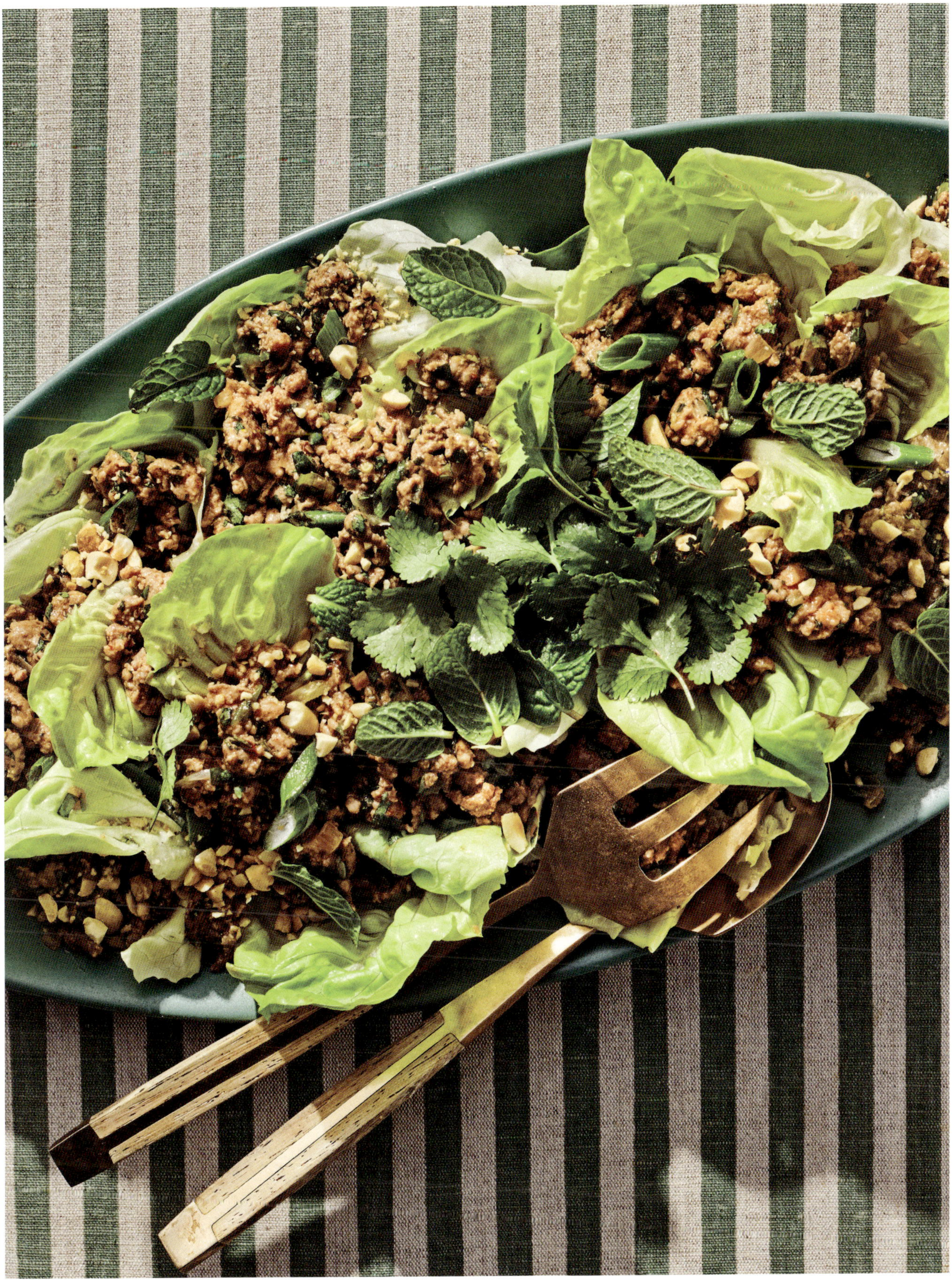

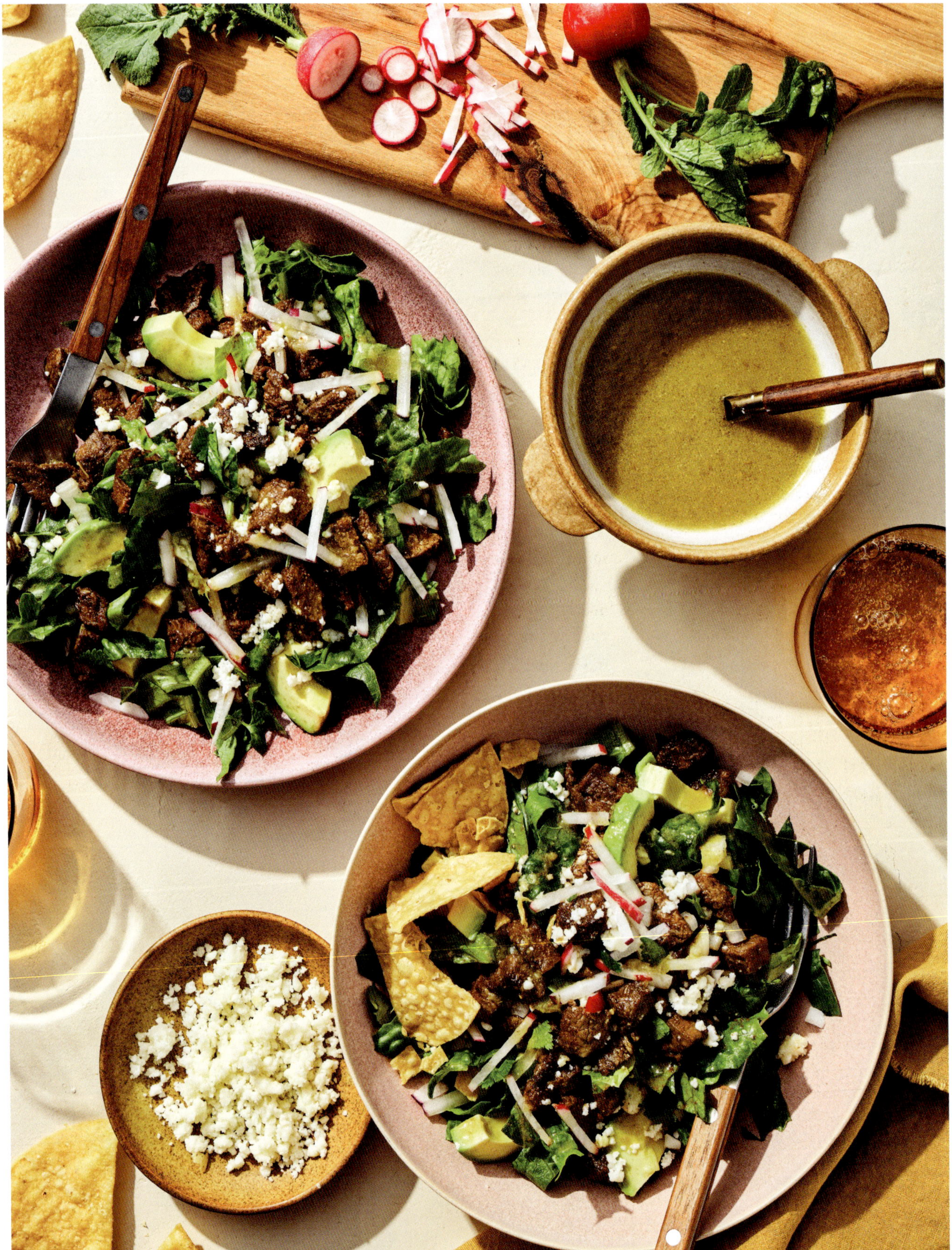

STEAK STREET TACO SALAD WITH SALSA VERDE VINAIGRETTE

MAKES 4 SERVINGS | **TOTAL TIME:** 30 MINUTES

DIETARY
GLUTEN-FREE
GRAIN-FREE (IF MODIFIED)
DAIRY-FREE (IF MODIFIED)
PALEO (IF MODIFIED)

As a self-proclaimed taco salad queen, I often skip dressing and drizzle everything with salsa. But this time, I've turned my favorite pantry staple—a jar of salsa—into a quick and zesty vinaigrette, perfect for when you want to use up the last bit in the jar. Complete with street-style steak, this is a taco lover's dream salad!

FOR THE SALSA VERDE VINAIGRETTE

⅓ cup salsa verde

¼ cup extra-virgin olive oil

½ teaspoon ground cumin

2 tablespoons freshly squeezed lime juice (about 1 lime)

½ teaspoon kosher salt

FOR THE STEAK

1½ pounds flap or skirt steak

2 teaspoons ground cumin

2 teaspoons chili powder

1 teaspoon garlic powder

1½ teaspoons kosher salt

½ teaspoon freshly ground black pepper

2 tablespoons avocado oil

FOR THE SALAD

8 cups thinly sliced romaine lettuce

½ cup finely diced white onion (about ½ small onion)

½ cup grated Cotija cheese (omit for dairy-free and paleo)

½ cup matchstick-cut red radishes

1 avocado, diced small

½ cup finely chopped fresh cilantro leaves

Corn tortilla chips (omit for paleo and grain-free)

MAKE THE SALSA VERDE VINAIGRETTE: In a small bowl or jar, whisk together the salsa verde, olive oil, cumin, lime juice, and salt. Set aside.

COOK THE STEAK: Slice the steak into a ½-inch dice and place in a medium bowl. Add the cumin, chili powder, garlic powder, salt, and pepper. Toss until steak is well coated.

IN a large skillet, heat the avocado oil over medium-high heat. Working in batches as necessary so as not to overcrowd the pan, add the steak and spread into a single layer. Cook, letting it brown on one side, about 4 minutes. Flip and continue cooking, stirring occasionally, until the steak is cooked through and slightly crisp around the edges, 4 to 5 more minutes. Using a slotted spoon, transfer the steak to a clean plate.

ASSEMBLE THE SALAD: Divide the lettuce among four bowls. Top with the diced steak, onion, Cotija (if using), radishes, avocado, and cilantro. Drizzle each salad with the salsa verde vinaigrette to taste. Serve with corn tortilla chips, if desired.

LEFTOVER salsa verde? Try my Skillet Migas Breakfast Frittata (page 43).

TANGY THAI CRUNCH SALAD WITH SEARED SALMON

MAKES 4 SERVINGS | **TOTAL TIME:** 35 MINUTES

DIETARY

- GLUTEN-FREE
- GRAIN-FREE
- DAIRY-FREE
- PALEO (IF MODIFIED)

Elevate your weeknight dinner with this refreshing and light salad. Fresh salmon is seared in nutty sesame oil until it's beautifully golden and tender. It's paired with a tangy slaw that's bursting with Thai flavors like zesty lime, a spicy pepper kick, and crunchy cabbage for a delightful meal that's both simple and satisfying.

FOR THE TANGY THAI DRESSING

1 tablespoon toasted sesame oil

1 tablespoon fish sauce

2 tablespoons rice vinegar

2 tablespoons freshly squeezed lime juice (about 1 lime)

3 tablespoons coconut aminos

2 Thai chiles, minced

2 garlic cloves, minced

1 teaspoon grated fresh ginger

1 tablespoon coconut sugar

FOR THE SLAW SALAD

3 cups finely shredded green cabbage (about ½ small head)

3 cups finely shredded purple cabbage (about ½ small head)

1 cup matchstick-cut carrots

4 Persian (mini) cucumbers, halved lengthwise and thinly sliced (about 2 cups)

¼ cup roughly chopped fresh cilantro leaves, plus more for garnish

¼ cup roughly chopped fresh mint leaves, plus more for garnish

¼ cup roughly chopped peanuts (sub cashews for paleo)

FOR THE SALMON

4 skin-on center-cut salmon fillets (6 to 8 ounces each), patted dry and pin bones removed

1 teaspoon kosher salt

½ teaspoon freshly ground black pepper

1 tablespoon toasted sesame oil

1 tablespoon avocado oil

MAKE THE DRESSING: In a small bowl or jar, whisk together the sesame oil, fish sauce, vinegar, lime juice, coconut aminos, chiles, garlic, ginger, and coconut sugar until well incorporated and the sugar is dissolved. Set aside.

PREPARE THE SLAW SALAD: In a large bowl, combine the green and purple cabbages, carrots, cucumbers, cilantro, and mint. Do not add the dressing until you're ready to serve. Set aside.

PREPARE THE SALMON: Season the salmon with the salt and pepper. In a large nonstick skillet, heat the sesame and avocado oils over medium-high heat. Add the salmon skin side down and cook, undisturbed, until golden and crisp, about 4 minutes. Flip and continue to cook, flesh side down, until the salmon is done to your liking and flakes easily with a fork, 4 to 5 more minutes. Transfer the fillets to a clean plate.

ASSEMBLE THE SALAD: Pour the dressing over the slaw and toss until well combined. Divide the slaw among four bowls. Top each bowl with a salmon fillet and some chopped nuts. Garnish with additional cilantro and mint.

LEFTOVER green cabbage? Try my Shortcut Chicken Pozole Verde (page 94) or Skillet Unstuffed Cabbage Rolls (page 200).

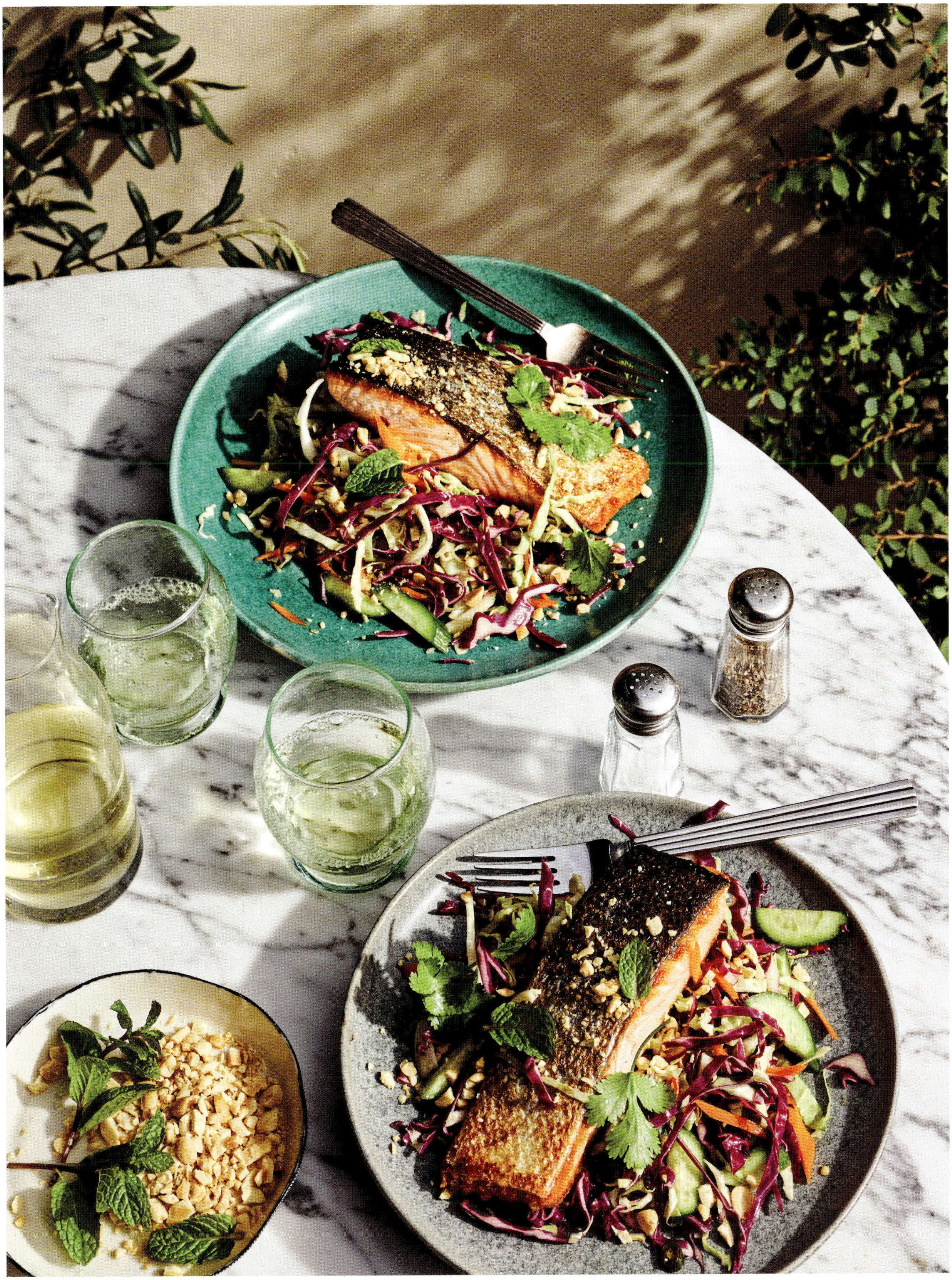

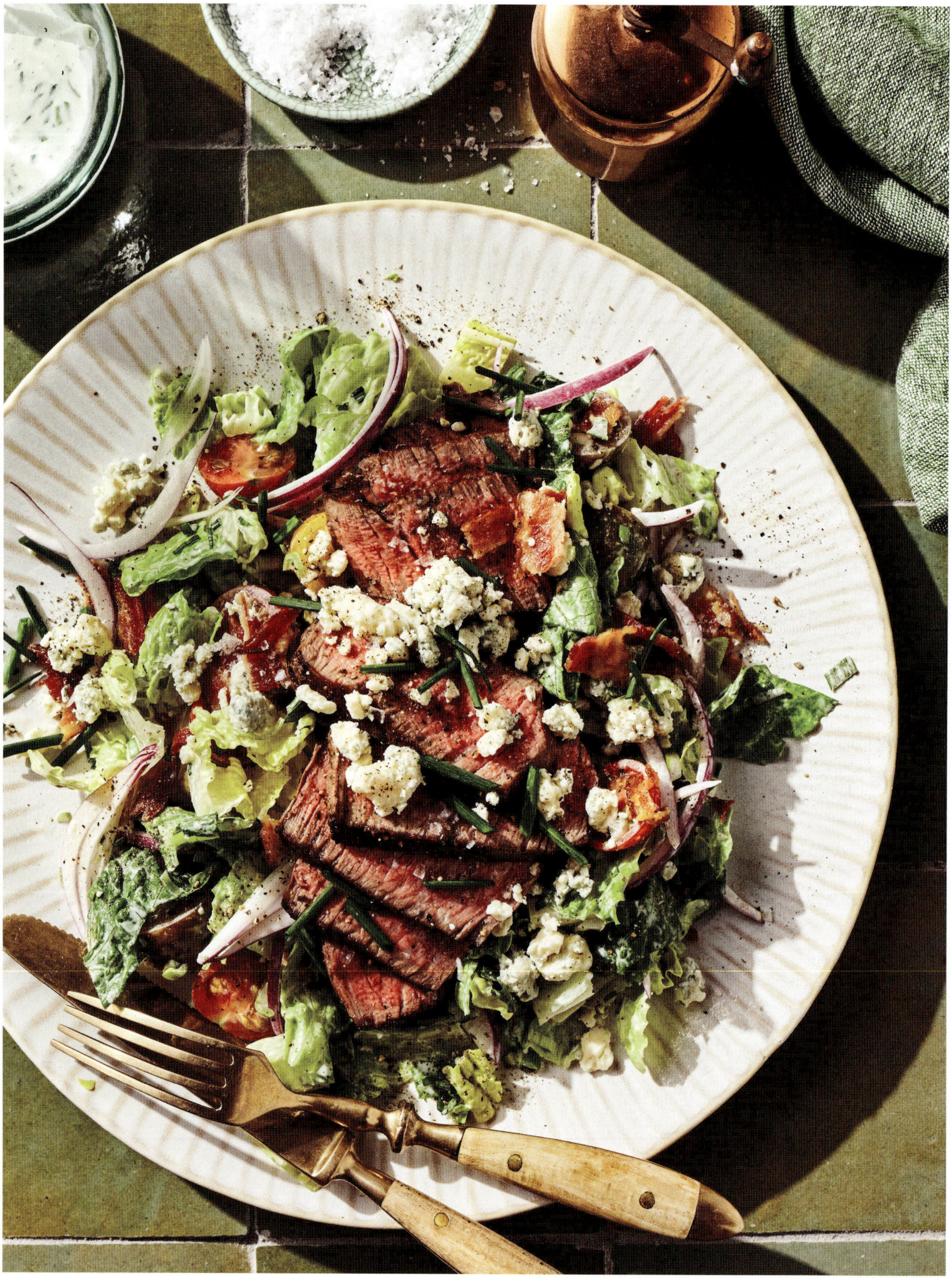

STEAKHOUSE CHOPPED SALAD

MAKES 4 SERVINGS | **TOTAL TIME:** 30 MINUTES

DIETARY
GLUTEN-FREE
GRAIN-FREE

This hearty salad is a fresh take on the classic wedge without the iceberg. Ready in just thirty minutes, it delivers all the flavors from your favorite steakhouse with minimal effort. Featuring crispy bacon, creamy blue cheese, ripe tomatoes, and juicy filet mignon, this weeknight-friendly meal feels truly restaurant-worthy.

FOR THE BLUE CHEESE DRESSING

2 garlic cloves, minced

¼ cup whole-milk plain Greek yogurt

2 tablespoons avocado oil mayo

¼ cup freshly squeezed lemon juice (about 2 lemons)

½ teaspoon kosher salt

¼ teaspoon freshly ground black pepper

½ cup crumbled blue cheese, divided

¾ cup chopped fresh chives, divided

FOR THE BACON AND STEAK

4 slices no-sugar-added bacon

4 filet mignon steaks (6 to 8 ounces each)

2 teaspoons kosher salt

½ teaspoon freshly ground black pepper

2 tablespoons avocado oil

FOR THE SALAD

8 cups sliced romaine lettuce (about 2 medium heads)

1 cup halved and thinly sliced red onion (about 1 small onion)

1 cup halved grape tomatoes

2 green onions, thinly sliced and roughly chopped (about ½ cup)

MAKE THE DRESSING: In a large bowl, combine the garlic, yogurt, mayo, lemon juice, salt, and pepper. Whisk until smooth. Add ⅓ cup of the blue cheese and ½ cup of the chives. Whisk to combine until the blue cheese starts to emulsify into the dressing but a few clumps remain. Set aside.

COOK THE BACON AND STEAK: Line a plate with paper towels. Place the bacon in a cold large skillet, preferably cast iron. Turn the heat to medium and cook until the bacon is crisp, about 4 minutes per side. Transfer the bacon to the prepared plate. Remove the skillet from the heat and wipe it down with a paper towel to remove the bacon grease. When the bacon is cool, crumble it and set it aside.

PAT the steaks dry with paper towels. Season all sides with the salt and pepper.

SET the skillet over medium-high heat. When hot, add the oil. Carefully add the steaks to the pan and cook until a deep brown crust forms, 3 to 4 minutes per side for medium-rare, 5 to 6 minutes per side for more well done. You will know that the steak is ready to flip when it easily releases from the pan. Transfer to a cutting board and let rest while you assemble the salad.

ASSEMBLE THE SALAD: Add the romaine, red onion, tomatoes, green onions, and crumbled bacon to the bowl with dressing and toss well to coat.

AFTER the steak has rested, cut into thin slices against the grain of the meat.

TO SERVE: Divide the salad among four bowls and top each with the sliced steak. Garnish with the remaining blue cheese crumbles and chives.

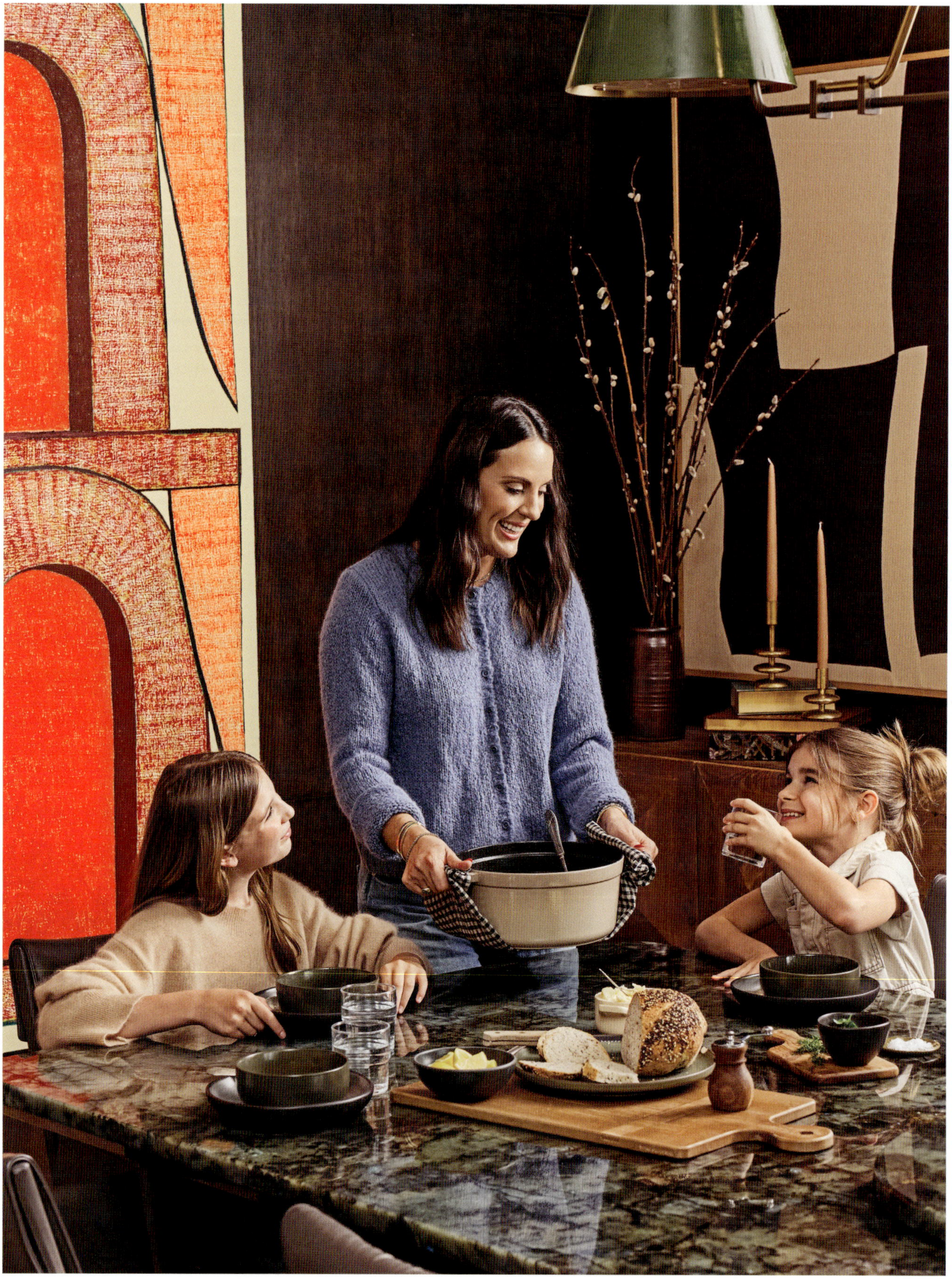

SIMPLE SOUPS

MARRY ME WHITE BEAN SOUP

MAKES 4 SERVINGS | **TOTAL TIME:** 40 MINUTES

DIETARY
GLUTEN-FREE
DAIRY-FREE (IF MODIFIED)
VEGETARIAN (IF MODIFIED)
MAKE AHEAD

This soup gets its name from the beloved "Marry Me" dishes that are so good, they just might earn you a marriage proposal! Inspired by the flavors of Marry Me Chicken, this cozy, flavor-packed soup features creamy cannellini beans, sun-dried tomatoes, pancetta, and a touch of coconut milk for richness. A hint of lemon and fresh basil keeps it bright and balanced, making it irresistibly delicious. Whether served with crusty bread or on its own, this bowl is sure to win hearts!

4 ounces diced pancetta (omit for vegetarian)

½ cup small-diced oil-packed sun-dried tomatoes, oil reserved

1 cup finely diced yellow onion (about ½ medium onion)

4 garlic cloves, minced

½ teaspoon crushed red pepper flakes

1 teaspoon kosher salt, plus more to taste

½ teaspoon freshly ground black pepper, plus more to taste

1 tablespoon tomato paste

¼ cup dry white wine

Two 15-ounce cans cannellini beans, drained and rinsed

2 cups low-sodium vegetable broth

1 cup unsweetened full-fat coconut milk or heavy cream

1 teaspoon dried oregano

1 bay leaf

1 parmesan cheese rind (omit for dairy-free)

Grated zest of ½ lemon

3 cups baby spinach

2 tablespoons freshly squeezed lemon juice (about 1 lemon)

½ cup thinly sliced fresh basil leaves, plus more for serving

Freshly grated parmesan cheese (omit for dairy-free)

IN a large pot or Dutch oven, cook the pancetta (if using) over medium heat, stirring occasionally, until the fat renders and the pancetta begins to crisp, about 5 minutes.

ADD 1 tablespoon oil from the sun-dried tomatoes to the pot, the sun-dried tomatoes, onion, garlic, pepper flakes, salt, and black pepper and cook, stirring, until the onion is tender, about 4 more minutes. Stir in the tomato paste until well combined.

ADD the wine and continue to cook, stirring and scraping up any browned bits off the bottom, until the wine has reduced by half, about 2 minutes.

ADD the beans, broth, milk, oregano, bay leaf, parmesan rind (if using), and lemon zest and bring the soup to a boil. Reduce the heat to a gentle simmer, about medium-low heat, cover, and cook for about 20 minutes, stirring occasionally, until the flavors have melded.

DISCARD the bay leaf and the parmesan rind. Stir in the spinach, lemon juice, and basil until the spinach just wilts. Taste and add more salt and black pepper as desired.

TO SERVE: Ladle the soup into bowls and top with basil and freshly grated parmesan (if using).

STORE in the fridge in an airtight container for 3 to 4 days, or in the freezer for up to 3 months without the garnishes. To reheat from the fridge, transfer to a pot over medium heat for 10 to 12 minutes, stirring occasionally, until warmed through, or microwave in 1-minute increments, stirring after each, until warmed through. Add more broth if needed. To reheat from frozen, thaw overnight in the fridge, then warm as directed. Top with fresh basil and freshly grated parmesan (if using) after reheating.

LEFTOVER sun-dried tomatoes? Try my Freezer-Friendly Mediterranean Breakfast Sandwiches (page 32) or Creamy Sun-Dried Tomato Basil Chicken (page 153).

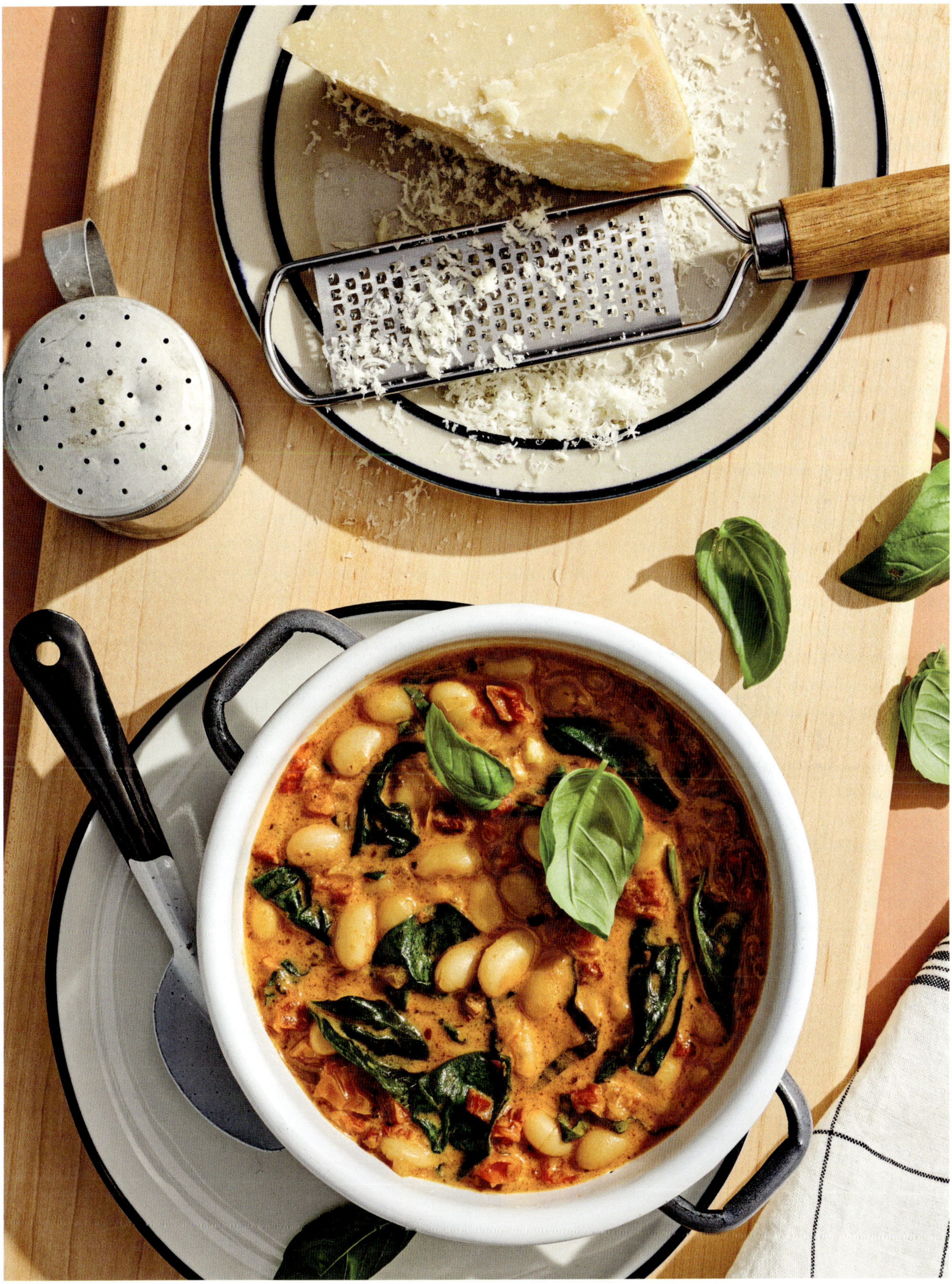

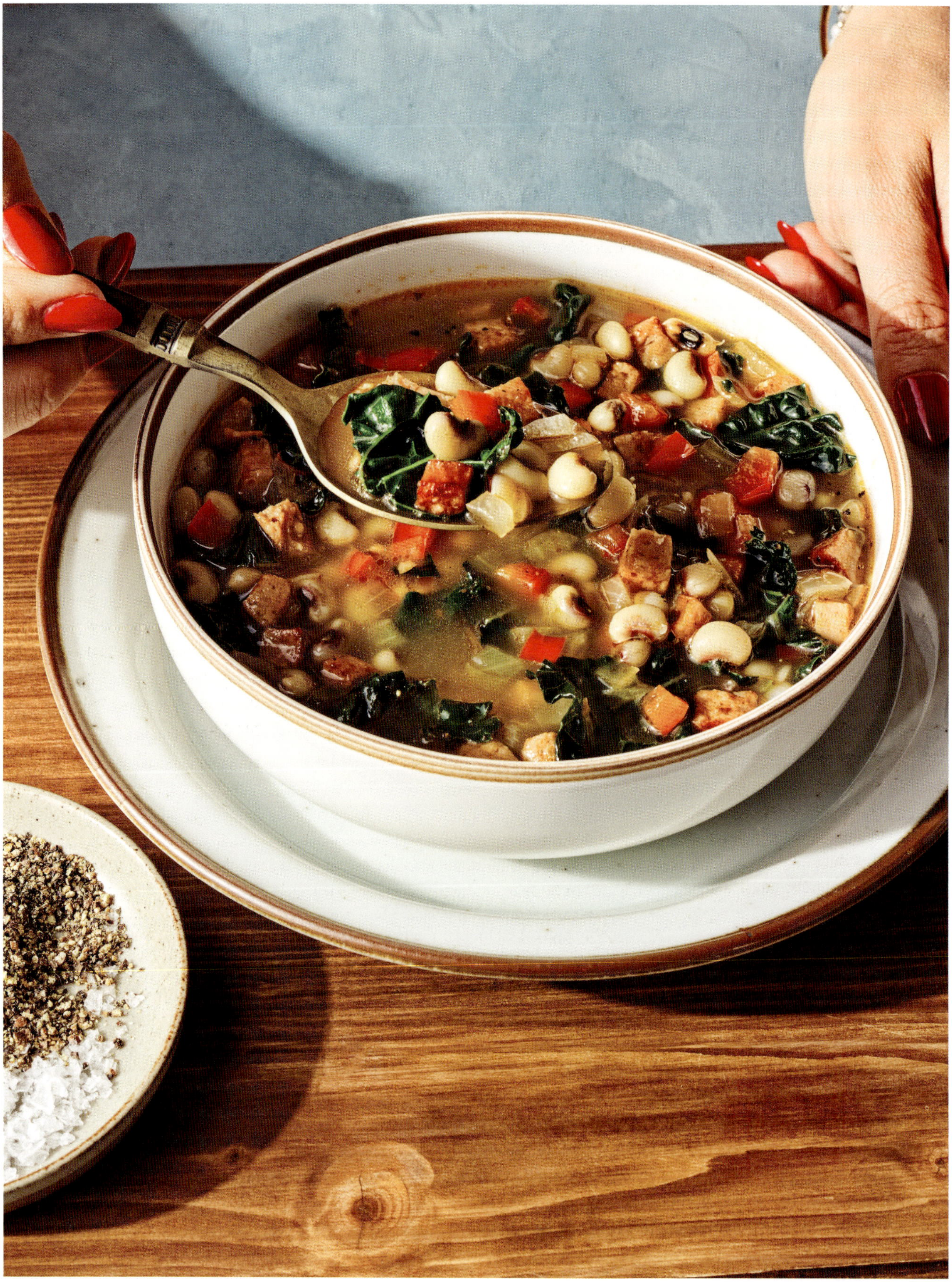

GOOD LUCK BLACK-EYED PEA SOUP

MAKES 6 SERVINGS | **TOTAL TIME:** 45 MINUTES

DIETARY
GLUTEN-FREE
GRAIN-FREE
DAIRY-FREE
MAKE AHEAD

This hearty, soul-warming soup is inspired by the Southern tradition of enjoying black-eyed peas for good luck in the new year—but it's delicious enough to enjoy any time of year. Smoky kielbasa, a touch of spice from jalapeño and chili powder, and a savory, aromatic broth make this a deeply satisfying one-pot meal. Using frozen black-eyed peas also keeps prep simple without sacrificing flavor!

2 tablespoons extra-virgin olive oil

12 ounces kielbasa sausage, cut into small dice

1 cup finely diced red bell pepper (about 1 small bell pepper)

1 cup finely diced yellow onion (about ½ medium onion)

½ cup seeded and finely diced jalapeño (about 1 large jalapeño)

4 garlic cloves, minced

1½ teaspoons kosher salt, plus more to taste

½ teaspoon freshly ground black pepper

2 teaspoons chili powder

1 teaspoon ground cumin

24 ounces frozen black-eyed peas (see note)

8 cups low-sodium chicken broth

2 teaspoons apple cider vinegar

1 bay leaf

4 cups de-ribbed and roughly chopped lacinato kale (about 1 bunch)

IN a large pot or Dutch oven, heat the oil over medium heat. Add the kielbasa and cook, stirring occasionally, until lightly browned, about 4 minutes.

ADD the bell pepper, onion, and jalapeño. Cook, stirring, until softened, 5 to 6 minutes. Stir in the garlic, salt, black pepper, chili powder, and cumin. Cook until fragrant, about 1 minute.

ADD the black-eyed peas, broth, vinegar, and bay leaf. Bring the soup to a gentle boil, then reduce the heat and simmer, covered, for about 20 minutes, or until the peas are tender and the flavors have melded.

DISCARD the bay leaf and stir in the kale and let cook until just wilted, 2 to 3 minutes. Taste and add more salt as desired. Ladle into bowls and serve.

STORE in the fridge in an airtight container for 3 to 4 days, or in the freezer for up to 3 months. To reheat from the fridge, transfer to a pot over medium heat for 10 to 12 minutes, stirring occasionally, until warmed through, or microwave in 1-minute increments, stirring after each, until warmed through. Add more broth if needed. To reheat from frozen, thaw overnight in the fridge, then warm as directed.

FROM MY KITCHEN TO YOURS

FOR DRIED BLACK-EYED PEAS: Be sure to soak them ahead of time. To soak, place 8 ounces (1¼ cups) dried peas in a large bowl and cover with water by several inches. Allow them to soak overnight (or at least 8 hours), then drain and rinse before adding to the soup. The soup cooking time may need to be extended by 10 to 15 minutes, until the peas are tender.

FOR CANNED BLACK-EYED PEAS: Substitute three 15-ounce cans, drained and rinsed. Reduce the simmering time by about 10 minutes, as canned peas are already fully cooked.

20-MINUTE WONTON SOUP

MAKES 4 SERVINGS | **TOTAL TIME:** 20 MINUTES

DIETARY
DAIRY-FREE
VEGETARIAN
MAKE AHEAD

I love keeping a bag of frozen wontons in my freezer for an easy dinner option. They're great with sautéed veggies, but I mostly use them for a quick and delicious soup that my whole family devours every time. Here's a fresh and easy recipe packed with flavor, thanks to garlic, ginger, lime, fish sauce, cilantro, and more!

1 tablespoon avocado oil

2 tablespoons toasted sesame oil

4 green onions, sliced on the diagonal, white and green parts kept separate

2 cups stemmed and thinly sliced shiitake mushrooms

1 teaspoon kosher salt, plus more to taste

2 heads baby bok choy, roughly chopped (about 2 cups)

2 garlic cloves, minced

2 teaspoons finely grated fresh ginger

1 tablespoon white miso paste

6 cups low-sodium vegetable broth (sub chicken broth for non-vegetarian)

2 tablespoons coconut aminos

1 tablespoon rice vinegar

1 teaspoon fish sauce

2 tablespoons freshly squeezed lime juice (about 1 lime)

One 12-ounce bag frozen vegetable wontons (sub chicken, pork, or beef)

Chili oil, optional for serving

2 tablespoons chopped fresh cilantro leaves

IN a large pot or Dutch oven, heat the avocado oil and toasted sesame oil over medium heat. Add the white parts of the green onions, mushrooms, and salt to the pot. Sauté until the veggies are tender, about 3 minutes.

ADD the baby bok choy, garlic, ginger, and miso paste. Stir to combine and sauté, stirring, until the bok choy is slightly tender, about 2 minutes.

STIR IN the broth, coconut aminos, vinegar, fish sauce, and lime juice and bring to a simmer. Add the wontons and cook until the wontons are tender, 2 to 6 minutes, depending on the size and brand. The wontons will float to the top when done.

TASTE and add more salt as desired. Serve in bowls with a drizzle of chili oil (if desired). Top with the reserved green parts of the green onions and the cilantro.

STORE in the fridge in an airtight container for 3 to 4 days, or in the freezer for up to 3 months without the garnishes. To reheat from the fridge, transfer to a pot over medium heat for 10 to 12 minutes, stirring occasionally, until warmed through, or microwave in 1-minute increments, stirring after each, until warmed through. To reheat from frozen, thaw overnight in the fridge, then warm as directed. Top with fresh green parts of the green onions and cilantro after reheating.

LEFTOVER miso paste? Try my Spicy Miso Chicken Salad (page 66).

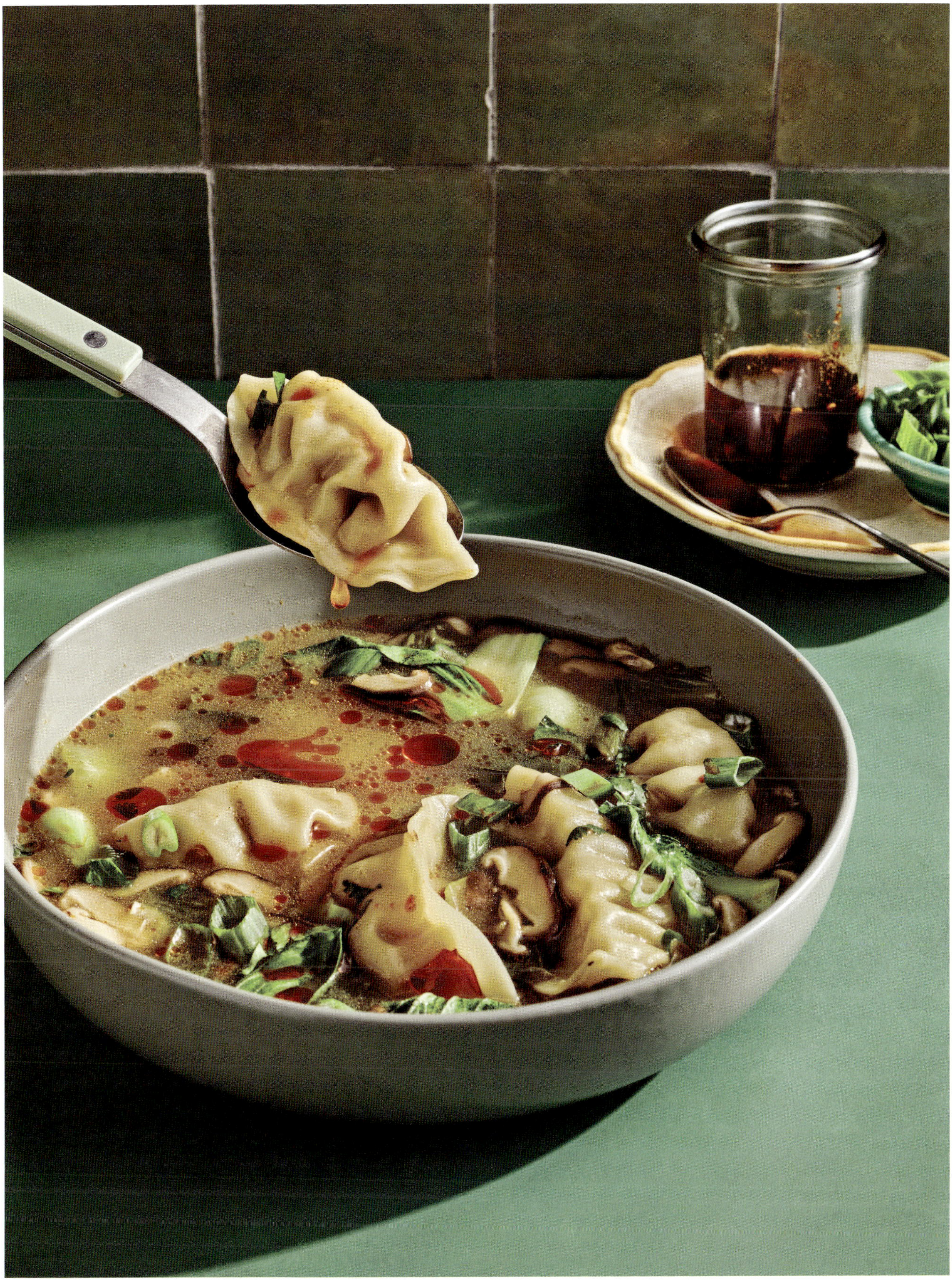

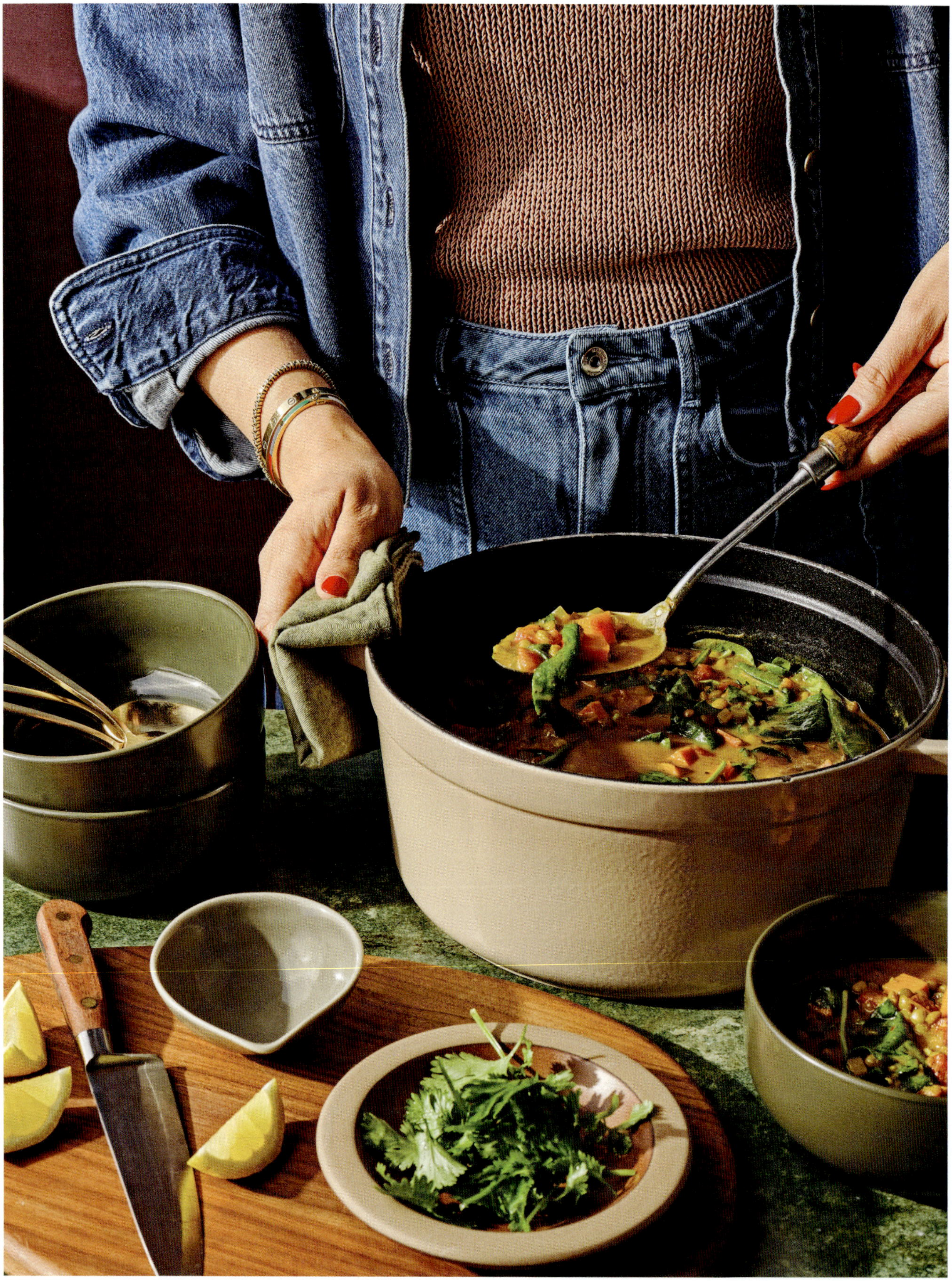

CURRIED LENTIL SOUP

MAKES 6 SERVINGS | **TOTAL TIME:** 45 MINUTES

DIETARY
GLUTEN-FREE
GRAIN-FREE
DAIRY-FREE
VEGETARIAN
MAKE AHEAD

This vibrant, veggie-packed curry soup is as nourishing as it is flavorful, offering a warm hug in every bowl. Sweet potatoes, lentils, and spinach are simmered in a spiced broth infused with curry powder, turmeric, and cumin, creating a dish that's both hearty and wholesome. A splash of coconut milk adds creamy richness, while fresh lemon juice brightens every bite. It's a comforting one-pot meal perfect for cozy evenings or a nutrient-rich lunch.

2 tablespoons extra-virgin olive oil

1 cup finely diced yellow onion (about ½ medium onion)

4 garlic cloves, minced

2 teaspoons kosher salt, plus more to taste

1 teaspoon freshly ground black pepper

½ teaspoon crushed red pepper flakes

2 cups medium-diced unpeeled sweet potato (about 1 large sweet potato)

1½ cups brown lentils, rinsed

1 tablespoon curry powder

1 teaspoon ground turmeric

1 teaspoon ground cumin

½ teaspoon smoked paprika

6 cups low-sodium vegetable broth

One 14.5-ounce can fire-roasted tomatoes

1 bay leaf

4 cups packed baby spinach

1 cup unsweetened full-fat coconut milk

2 tablespoons freshly squeezed lemon juice (about 1 lemon)

Fresh cilantro leaves, for serving

IN a large pot or Dutch oven, heat the oil over medium heat. Add the onion, garlic, salt, black pepper, and pepper flakes. Cook, stirring, until the onions are tender, about 5 minutes.

ADD the sweet potato, lentils, curry powder, turmeric, cumin, and paprika. Continue to cook, stirring, until the spices are fragrant and lightly toasted, about 2 minutes.

ADD the broth, tomatoes, and bay leaf. Bring to a rapid simmer, then reduce the heat to a gentle simmer, about medium-low heat. Cover and cook until the lentils and sweet potatoes are tender, about 25 minutes, stirring occasionally.

ADD the spinach and coconut milk. Stir until well combined and the spinach has just wilted. Let simmer, uncovered, for 5 minutes to allow the flavors to meld together.

REMOVE from the heat and stir in the lemon juice. Discard the bay leaf. Taste and add more salt as desired.

TO SERVE: Ladle the soup into bowls and garnish with cilantro.

STORE in the fridge in an airtight container for 3 to 4 days, or in the freezer for up to 3 months without the garnishes. To reheat from the fridge, transfer to a pot over medium heat for 10 to 12 minutes, stirring occasionally, until warmed through, or microwave in 1-minute increments, stirring after each, until warmed through. Add more broth if needed. To reheat from frozen, thaw overnight in the fridge, then warm as directed. Top with fresh cilantro after reheating.

GROUND BEEF AND BARLEY STEW

MAKES 8 SERVINGS | **TOTAL TIME:** 50 MINUTES

DIETARY
DAIRY-FREE
MAKE AHEAD

Cozy, comforting, and perfect for busy weeknights, this stew is my quicker take on a classic. Typically made with tender chunks of beef simmered with hearty barley, veggies, and rich broth, in this version I've swapped in ground beef to make it come together faster, without sacrificing any of that slow-cooked flavor. It's a family-friendly dinner that's both nourishing and easy to make—perfect for those chilly fall evenings!

2 tablespoons extra-virgin olive oil

1 cup finely diced yellow onion (about ½ medium onion)

1 cup thinly sliced celery (about 2 stalks)

1 cup medium-diced carrot (about 1 large carrot)

1 pound ground beef (90/10)

3 garlic cloves, minced

2 teaspoons kosher salt

1 teaspoon freshly ground black pepper

1½ teaspoons smoked paprika

1 teaspoon dried oregano

2 tablespoons tamari or soy sauce

2 tablespoons tomato paste

1 tablespoon balsamic vinegar

4 cups low-sodium beef broth

One 14.5-ounce can no-salt-added diced tomatoes

1 cup pearled barley

1 teaspoon finely chopped fresh rosemary leaves or ½ teaspoon dried

2 teaspoons finely chopped fresh thyme leaves or 1 teaspoon dried

1 bay leaf

Fresh thyme leaves, for garnish

IN a large pot or Dutch oven, heat the oil over medium heat. Add the onion, celery, and carrot and cook, stirring, until the veggies soften, about 6 minutes.

ADD the ground beef and continue to cook, breaking up the meat with the edge of a spoon, until the beef is cooked through and no longer pink, about 7 minutes. Drain off the excess fat and return the beef to the pot.

ADD the garlic, salt, pepper, paprika, oregano, tamari, tomato paste, and vinegar. Stir until well combined with the ground beef mixture and the tomato paste toasts a bit, about 2 minutes.

WHILE stirring, add the broth, tomatoes, barley, rosemary, thyme, and bay leaf and bring to a boil. Reduce the heat to a gentle simmer, about medium-low heat, cover, and cook until the barley is tender, 25 to 30 minutes.

REMOVE the stew from the heat and discard the bay leaf. Let cool for 5 minutes to thicken slightly before serving. To serve, ladle into bowls and sprinkle with fresh thyme.

STORE in the fridge in an airtight container for 3 to 4 days, or in the freezer for up to 3 months. To reheat from the fridge, transfer to a pot over medium heat for 10 to 12 minutes, stirring occasionally, until warmed through, or microwave in 1-minute increments, stirring after each, until warmed through. Add more broth if needed. To reheat from frozen, thaw overnight in the fridge, then warm as directed. Top with fresh thyme after reheating.

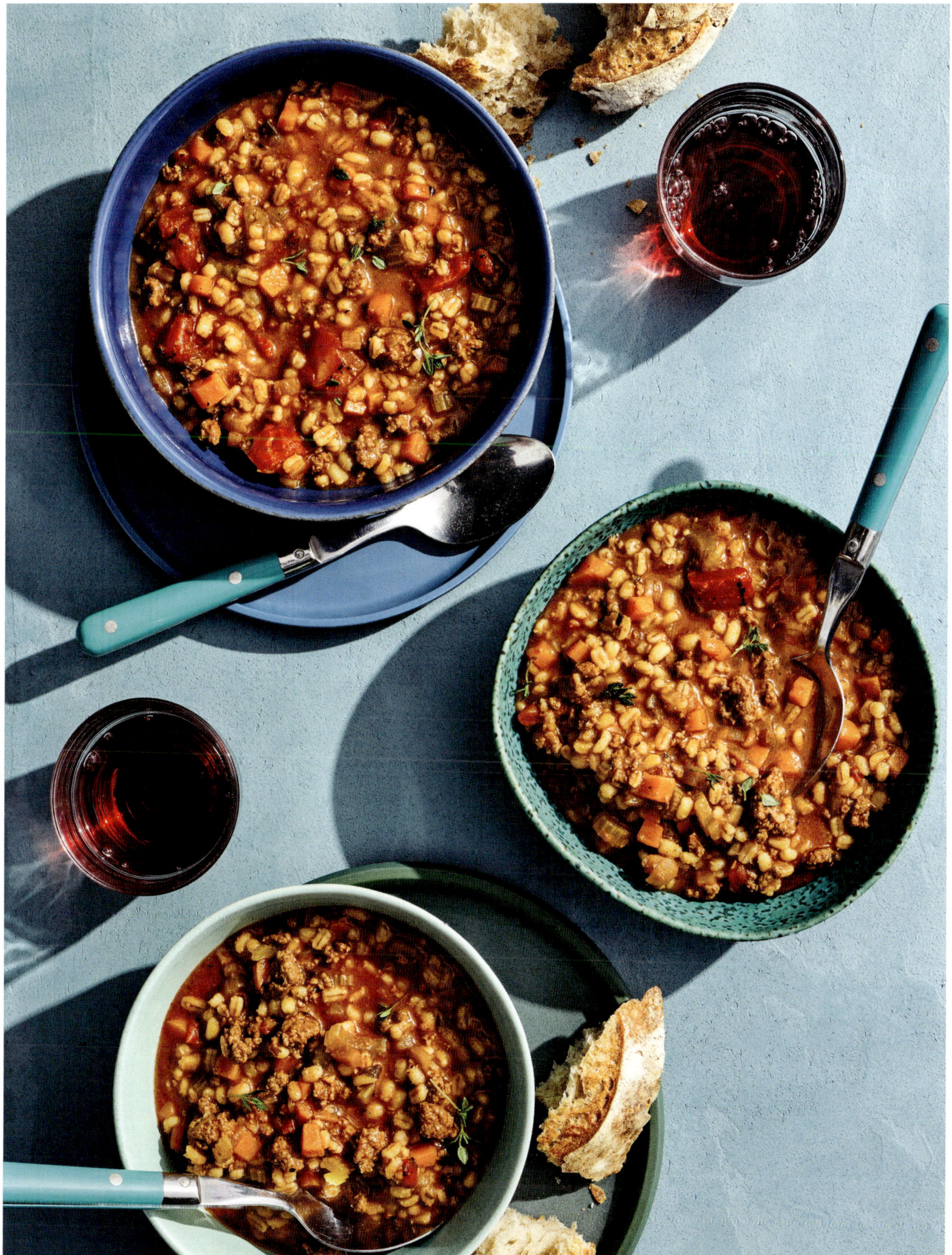

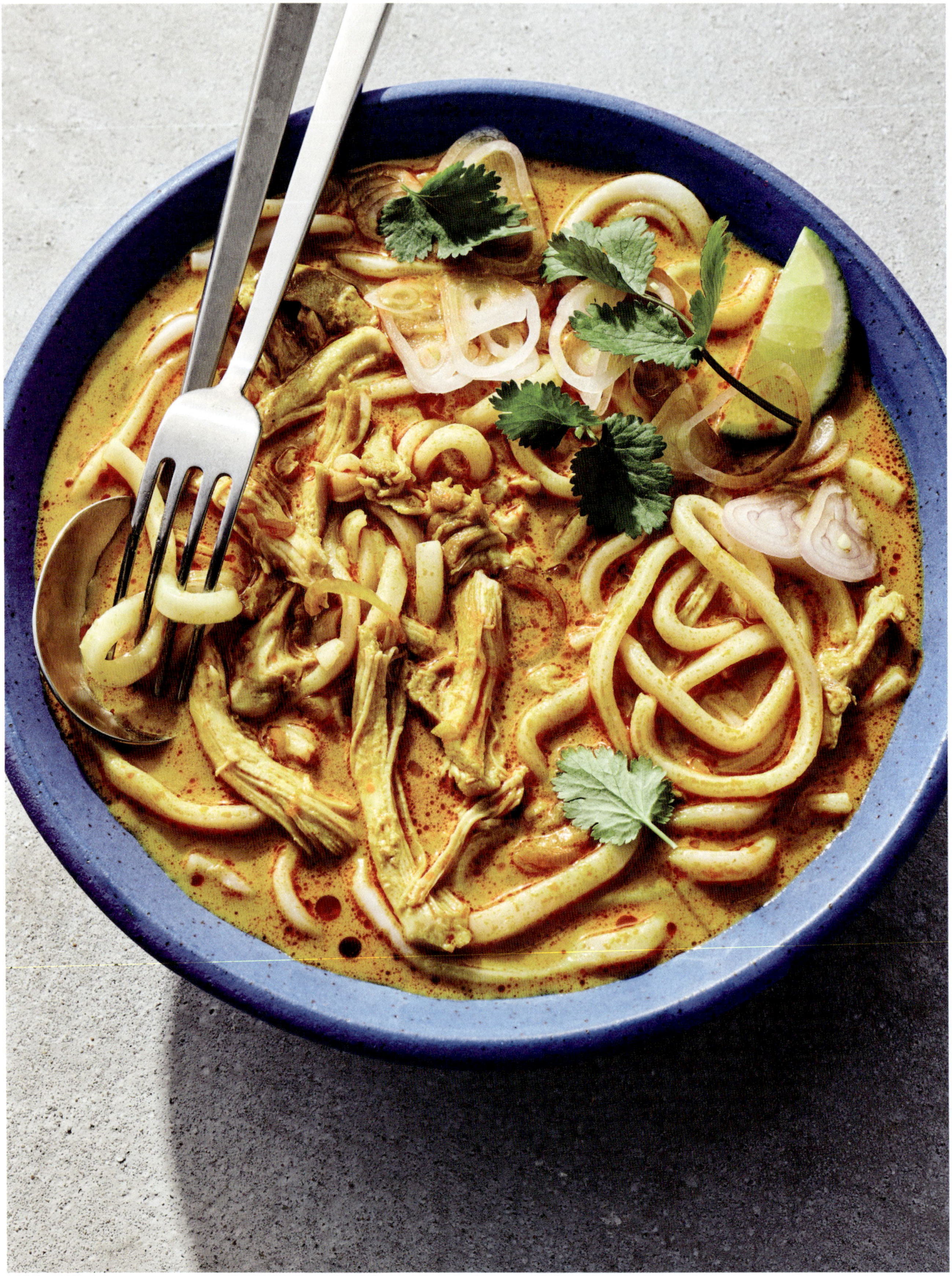

CHICKEN KHAO SOI–INSPIRED SOUP

MAKES 4 SERVINGS | **TOTAL TIME:** 40 MINUTES

DIETARY
GLUTEN-FREE
DAIRY-FREE
MAKE AHEAD

Get ready to savor this vibrant soup! Made with a blend of red curry paste and aromatic spices like curry powder and turmeric, it's a quick way to enjoy Thai-inspired flavors at home. Imagine a bowl filled with tender chicken and noodles, all coming together in a spicy golden broth.

2 tablespoons avocado oil

1 pound boneless, skinless chicken thighs, trimmed of excess fat and patted dry

1 teaspoon kosher salt

½ teaspoon freshly ground black pepper

2 large shallots, halved lengthwise and thinly sliced (about 1 cup)

4 garlic cloves, minced

2 teaspoons minced fresh ginger

1 teaspoon ground turmeric

2 teaspoons ground curry powder

1 teaspoon ground coriander

1 tablespoon Thai red curry paste

4 cups low-sodium chicken broth

1 cup unsweetened full-fat coconut milk

2 tablespoons fish sauce

2 tablespoons coconut aminos

1 tablespoon coconut sugar

Grated zest of ½ lime

9 ounces Cantonese egg or udon noodles

2 tablespoons freshly squeezed lime juice (about 1 lime)

¼ cup finely chopped fresh cilantro leaves

FOR SERVING

1 shallot, thinly sliced

Fresh cilantro leaves

Lime wedges

BRING a medium pot of water to a boil.

MEANWHILE, in a large pot or Dutch oven, heat the oil over medium heat. Add the chicken, salt, and pepper and cook, stirring occasionally, until the chicken begins to brown on the edges, about 5 minutes. The chicken does not need to be cooked through, as it will finish cooking in the broth.

ADD the shallots, garlic, and ginger. Cook, stirring, until the shallots are tender, about 3 minutes.

ADD the turmeric, curry powder, coriander, and curry paste and continue to cook, stirring, toasting the spices, about 2 minutes.

STIR in the broth until it is incorporated with the other ingredients. Add the coconut milk, fish sauce, coconut aminos, coconut sugar, and lime zest and stir to combine. Bring to a rapid simmer. Reduce the heat to a gentle simmer, about medium-low heat, cover, and cook until the chicken is cooked through and the flavors have melded, 12 to 14 minutes.

MEANWHILE, add the noodles to the pot of boiling water. Cook according to package directions. Drain and set aside.

USING tongs, remove the chicken thighs from the broth and transfer to a cutting board. Using two forks, shred the chicken thighs. Add the meat back to the broth along with the lime juice and cilantro. Stir to combine.

TO SERVE: Divide the noodles among four bowls. Ladle the soup over the noodles. Garnish each bowl with some shallot slices, cilantro, and a wedge of lime for squeezing.

STORE the soup separate from the noodles in the fridge in an airtight container for 3 to 4 days, or in the freezer for up to 3 months without the garnishes. To reheat from the fridge, transfer to a pot over medium heat for 10 to 12 minutes, stirring occasionally, until warmed through, or microwave in 1-minute increments, stirring after each, until warmed through. To reheat from frozen, thaw overnight in the fridge, then warm as directed. Ladle over the noodles and top with fresh shallot, cilantro, and a wedge of lime after reheating.

LEFTOVER red curry paste? Try my Thai Red Curry Shrimp Noodles (page 110), Tangy Thai Braised Chicken (page 162), or Red Curry Pork Stir-Fry (page 191).

LEMONY CHICKEN AND CHICKPEA STEW

DIETARY
DAIRY-FREE
MAKE AHEAD

MAKES 6 SERVINGS | **TOTAL TIME:** 35 MINUTES

This Greek-inspired chicken and chickpea stew brings together bright lemon, oregano, and dill for a fresh and flavorful meal. It's a protein-packed, wholesome dinner that's perfect for meal prep or any night of the week. I'm always looking for ways to add chickpeas to my meals, and this stew is one of my favorites—delicious, hearty, and satisfying every time!

2 tablespoons extra-virgin olive oil
1 cup finely diced yellow onion (about ½ medium onion)
1 cup small-diced celery (about 2 stalks)
¾ cup small-diced carrot (about 1 carrot)
4 garlic cloves, minced
2 teaspoons kosher salt, plus more to taste
1 teaspoon freshly ground black pepper
½ teaspoon crushed red pepper flakes
½ teaspoon paprika
½ teaspoon ground turmeric
1 teaspoon ground coriander
One 15-ounce can chickpeas, drained and rinsed
4 cups low-sodium chicken broth
2 bay leaves
Grated zest of ½ lemon
¼ cup Israeli or pearl couscous
1 tablespoon finely chopped fresh oregano leaves
4 cups shredded cooked chicken (I use rotisserie)
2 tablespoons freshly squeezed lemon juice (about 1 lemon)
2 tablespoons finely chopped fresh parsley leaves
2 tablespoons finely chopped fresh dill leaves, plus more for serving

IN a large pot or Dutch oven, heat the oil over medium heat. Add the onion, celery, carrot, garlic, salt, and black pepper and cook, stirring, until the veggies are tender, about 8 minutes.

ADD the pepper flakes, paprika, turmeric, and coriander and continue to cook, stirring, toasting the spices, about 2 minutes.

ADD the chickpeas, broth, bay leaves, and lemon zest and bring to a rapid simmer. Reduce the heat to a gentle simmer, about medium-low heat, and stir in the couscous and oregano. Cover and cook until the chickpeas and couscous are tender, about 10 minutes.

ADD the chicken, lemon juice, parsley, and dill and stir to combine. Let simmer, uncovered, to warm the chicken and allow the flavors to meld, about 5 minutes.

DISCARD the bay leaves. Taste and add more salt as desired. To serve, ladle into bowls and top with additional dill.

STORE in the fridge in an airtight container for 3 to 4 days, or in the freezer for up to 3 months. To reheat from the fridge, transfer to a pot over medium heat for 10 to 12 minutes, stirring occasionally, until warmed through, or microwave in 1-minute increments, stirring after each, until warmed through. Add more broth if needed. To reheat from frozen, thaw overnight in the fridge, then warm as directed. Top with additional fresh dill after reheating.

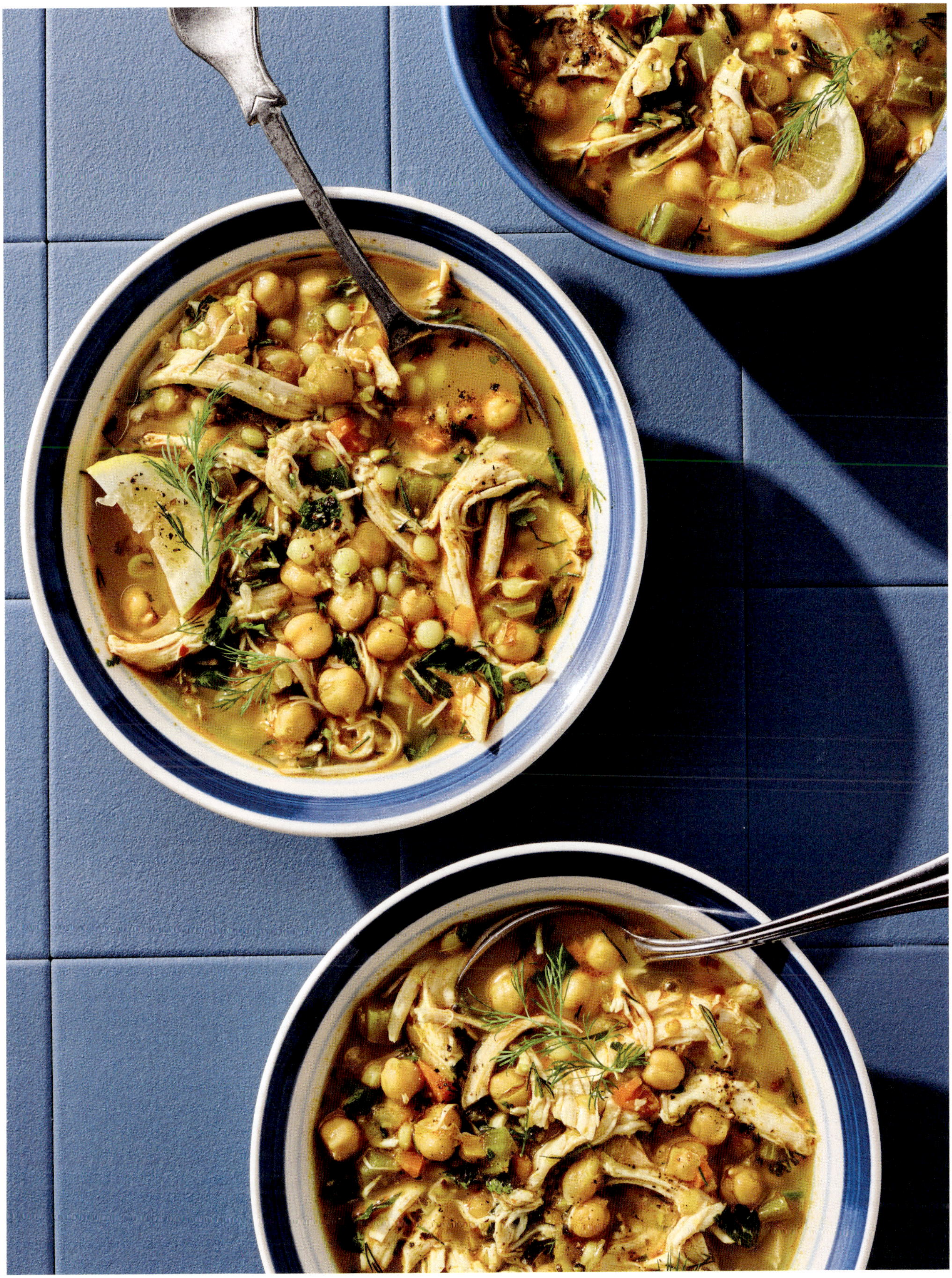

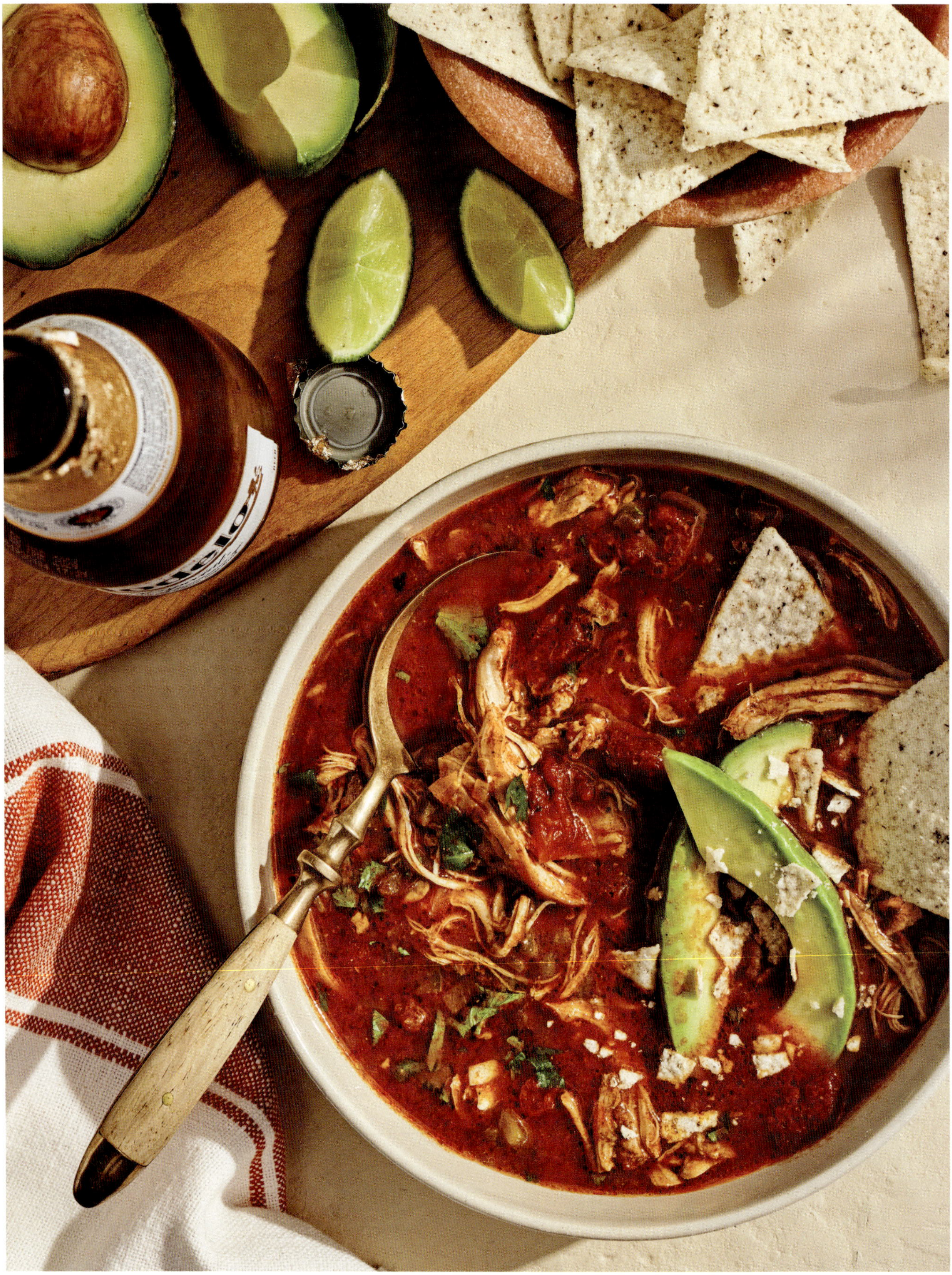

SLOW COOKER OR PRESSURE COOKER CHICKEN, LIME, AND AVOCADO SOUP

MAKES 6 SERVINGS | **TOTAL TIME:** 4 TO 8 HOURS (SLOW COOKER) OR 25 MINUTES (PRESSURE COOKER)

DIETARY
GLUTEN-FREE
GRAIN-FREE
DAIRY-FREE
PALEO
MAKE AHEAD

This soup is the perfect blend of light and bright flavors effortlessly coming together in one pot. Just toss the ingredients into your slow cooker or pressure cooker, set it, and let the magic happen. The result is a deliciously comforting soup with a citrusy kick, but the real star is the creamy bites of avocado that make each spoonful irresistible.

2 pounds boneless, skinless chicken thighs, trimmed of excess fat and patted dry

1 cup finely diced yellow onion (about ½ medium onion)

½ cup seeded and finely diced jalapeño (about 1 large jalapeño)

3 garlic cloves, minced

One 15-ounce jar no-sugar-added red enchilada sauce

One 14.5-ounce can fire-roasted diced tomatoes

One 4-ounce can mild diced green chiles

4 cups low-sodium chicken broth

Grated zest of ½ lime

2 teaspoons chili powder

1 teaspoon ground cumin

1 teaspoon dried oregano

2 teaspoons kosher salt

1 teaspoon freshly ground black pepper

¼ cup finely chopped fresh cilantro leaves

¼ cup freshly squeezed lime juice (about 2 limes)

FOR SERVING

2 avocados, thinly sliced

Grain-free tortilla chips, optional

SLOW COOKER METHOD

IN a slow cooker, combine the chicken, onion, jalapeño, garlic, enchilada sauce, tomatoes, green chiles, broth, lime zest, chili powder, cumin, oregano, salt, and black pepper. Stir to combine.

COVER and cook on high for 4 hours or, preferably, on low for 8 hours.

WHEN the cook time is complete, using tongs, transfer the chicken to a sheet pan. Using two forks, shred the chicken. Return it to the slow cooker along with the cilantro and lime juice. Stir to combine.

TO SERVE: Ladle the soup into bowls and top with plenty of avocado. Crush some tortilla chips on top (if using).

PRESSURE COOKER METHOD

IN a pressure cooker, combine the chicken, onion, jalapeño, garlic, enchilada sauce, tomatoes, green chiles, broth, lime zest, chili powder, cumin, oregano, salt, and black pepper. Stir to combine.

LOCK the lid on the pressure cooker and ensure the vent is sealed. Press the "manual" or "pressure cook" button (depending on your model) and set the time to 15 minutes.

WHEN the cook time is complete, quick-release the pressure. When all the pressure has been released, carefully remove the lid. Using tongs, transfer the chicken to a sheet pan. Using two forks, shred the chicken. Return it to the pressure cooker along with the cilantro and lime juice. Stir to combine.

TO SERVE: Ladle the soup into bowls and top with plenty of avocado. Crush some tortilla chips on top (if using).

FROM MY KITCHEN TO YOURS

STORAGE NOTE: Store leftovers in the fridge in an airtight container for 3 to 4 days, or in the freezer for up to 3 months without the garnishes. To reheat from the fridge, transfer to a pot over medium heat for 10 to 12 minutes, stirring occasionally, until warmed through, or microwave in 1-minute increments, stirring after each, until warmed through. To reheat from frozen, thaw overnight in the fridge, then warm as directed. Top with fresh avocado and tortilla chips (if using).

KIMCHI RAMEN

MAKES 2 SERVINGS | **TOTAL TIME:** 20 MINUTES

DIETARY
DAIRY-FREE
VEGETARIAN
GLUTEN-FREE (IF MODIFIED)

This ramen is a cozy, twenty-minute bowl of rich, umami-packed flavor. With its fragrant broth and vibrant vegetables, it's the ultimate warm-up meal that's both quick and deeply satisfying. Kimchi is the real star here, infusing the broth with a tangy, fermented kick that's slightly sour and adds layers of complexity. As the noodles soften, they absorb the lightly spicy, savory broth, making each bite full of comforting flavor.

- 2 tablespoons avocado oil
- 4 green onions, thinly sliced, white and green parts kept separate
- 4 cups stemmed and thinly sliced shiitake mushrooms
- 3 garlic cloves, minced
- 2 teaspoons finely grated fresh ginger
- ½ teaspoon kosher salt
- 1 teaspoon toasted sesame oil
- 1 tablespoon gluten-free gochujang (see note)
- 4 cups low-sodium vegetable or chicken broth
- 2 tablespoons coconut aminos
- 1 teaspoon coconut sugar
- 1 cup roughly chopped cabbage kimchi
- Two 6-ounce packages ramen noodles, minus the seasoning packets (sub gluten-free brown rice ramen for gluten-free)
- 2 jammy eggs, optional for serving (see note)
- 1 teaspoon toasted sesame seeds, for serving

IN a large, deep skillet, heat the avocado oil over medium heat. Add the white parts of the green onions, the mushrooms, garlic, ginger, and salt. Cook, stirring, until the onions begin to soften, about 3 minutes.

ADD the sesame oil and gochujang and stir to combine. While stirring, add the broth, coconut aminos, and coconut sugar. Stir in the kimchi and bring to a rapid simmer.

REDUCE the heat to a gentle simmer and nestle in the ramen noodles. Cook, undisturbed, for 2 to 3 minutes, until the noodles soften and separate when tossed. Continue cooking until the noodles are tender, about 2 more minutes.

STIR in the green parts of the green onions and serve immediately. To serve, divide the noodles and broth between two bowls, and top with the jammy eggs (if using) and toasted sesame seeds. The longer you let the noodles sit in the broth, the more they absorb the liquid, so to ensure your bowls are nice and soupy, enjoy immediately. If needed, reheat with additional broth.

FROM MY KITCHEN TO YOURS

FOR GOCHUJANG: Gochujang, a fermented Korean chile paste, is often made with wheat, which helps it firm up and can make gluten-free options difficult to find. However, the Coconut Secret brand, made with coconut aminos, is available online and at many grocers.

FOR JAMMY EGGS: Bring a small pot of water to a boil. Gently lower 2 eggs into the pot and allow them to simmer for 6½ minutes. While the eggs are cooking, prepare an ice water bath in a medium bowl. When the eggs are done, use a slotted spoon to transfer the eggs to the ice water bath and rest for 5 minutes. Once cooled, peel, slice in half, and place on top of your soup for a rich, silky bite.

LEFTOVER kimchi or gochujang? Try my Sweet and Savory Korean-Style Beef Bowls (page 196).

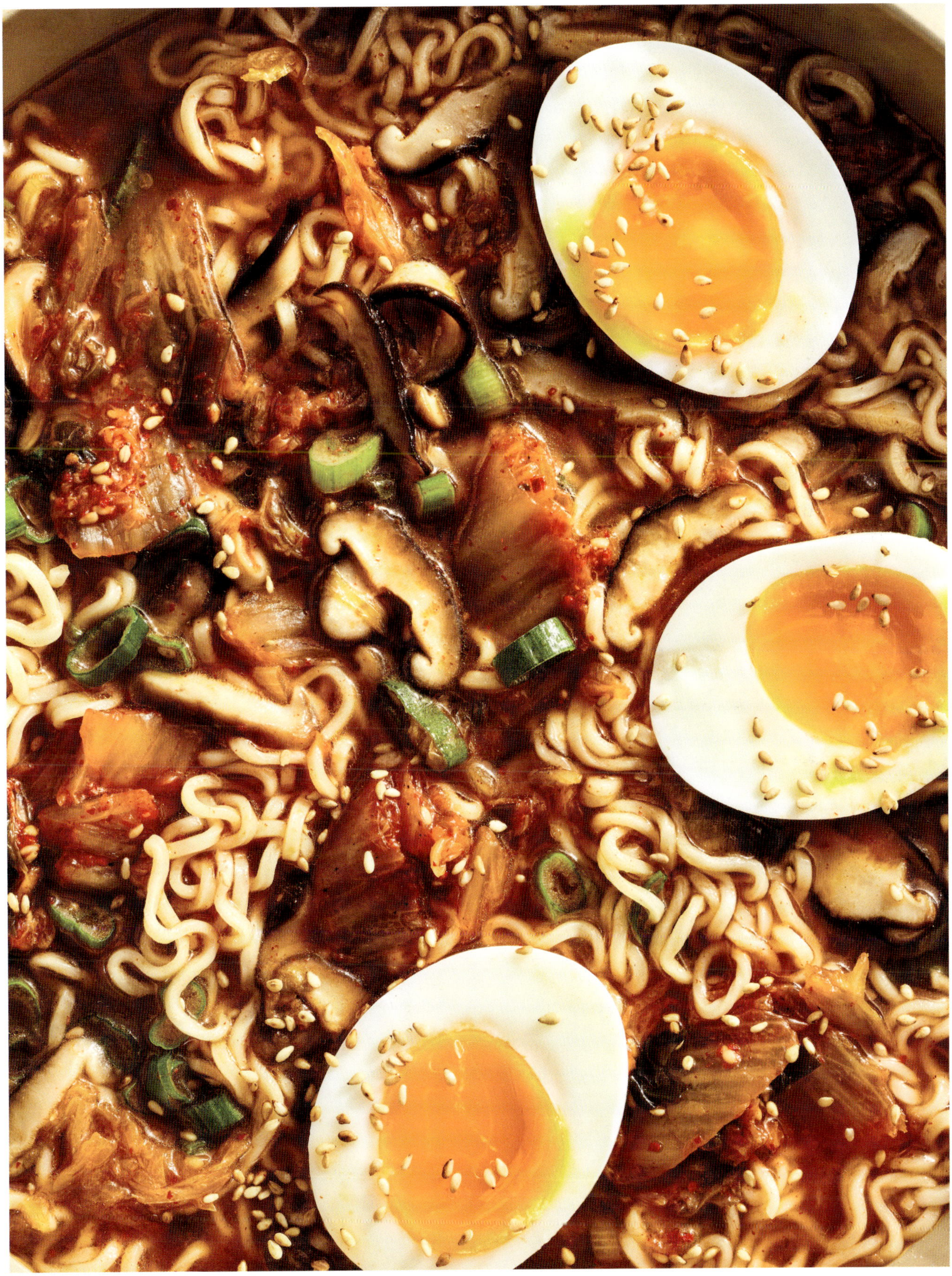

SHORTCUT CHICKEN POZOLE VERDE

MAKES 6 SERVINGS | **TOTAL TIME**: 45 MINUTES

DIETARY
GLUTEN-FREE
DAIRY-FREE
MAKE AHEAD

Pozole is one of my favorite traditional Mexican dishes. While this isn't your traditional pozole, it allows you to enjoy the flavors you crave quickly any night of the week. All you need is a handful of ingredients, one pot, and a blender.

FOR THE POZOLE

2 tablespoons avocado oil

1½ cups medium-diced white onion (about ¾ medium onion)

½ cup seeded and finely diced jalapeño (about 1 large jalapeño), optional

2 cups medium-diced poblano pepper (about 2 medium poblanos)

4 garlic cloves, minced

2 teaspoons kosher salt, plus more to taste

½ teaspoon crushed red pepper flakes

1 teaspoon ground cumin

2 cups loosely packed fresh cilantro leaves and tender stems

6 cups low-sodium chicken broth, divided

One 15-ounce jar green enchilada sauce

1½ pounds boneless, skinless chicken breasts, trimmed of excess fat and patted dry

Two 15-ounce cans white hominy, drained and rinsed

2 tablespoons freshly squeezed lime juice (about 1 lime)

FOR SERVING

½ cup finely diced white onion (about ½ small onion)

1 cup thinly sliced radishes (about 1 bunch)

1½ cups finely shredded green cabbage (about ¼ small head)

1 avocado, cubed

¼ cup finely chopped fresh cilantro leaves

Lime wedges

MAKE THE POZOLE: In a large pot or Dutch oven, heat the oil over medium-high heat. Add the onion, jalapeño (if using), poblano, garlic, salt, pepper flakes, and cumin. Sauté until the veggies are tender, 5 to 7 minutes.

TRANSFER the sautéed veggies to a blender. Add the cilantro and 1 cup of the broth. Blend until smooth.

CAREFULLY pour the blended mixture back into the pot over medium-high heat. Add the remaining 5 cups broth and the enchilada sauce. Bring to a boil. Reduce the heat to a simmer.

CUT the chicken breasts in half and add them to the soup along with the hominy. Cover and cook, simmering lightly, until the chicken is cooked through and the hominy is tender, about 20 minutes.

USING tongs, carefully remove the chicken from the soup and transfer it to a cutting board. Using two forks, shred the chicken. Return it to the soup along with the lime juice and stir to combine.

SIMMER, uncovered, for 5 minutes. Remove from the heat. Taste and add more salt as desired.

TO SERVE: Ladle the soup into large bowls and garnish as desired with onion, radish, cabbage, avocado, cilantro, and a lime wedge for squeezing.

STORE in the fridge in an airtight container for 3 to 4 days, or in the freezer for up to 3 months without the garnishes. To reheat from the fridge, transfer to a pot over medium heat for 10 to 12 minutes, stirring occasionally, until warmed through, or microwave in 1-minute increments, stirring after each, until warmed through. To reheat from frozen, thaw overnight in the fridge, then warm as directed. Top with fresh onion, radish, cabbage, avocado, cilantro, and a lime wedge for squeezing after reheating.

LEFTOVER cabbage? Try my Tangy Thai Crunch Salad with Seared Salmon (page 70).

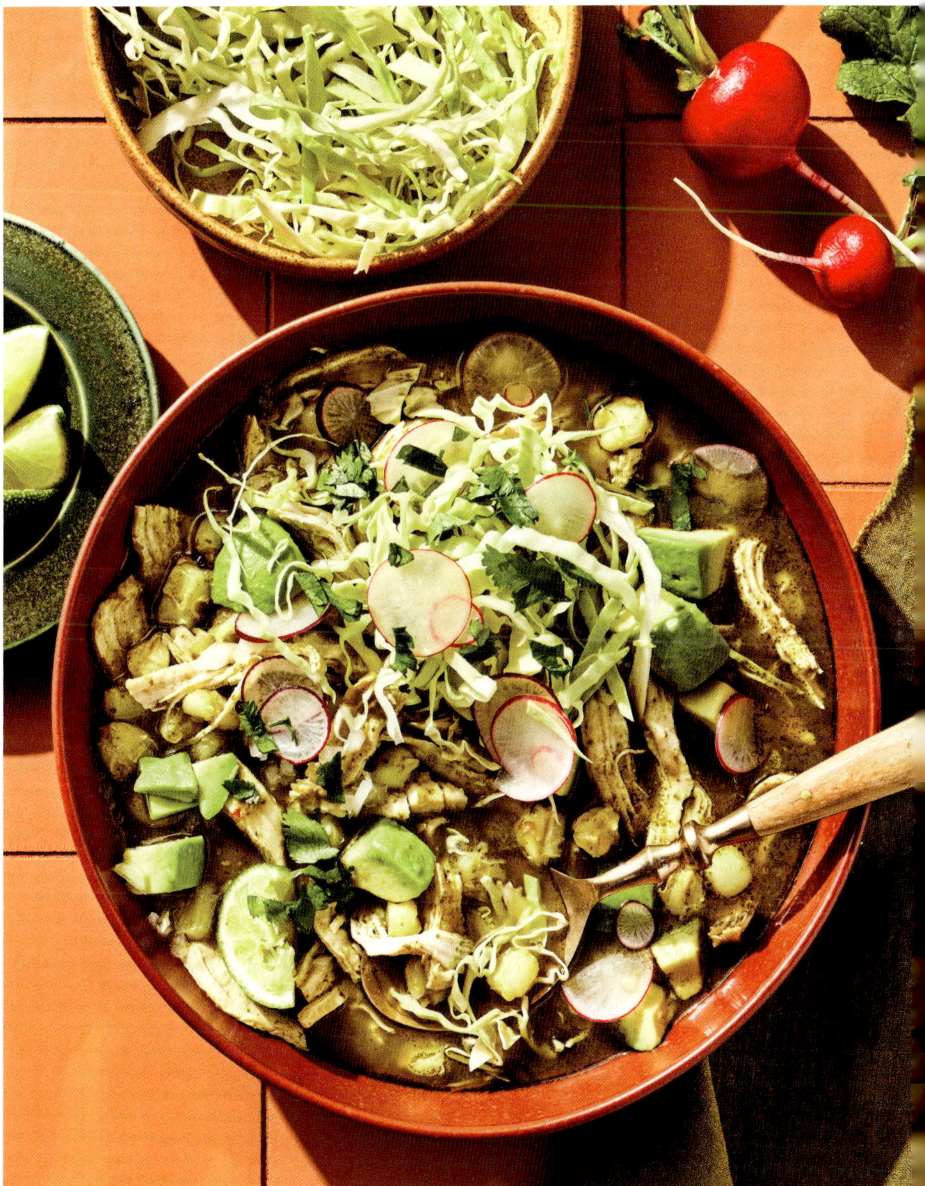

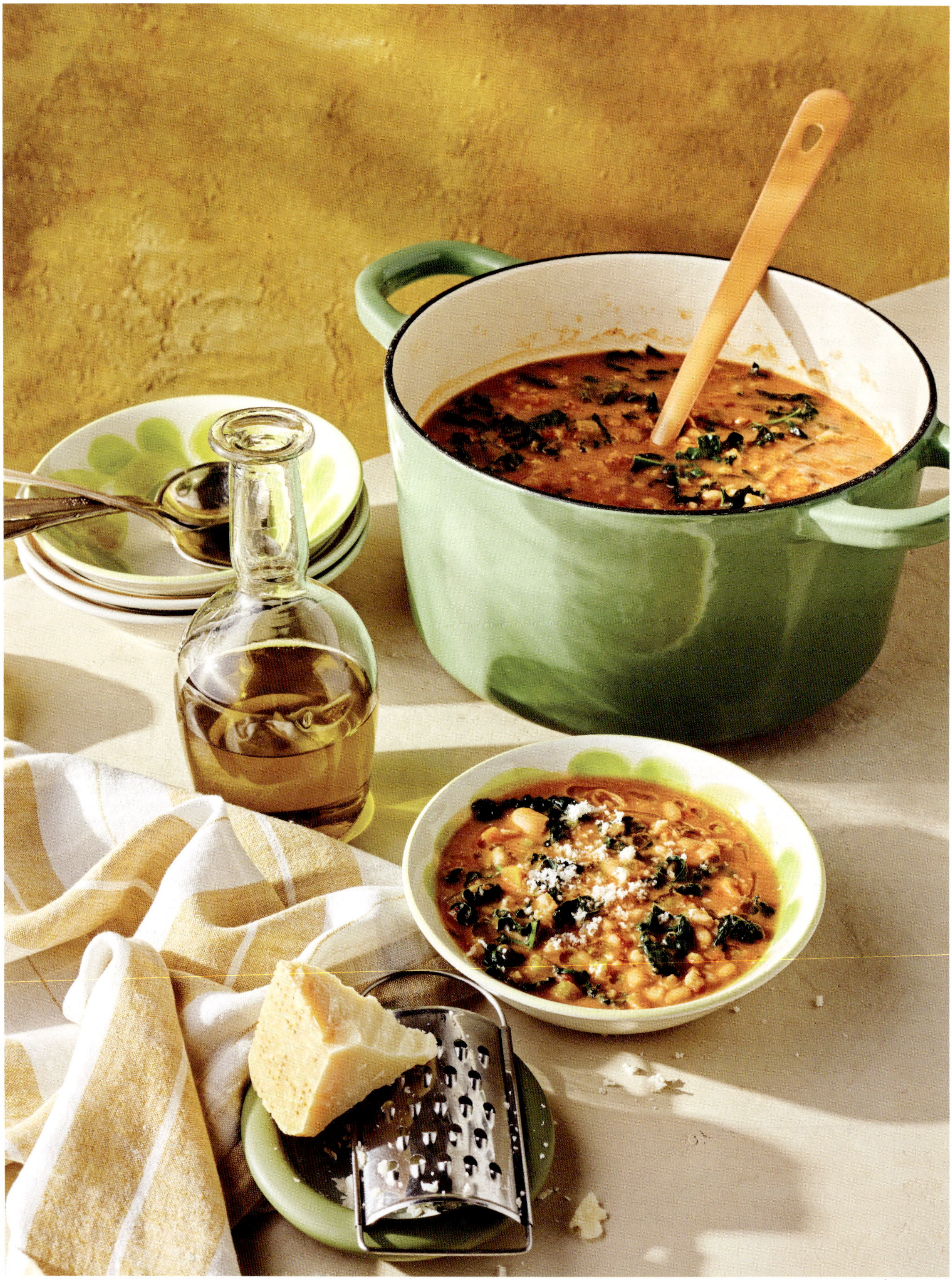

TUSCAN FARRO SOUP

MAKES 8 SERVINGS | **TOTAL TIME:** 55 MINUTES

DIETARY
GLUTEN-FREE
DAIRY-FREE (IF MODIFIED)
VEGETARIAN (IF MODIFIED)
MAKE AHEAD

This hearty Tuscan Farro Soup is a nourishing dish made with fiber-rich farro and tender vegetables in a flavorful broth. Perfect for cozy nights or meal prep, it brings the essence of Italian countryside cooking to your table.

- 4 ounces diced pancetta (omit for vegetarian and sub 2 tablespoons of extra-virgin olive oil)
- 1 cup small-diced celery (about 2 stalks)
- ¾ cup small-diced carrot (about 1 carrot)
- 1 cup small-diced yellow onion (about 1 small onion)
- 4 garlic cloves, minced
- 1½ teaspoons kosher salt, plus more to taste
- ½ teaspoon freshly ground black pepper
- ½ teaspoon crushed red pepper flakes
- 1 tablespoon tomato paste
- One 14.5-ounce can crushed tomatoes
- 8 cups low-sodium vegetable broth
- 1 teaspoon Italian seasoning
- 2 fresh rosemary sprigs
- 1 cup dry pearled farro, rinsed
- Two 15-ounce cans cannellini beans, drained and rinsed
- 4 cups de-ribbed and roughly chopped lacinato kale (about 1 bunch)
- 2 tablespoons freshly squeezed lemon juice (about 1 lemon)
- Extra-virgin olive oil, for serving
- Freshly grated parmesan cheese (omit for dairy-free)

LINE a plate with paper towels. In a large pot or Dutch oven, cook the pancetta over medium-high heat, stirring occasionally, until the fat renders and the pancetta begins to crisp, about 5 minutes. Using a slotted spoon, remove the pancetta from the pot and transfer to the prepared plate. Set aside. Reserve 2 tablespoons of fat in the pot.

ADD the celery, carrot, onion, garlic, salt, black pepper, and pepper flakes in the pot and cook over medium-high heat, stirring, until the veggies are tender, about 6 minutes.

STIR in the tomato paste until it is incorporated into the veggies. Add the crushed tomatoes, broth, Italian seasoning, and rosemary. Stir and bring to a rapid simmer. Add the farro and cannellini beans and reduce the heat to a gentle simmer, about medium-low heat.

COVER and cook, lightly simmering, until the farro is tender, about 25 minutes.

WHEN the farro is tender, reduce the heat to low. Remove and discard the rosemary sprigs. Carefully ladle about 2 cups of the soup into a blender. Blend that portion of the soup until smooth and creamy. (Alternatively, ladle the soup into a wide-mouth jar and blend with an immersion blender.) Add the blended soup back into the pot along with the cooked pancetta, kale, and lemon juice and stir to combine. Continue to cook on low, uncovered, to allow the soup to thicken slightly and the kale to wilt, about 10 more minutes.

TO SERVE: Ladle the soup into bowls and garnish with a drizzle of olive oil and a sprinkle of freshly grated parmesan (if using).

STORE in the fridge in an airtight container for 3 to 4 days, or in the freezer for up to 3 months. To reheat from the fridge, transfer to a pot over medium heat for 10 to 12 minutes, stirring occasionally, until warmed through, or microwave in 1-minute increments, stirring after each, until warmed through. Add more broth if needed. To reheat from frozen, thaw overnight in the fridge, then warm as directed. Top with a drizzle of olive oil and fresh parmesan (if using) after reheating.

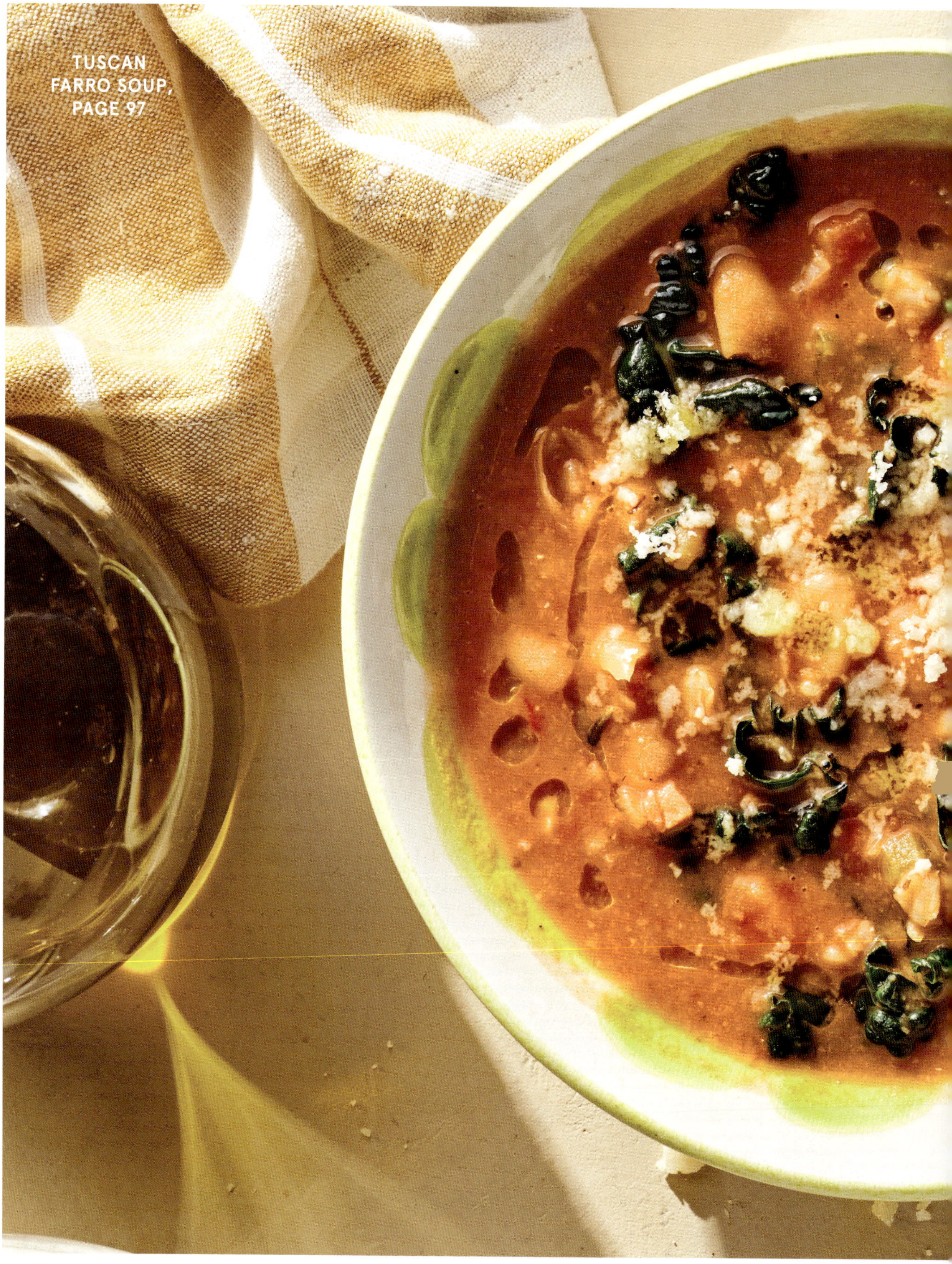

TUSCAN FARRO SOUP, PAGE 97

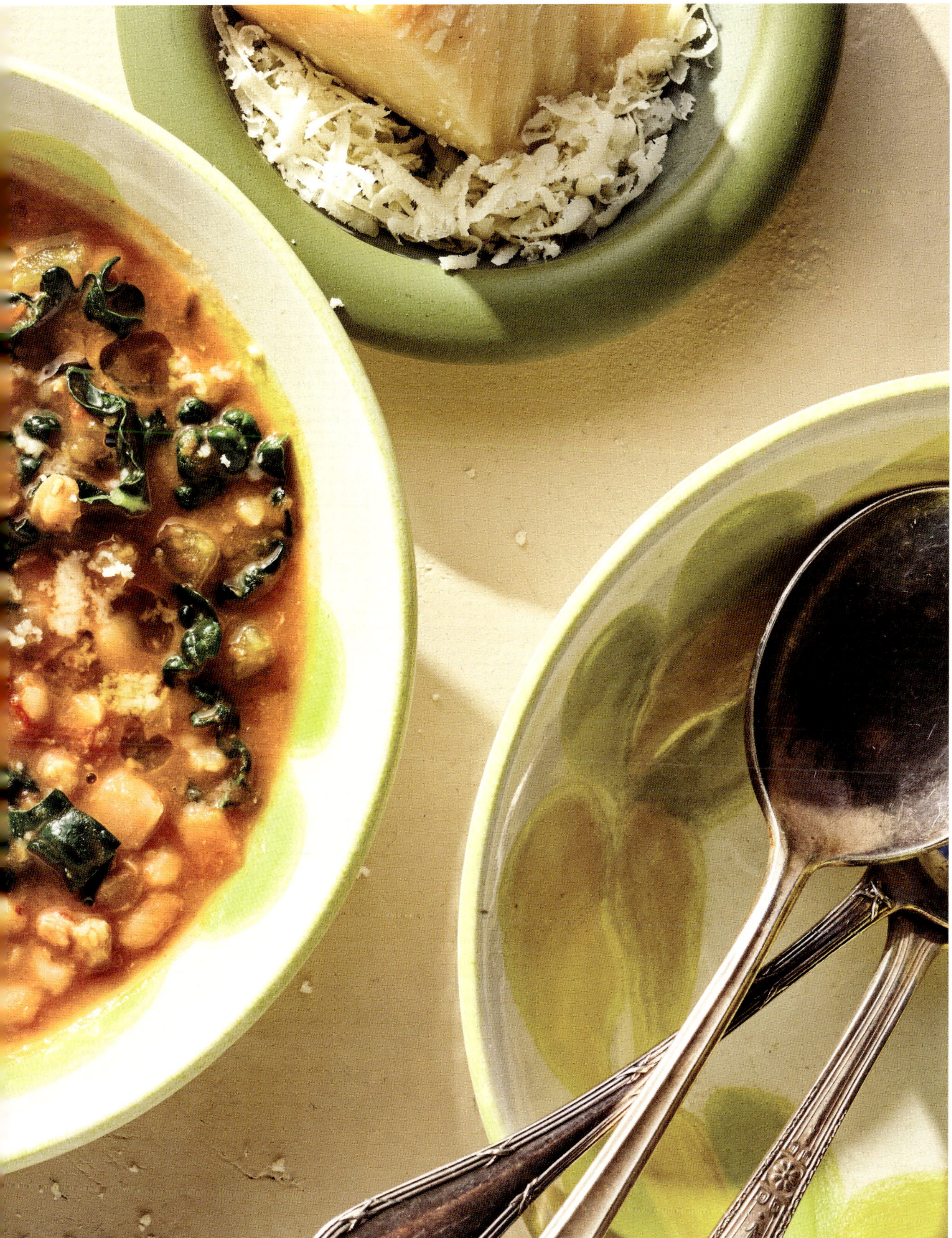

SLOW COOKER OR PRESSURE COOKER GREEN CHILE STEW

MAKES 6 SERVINGS | **TOTAL TIME:** 4 TO 8 HOURS (SLOW COOKER) OR 45 MINUTES (PRESSURE COOKER)

DIETARY
GLUTEN-FREE
GRAIN-FREE (IF MODIFIED)
DAIRY-FREE (IF MODIFIED)
PALEO (IF MODIFIED)
MAKE AHEAD

This hearty stew is my mother-in-law's signature recipe for feeding a crowd—and for good reason! A beloved New Mexican staple, it's packed with comforting flavors and is surprisingly simple to make. In my version, I let the slow cooker or pressure cooker do all the work. I just toss in the ingredients, set the cooker, and let the magic happen. Perfect for chilly evenings, this hearty stew is the ultimate cozy-up meal after a long day.

2 teaspoons kosher salt
1 teaspoon freshly ground black pepper
2 teaspoons ground cumin
1 teaspoon dried oregano
2 pounds pork shoulder or tenderloin, silver skin removed, cut into ½-inch dice
2 cups small-diced yellow onion (about 1 medium onion)
4 garlic cloves, minced
1 pound yellow potatoes, cut into ½-inch dice
One 16-ounce jar flame-roasted medium or mild Hatch green chiles (see note)
2 cups low-sodium chicken broth
1 cup frozen corn (omit for grain-free and paleo)
2 tablespoons freshly squeezed lime juice (about 1 lime)
Fresh cilantro leaves, for serving
Shredded Monterey Jack cheese (omit for dairy-free and paleo)

SLOW COOKER METHOD

IN a small bowl, combine the salt, black pepper, cumin, and oregano.

IN a slow cooker, combine the diced pork and half of the seasoning blend. Toss and massage the spices into the meat to adhere. Add the onion, garlic, potatoes, chiles, broth, and the rest of the spice blend. Stir until well combined, cover, and let cook on high for 4 hours or, preferably, low for 8 hours until the pork is cooked through and the potatoes are tender.

WHEN the cook time is complete, stir in the corn (if using) and lime juice. Cover and continue to cook until the corn has thawed, about 5 more minutes.

TO SERVE: Ladle the soup into bowls. Top with cilantro and Monterey Jack, if desired.

PRESSURE COOKER METHOD

IN a small bowl, combine the salt, black pepper, cumin, and oregano.

IN a pressure cooker, combine the diced pork and half of the seasoning blend. Toss and massage the spices into the meat to adhere. Add the onion, garlic, potatoes, chiles, broth, and the rest of the spice blend. Stir until well combined.

LOCK the lid on the pressure cooker and ensure the vent is sealed. Press the "manual" or "pressure cook" button (depending on your model) and set the time to 35 minutes.

WHEN the cook time is complete, quick-release the pressure. When all the pressure has been released, carefully remove the lid. The pork should be cooked through and the potatoes tender. Stir in the corn (if using) and lime juice and let rest, uncovered, until the corn has thawed, about 5 minutes.

TO SERVE: Ladle the soup into bowls. Top with cilantro and Monterey Jack, if desired.

FROM MY KITCHEN TO YOURS

ON HATCH GREEN CHILES: Hatch green chiles are a variety of chile pepper grown in the Hatch Valley of New Mexico, and they're prized for their smoky, slightly sweet, and mildly spicy flavor. They're typically roasted to enhance their unique taste. In this recipe, I use roasted green chiles and adjust based on what's in season—fresh, frozen, or jarred. When using jarred, I use the 505 Southwestern brand. If substituting fresh or frozen chiles for the jarred ones, use 2 cups diced roasted green chiles. Be sure to use mild or medium chiles, as the hot variety can be overwhelmingly spicy.

STORAGE NOTE: Store leftovers in the fridge in an airtight container for 3 to 4 days, or in the freezer for up to 3 months without the garnishes. To reheat, transfer to a pot over medium heat for 10 to 12 minutes, until warmed through, stirring occasionally, or microwave in 1-minute increments, stirring after each, until warmed through. Top with fresh cilantro and Monterey Jack, if desired, after reheating.

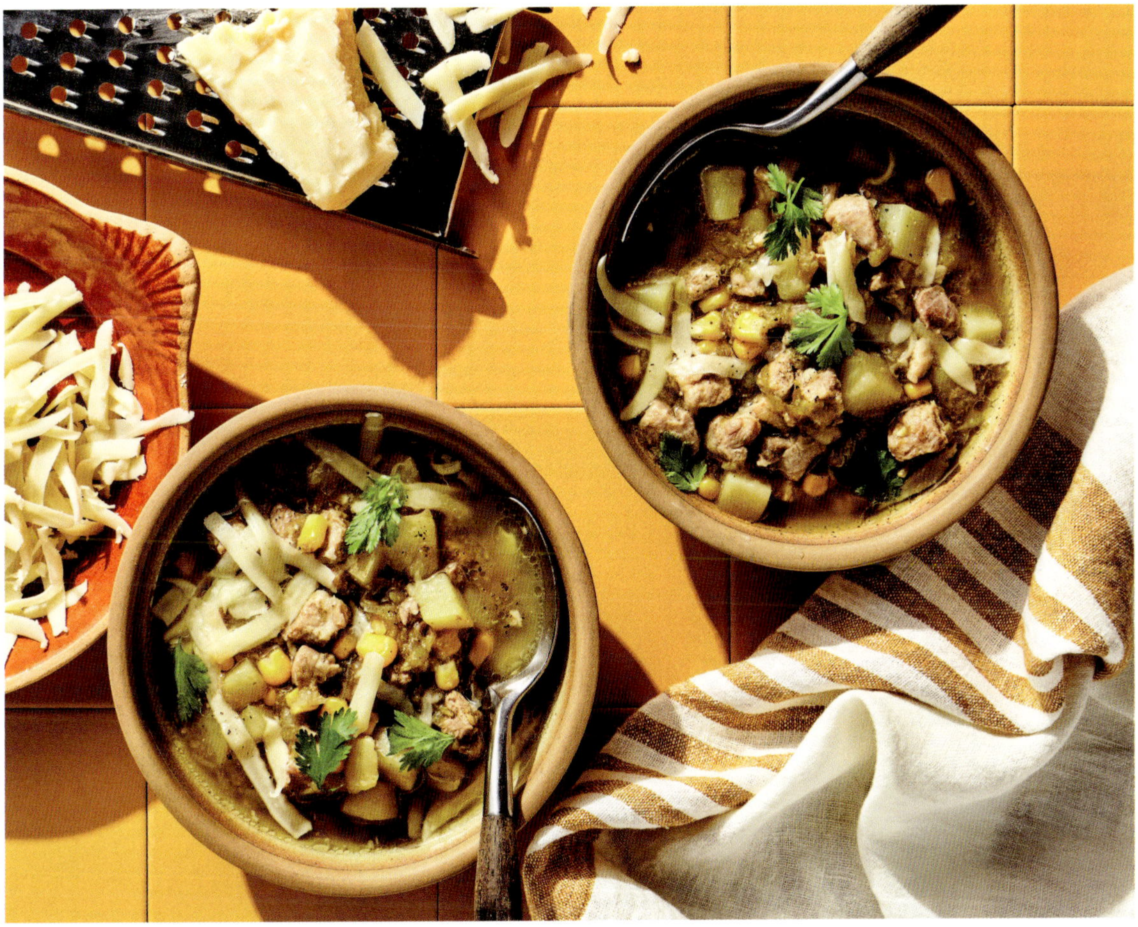

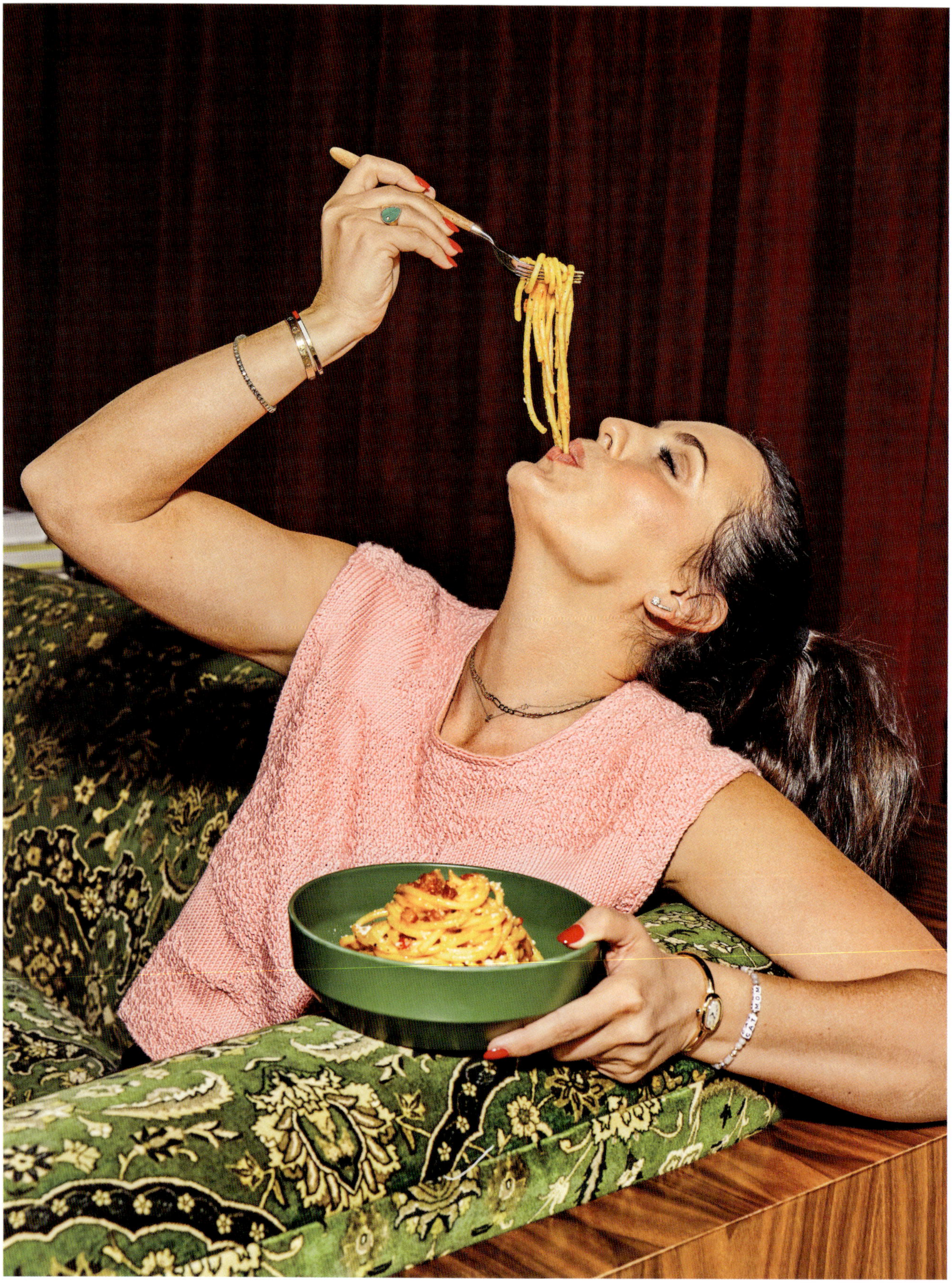

PASTA AND NOODLES

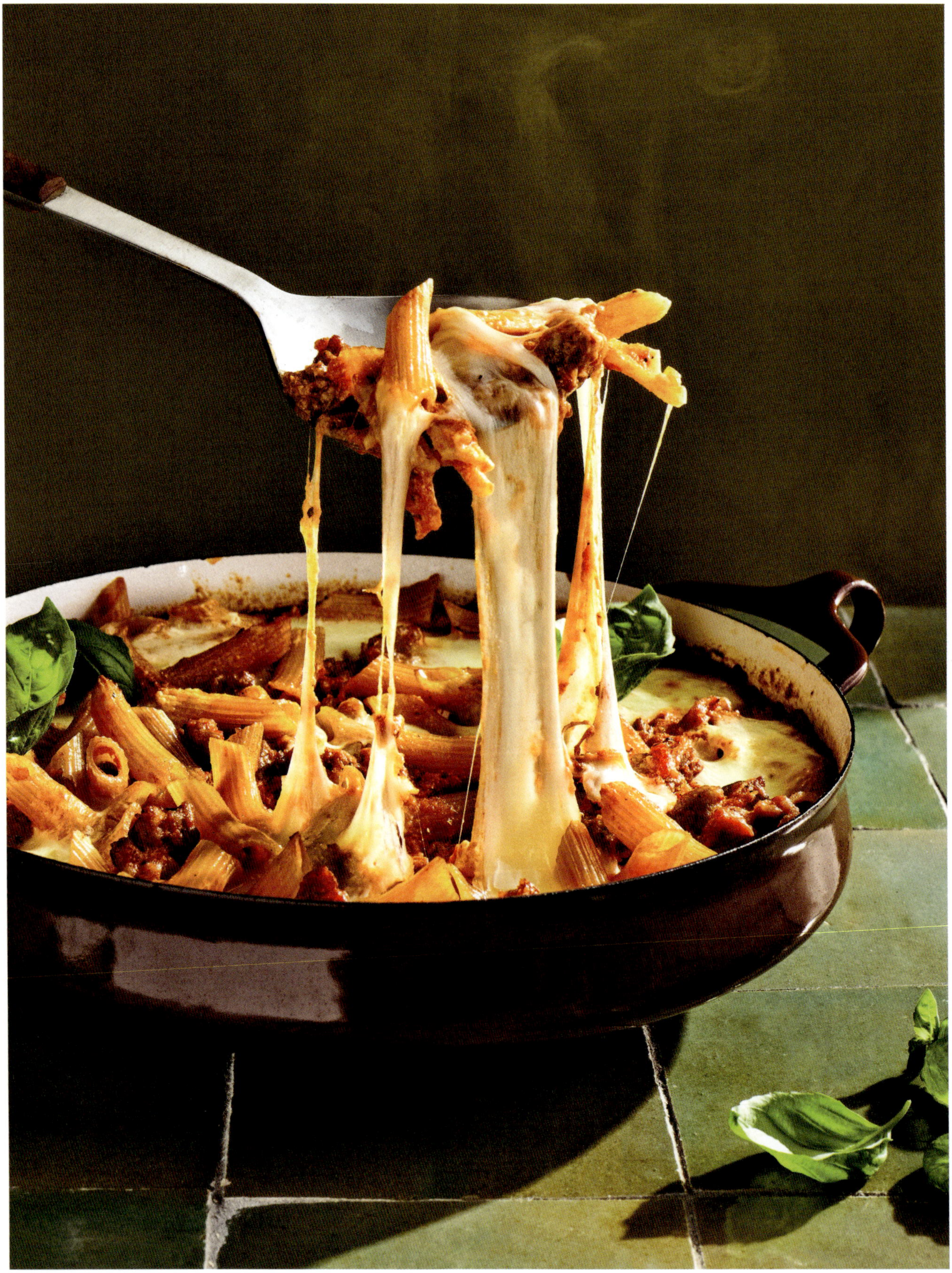

SKILLET-BAKED ZITI WITH SAUSAGE AND RICOTTA

MAKES 6 SERVINGS | **TOTAL TIME:** 50 MINUTES

DIETARY
GLUTEN-FREE
MAKE AHEAD

This family weeknight favorite is like the cozy hug of traditional baked ziti without the fuss. All the cheesy, saucy goodness simmered up in just one pot and finished in the oven, ready to satisfy your cravings with minimal effort!

- 1 tablespoon extra-virgin olive oil
- 1 pound bulk mild or hot Italian sausage
- 1 cup finely diced yellow onion (about ½ medium onion)
- 3 garlic cloves, minced
- 1 teaspoon Italian seasoning
- 1 teaspoon kosher salt
- ½ teaspoon freshly ground black pepper
- 2 cups jarred marinara sauce
- ¼ cup dry white wine
- ¾ cup low-sodium beef broth
- ½ cup whole-milk ricotta
- ½ cup shredded parmesan cheese
- 8 ounces gluten-free brown rice ziti or penne (see note)
- 5 ounces fresh mozzarella cheese
- Torn fresh basil leaves, for serving

POSITION a rack in the center of the oven and preheat the oven to 375°F.

IN a large, deep oven-safe skillet or 3.5-quart braiser with fitted lid, heat the oil over medium-high heat. Add the sausage and cook, breaking up the meat with the edge of a spoon, until cooked through and no longer pink, about 7 minutes.

ADD the onion and garlic. Cook until tender, about 4 minutes. Drain off the excess fat and return the sausage and vegetables to the pan. Reduce the heat to medium-low and add the Italian seasoning, salt, pepper, marinara, wine, broth, ricotta, and parmesan. Stir until well combined. Add the ziti and toss until evenly coated in the sauce. Spread into an even layer.

TEAR the mozzarella into 1-inch pieces and evenly distribute it over the top of the pasta. Cover the skillet with a lid, transfer to the oven, and bake for 20 minutes.

REMOVE the lid and continue to bake until the mozzarella is bubbly and the pasta is tender, about 15 more minutes.

GARNISH with fresh basil. Let cool slightly before serving. Store leftovers in an airtight container in the fridge for up to 4 days. Reheat in the microwave or in a 350°F oven until warmed through, adding a splash of broth to help rehydrate the pasta if needed.

FROM MY KITCHEN TO YOURS

FREEZER NOTE: Bake fully as directed and let cool. Transfer to a freezer- and oven-safe dish (so it's no longer in the skillet), press plastic wrap directly onto the surface so no air touches it, then wrap tightly in heavy-duty foil and freeze for up to 2 months. Thaw overnight in the refrigerator, remove and discard the wrap and foil, then bake, covered with a tight-fitting lid, at 350°F until hot and bubbly, about 30 minutes.

PASTA NOTE: You can use regular pasta for this dish. If using gluten-free pasta, I recommend using brown rice pasta only, as the starches from the rice pasta will help thicken the dish. A legume- or corn-based gluten-free pasta will not work in this recipe.

CALABRIAN CARBONARA

MAKES 2 SERVINGS | **TOTAL TIME:** 30 MINUTES

DIETARY
GLUTEN-FREE (IF MODIFIED)

After a long week, there's nothing better than a simple, classic pasta dish to ease into the weekend. This is my take on carbonara—rich and comforting with a little twist. The key to carbonara's luscious sauce is gently cooked eggs, which create a velvety texture that clings to the pasta without the need for cream. A spoonful of chopped Calabrian peppers adds just the right amount of heat to wake up your taste buds without overpowering the dish. This recipe is simple, a little spicy, and always a winner.

Kosher salt

8 ounces spaghetti or bucatini pasta (sub gluten-free brown rice spaghetti for gluten-free)

4 large eggs, at room temperature

¾ cup freshly grated pecorino Romano cheese, plus more for serving

1 teaspoon coarsely ground black pepper, plus more for serving

1 to 2 tablespoons jarred chopped Calabrian peppers (see note)

4 ounces pancetta or bacon, cut into small cubes

BRING a large pot of water to a boil. When the water comes to a boil, add plenty of salt (I use about 1 tablespoon) and the pasta and cook until al dente according to the package directions.

MEANWHILE, in a medium bowl, combine the eggs, pecorino Romano, black pepper, and Calabrian peppers. Whisk until well combined. Set aside.

IN a large, deep skillet, cook the pancetta over medium heat, stirring occasionally, until the fat renders and the pancetta begins to crisp, about 5 minutes. When crisp, reduce the heat to low and keep warm while you wait for the pasta to finish.

WHEN the pasta is cooked, drain and immediately add the pasta to the skillet with the pancetta over low heat. Toss until well combined with the pancetta and its fat.

REMOVE the pan from the heat and pour the egg mixture into the pan. Continuously toss to lightly cook the eggs (taking care not to overcook and scramble) and coat the pasta with the egg mixture. The pasta should be well coated and glossy after tossing for 2 to 3 minutes. Taste and add salt as desired.

DIVIDE between two bowls and top with more grated pecorino Romano and black pepper.

FROM MY KITCHEN TO YOURS

Calabrian peppers are spicy, smoky peppers from southern Italy. They are incredibly versatile and pack just the right amount of heat without being overpowering. One of the most common ways to find them is chopped and packed in oil and vinegar, which gives you little bits of pepper and plenty of flavor in every bite. You can find it in most grocery stores in the condiment aisle or near the pickles and olives. If you're sensitive to heat, I'd recommend using just 1 tablespoon of the Calabrian chiles in this recipe.

LEFTOVER chopped Calabrian peppers? Try my Calabrian Chile Meatball Orzo Skillet (page 173).

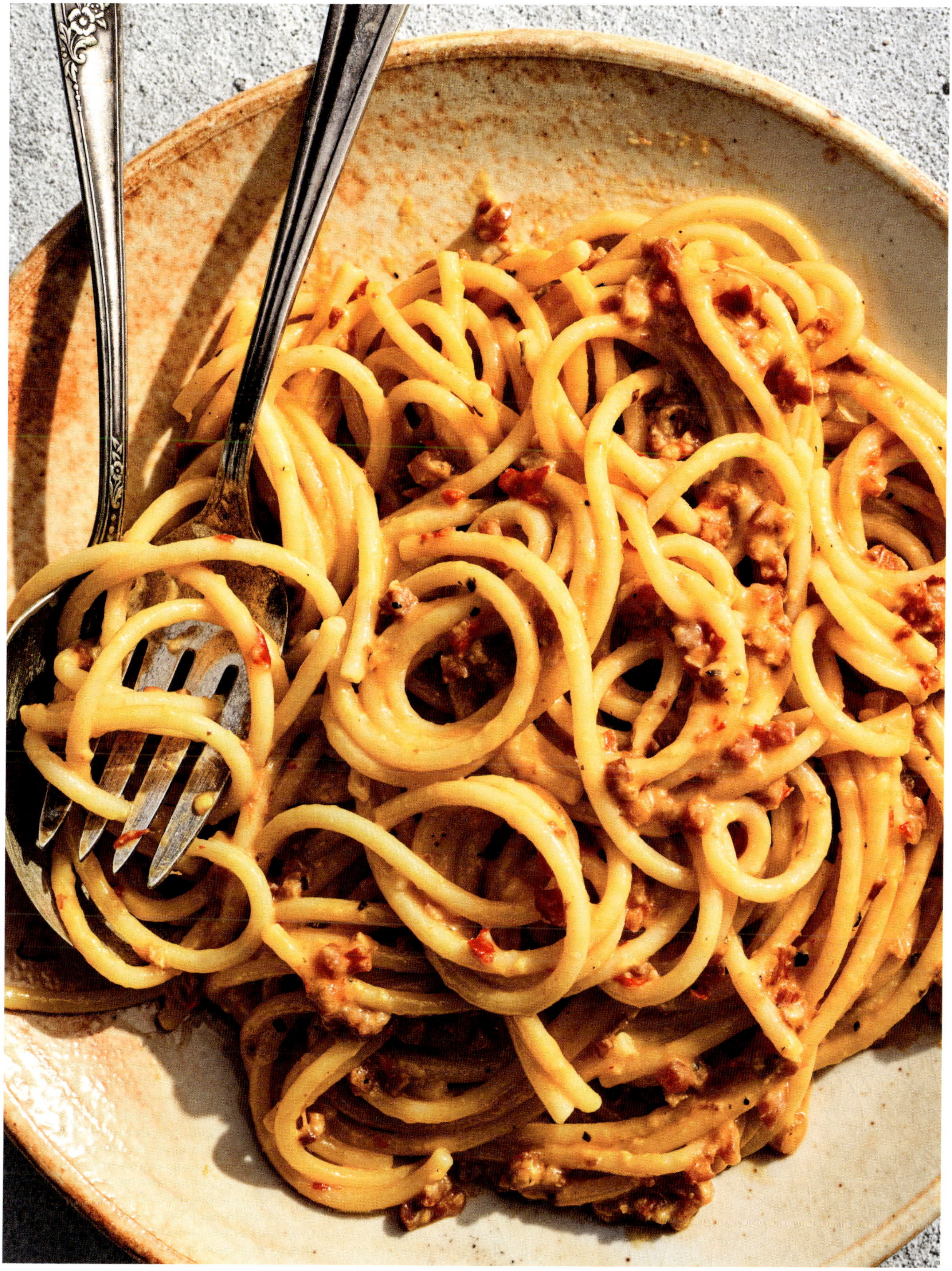

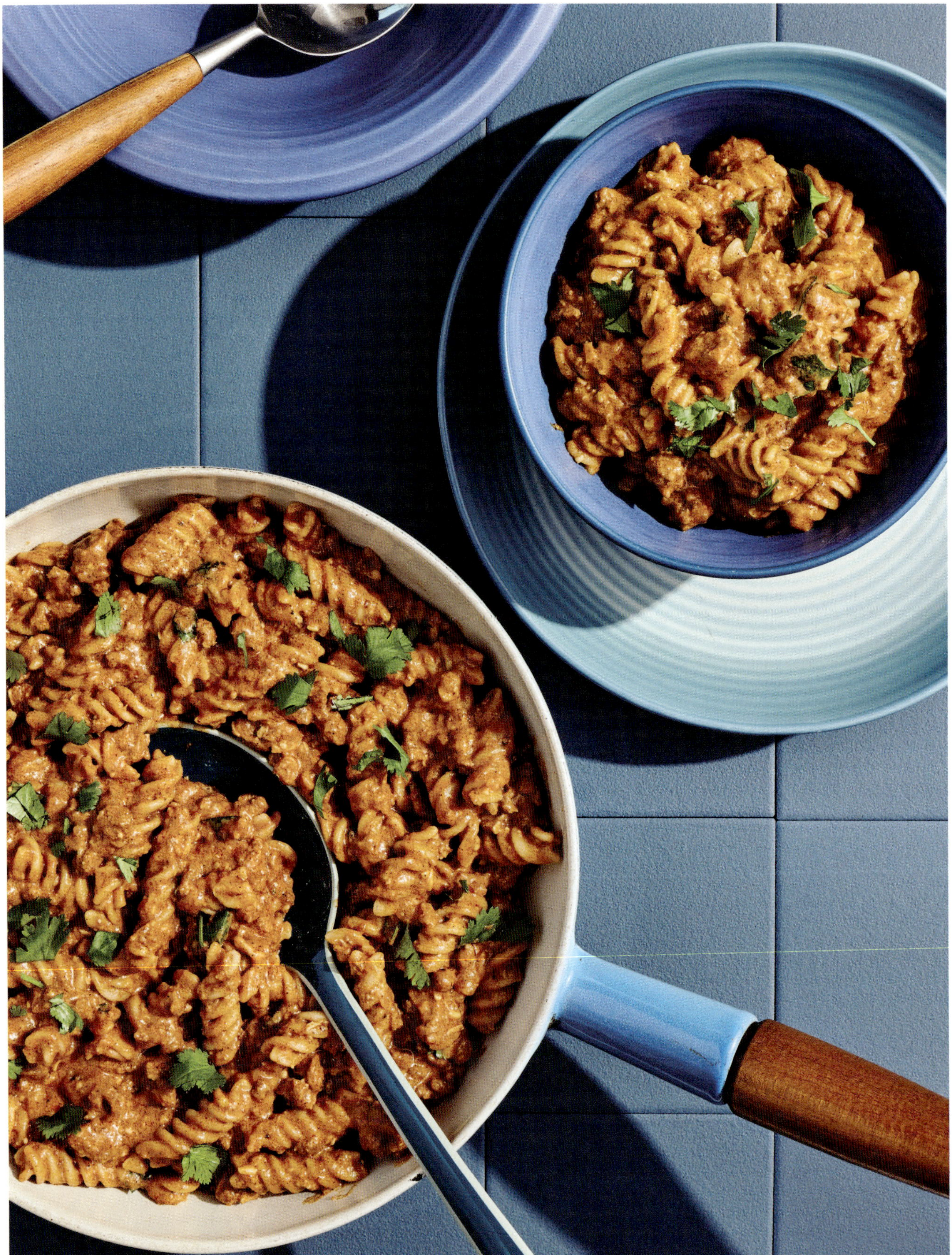

ONE-POT CHEESY ENCHILADA HELPER

MAKES 6 SERVINGS | **TOTAL TIME:** 35 MINUTES

DIETARY
GLUTEN-FREE
MAKE AHEAD

Get ready to dive into a flavor-packed fiesta! This dish is like your favorite Hamburger Helper, but with a twist. Ground beef, creamy cheese, and saucy enchilada sauce all mingle in one pot for a meal that's easy, cheesy, and oh so satisfying. Say hello to your new go-to dinner, especially for feeding a busy family!

2 tablespoons avocado oil
1 cup small-diced yellow onion (about 1 small onion)
2 garlic cloves, minced
1 pound ground beef (90/10)
1 teaspoon kosher salt
½ teaspoon freshly ground black pepper
1 teaspoon chili powder
1 teaspoon ground cumin
8 ounces gluten-free brown rice fusilli pasta
One 15-ounce can red enchilada sauce
2 cups low-sodium beef broth
½ cup whole-milk plain Greek yogurt
1 cup shredded Mexican blend cheese
1 tablespoon freshly squeezed lime juice (about ½ lime)
¼ cup chopped fresh cilantro leaves

IN a large, deep skillet, heat the oil over medium-high heat. Add the onion and garlic and cook, stirring, until the onion is tender, about 3 minutes.

ADD the ground beef and cook, breaking up the meat with the edge of a spoon, until the beef is browned and cooked through, about 7 minutes. Drain off the excess fat and return the beef to the pan.

ADD the salt, pepper, chili powder, and cumin. Cook, stirring, until the mixture is well combined and the spices are fragrant, about 2 minutes.

ADD the pasta, enchilada sauce, and broth. Stir to combine and bring to a rapid simmer. Reduce the heat to a gentle simmer, about medium-low heat. Cook, uncovered, and stirring often, until the pasta is tender and most of the liquid has been absorbed, 12 to 15 minutes.

REDUCE the heat to low. Stir in the yogurt, cheese, and lime juice. Cook, stirring, until the cheese has melted and is well combined.

REMOVE from the heat and finish by stirring in the cilantro.

STORE leftovers in an airtight container in the fridge for up to 3 days. Reheat in a saucepan or skillet over medium heat with a splash of broth to loosen the sauce, stirring occasionally, or microwave in 1-minute increments, stirring between, until warmed through.

THAI RED CURRY SHRIMP NOODLES

MAKES 4 SERVINGS | **TOTAL TIME:** 30 MINUTES

DIETARY
GLUTEN-FREE
DAIRY-FREE
MAKE AHEAD

These quick and easy Thai-inspired noodles are a hit with my kids, thanks to their mild but flavorful sauce. Red curry paste gives the dish a gentle spice that's balanced by creamy coconut milk, making it perfect for family dinners. Ready in just thirty minutes, this gluten-free and dairy-free meal combines tender shrimp with fragrant herbs and vibrant vegetables for a dish everyone will love.

8 ounces wide rice noodles
Kosher salt
2 tablespoons avocado oil
2 cups thinly sliced red bell pepper (about 1 large pepper)
1 cup thinly sliced white onion (about 1 small onion)
3 garlic cloves, minced
½ teaspoon freshly ground black pepper
2 tablespoons Thai red curry paste
1 cup unsweetened full-fat coconut milk
2 tablespoons coconut aminos
1 tablespoon fish sauce
2 teaspoons coconut sugar
Grated zest of ½ lime
2 tablespoons freshly squeezed lime juice (about 1 lime)
1 pound peeled, deveined, tail-off shrimp (36/40 count), patted dry
½ cup roughly chopped fresh cilantro leaves
1 cup roughly chopped Thai or regular basil leaves

LEFTOVER red curry paste? Try my Chicken Khao Soi-Inspired Soup (page 87), Tangy Thai Braised Chicken (page 162), or Red Curry Pork Stir-Fry (page 191).

BRING a large pot of water to a boil. Add the the rice noodles and plenty of salt (I use about 1 tablespoon) to the boiling water and cook until al dente according to the package directions. When the pasta is cooked, drain and rinse with cold water. Set aside.

IN a large, deep skillet, heat the oil over medium-high heat. Add the bell pepper, onion, garlic, 1½ teaspoons kosher salt, and black pepper. Cook, stirring, until the veggies are tender, 3 to 4 minutes.

ADD the curry paste and continue to cook, stirring, until fragrant and toasted, about 2 minutes.

POUR in the coconut milk, coconut aminos, fish sauce, coconut sugar, lime zest, and lime juice. Stir until well combined and bring to a simmer. Let simmer, stirring often, to allow the sauce to thicken slightly, 2 to 3 minutes.

REDUCE the heat to a gentle simmer, about medium-low heat. Add the shrimp and stir to coat well with the sauce. Cook until the shrimp are cooked through and no longer opaque, 3 to 4 minutes.

RINSE the noodles under cold water once more to ensure they are not sticky, then transfer to the skillet. Add the cilantro and basil. Gently toss until the noodles are well coated in the sauce, about 2 more minutes.

TO SERVE: Use tongs to transfer the noodles, shrimp, and vegetables to bowls and pour additional sauce on top.

STORE leftovers in an airtight container in the fridge for up to 3 days. Reheat in a saucepan or skillet over medium heat with a splash of broth to loosen the sauce, stirring occasionally until warmed through.

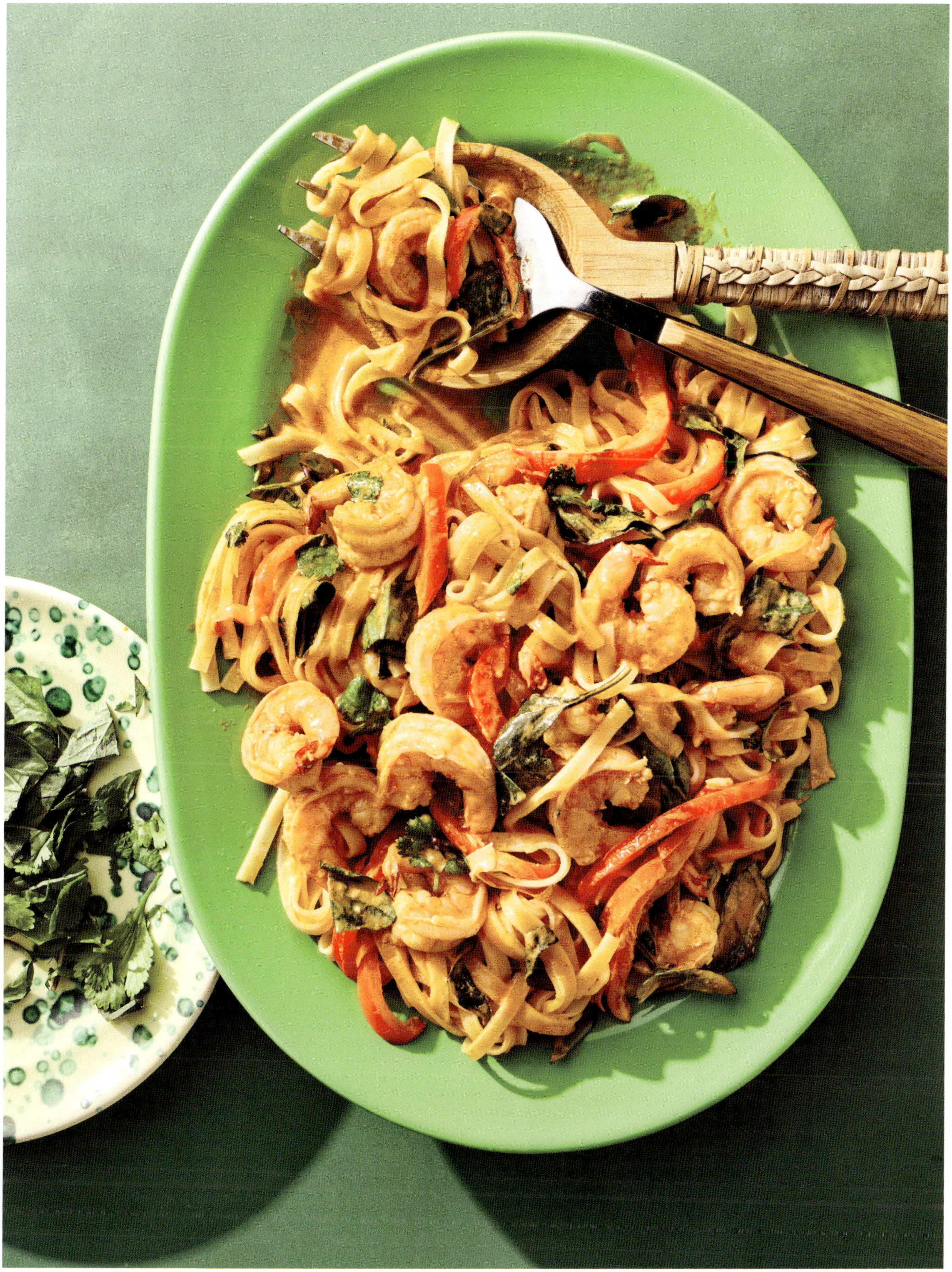

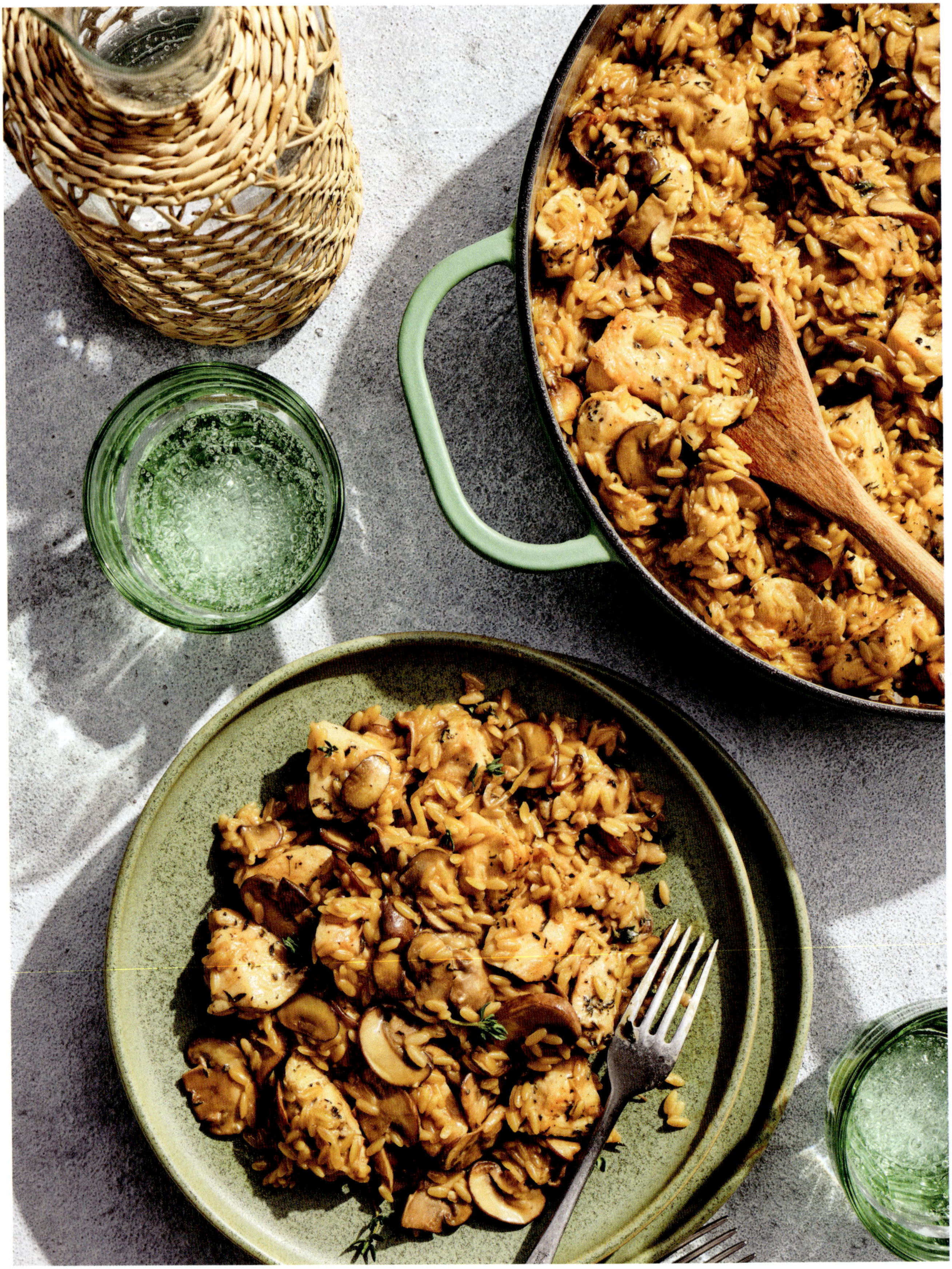

ONE-POT CHICKEN MARSALA ORZO

MAKES 4 SERVINGS | **TOTAL TIME:** 35 MINUTES

DIETARY
GLUTEN-FREE (IF MODIFIED)
MAKE AHEAD

This one-pot orzo dish has all the flavors of a traditional chicken Marsala but comes together in one pan in thirty-five minutes. With savory mushrooms, fragrant thyme, a splash of marsala, and a creamy finish from the crème fraîche, this dish is easy enough for a weeknight but impressive enough for company.

- 1 pound boneless, skinless chicken breasts, trimmed of excess fat, patted dry, and cut into 1-inch pieces
- 2 teaspoons kosher salt, divided
- ½ teaspoon freshly ground black pepper
- 1 teaspoon onion powder
- ½ teaspoon dried thyme
- 3 tablespoons extra-virgin olive oil, divided
- 1 tablespoon unsalted butter
- 3 cups stemmed and thinly sliced cremini mushrooms
- ½ cup halved and thinly sliced shallot (about 1 large shallot)
- 4 garlic cloves, minced
- 2 teaspoons fresh thyme leaves, plus more for serving
- ¾ cup marsala wine
- 1 cup orzo (sub brown rice orzo or other small pasta for gluten-free)
- 2 cups low-sodium chicken broth
- Grated zest of ½ lemon
- 1 tablespoon freshly squeezed lemon juice (about ½ lemon)
- ⅓ cup crème fraîche

IN a medium bowl, combine the chicken, 1 teaspoon of the salt, the pepper, onion powder, and dried thyme. Toss to evenly season the chicken.

IN a large, deep skillet or 3.5-quart braiser with fitted lid, heat 2 tablespoons of the oil over medium-high heat. Add the chicken in a single layer and cook for 3 to 4 minutes per side until completely cooked through. Transfer to a clean plate and set aside.

TO the same skillet, add the remaining 1 tablespoon oil and the butter. When the butter has melted, add the mushrooms and shallot. Cook, undisturbed, for 5 minutes to allow the mushrooms to get a good sear. Cook, stirring, for an additional 2 to 3 minutes, until the mushrooms are a deep golden brown.

REDUCE the heat to medium. Add the garlic, the remaining 1 teaspoon of salt, and the fresh thyme. Cook for 1 minute, until the garlic is fragrant. Add the marsala and stir, scraping up any browned bits off the bottom of the pan. Cook until the marsala has reduced by half, about 1 minute.

ADD the orzo, broth, and lemon zest. Stir to combine. Bring to a rapid simmer, then reduce heat to a gentle simmer, about medium-low heat, and cook for 8 minutes, stirring frequently, until most of the liquid has been absorbed and the orzo is almost done.

REDUCE the heat to low and add the chicken and any of its juices, the lemon juice, and the crème fraîche. Stir until well combined. Cover and cook until the chicken is warmed through and the orzo is al dente, 2 to 3 more minutes.

TO SERVE: Scoop the orzo and chicken into bowls and garnish with extra fresh thyme leaves.

STORE leftovers in an airtight container in the fridge for up to 3 days. Reheat in a saucepan or skillet over medium heat with a splash of broth to loosen the sauce, stirring occasionally, or microwave in 1-minute increments, stirring between, until warmed through.

SAUSAGE, FENNEL, AND LEMON PASTA

MAKES 4 SERVINGS | **TOTAL TIME:** 30 MINUTES

DIETARY
GLUTEN-FREE (IF MODIFIED)

This pasta keeps things light with a fresh twist. Tangy Greek yogurt, tart lemon, and white wine add balance and brightness, while the sausage and fennel seeds bring an elevated, five-star flavor. This simple yet sophisticated dish is perfect for weeknights. Pair with a crisp side salad for a complete dreamy dinner.

Kosher salt

12 ounces mezze maniche rigate or rigatoni pasta (sub brown rice pasta for gluten-free)

1 tablespoon extra-virgin olive oil

1 pound bulk mild or hot Italian sausage

½ cup finely diced shallot (about 1 large shallot)

8 cups baby kale (about 5 ounces)

2 garlic cloves, minced

1 teaspoon fennel seeds, coarsely chopped

½ teaspoon crushed red pepper flakes, plus more for serving

½ cup dry white wine or low-sodium chicken broth

Grated zest of ½ lemon

2 tablespoons freshly squeezed lemon juice (about 1 lemon)

⅔ cup whole-milk plain Greek yogurt

¼ cup grated parmesan cheese, plus more for serving

½ teaspoon freshly ground black pepper

¼ cup finely chopped fresh parsley leaves

BRING a large pot of water to a boil. Add plenty of salt (I use about 1 tablespoon) and the pasta to the boiling water and cook until al dente according to the package directions. When the pasta is cooked, reserve 1 cup of the starchy pasta water, then drain the pasta. Set aside.

WHILE the pasta is cooking, in a large, deep skillet, heat the oil over medium-high heat. Add the sausage and cook, breaking up the meat with the edge of a spoon, until cooked through and no longer pink, about 7 minutes. Drain off the excess fat and return the sausage to the pan.

ADD the shallot and cook until softened, about 3 minutes. Stir in the kale, garlic, fennel seeds, and pepper flakes. Cook for 1 to 2 minutes, stirring occasionally, until the garlic is fragrant and the kale has wilted.

POUR in the wine (or broth) and continue to cook, scraping up any browned bits off the bottom of the pan, until it has reduced by half, about 2 minutes. Stir in ½ cup of the reserved pasta water, the lemon zest, and the lemon juice.

REDUCE the heat to low and add the yogurt, parmesan, 1 teaspoon kosher salt, and black pepper. Stir until the sauce becomes creamy and smooth. Be careful not to let the sauce boil, as this will cause the yogurt to curdle.

ADD the cooked pasta to the skillet, tossing to coat the pasta evenly in the sauce. If the sauce is too thick, add more pasta water ¼ cup at a time as needed.

STIR in the parsley. Serve the pasta immediately with extra parmesan and pepper flakes on top.

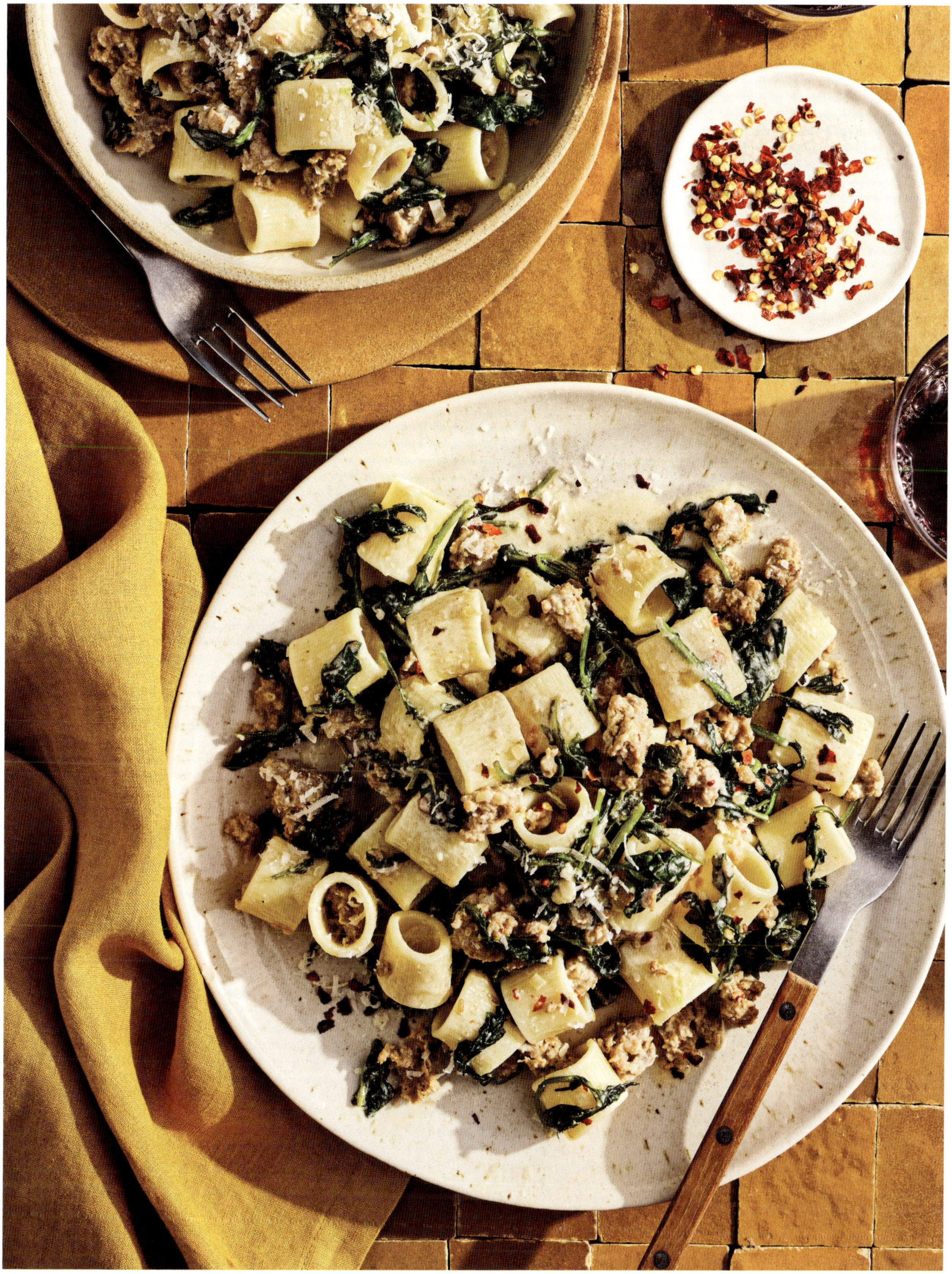

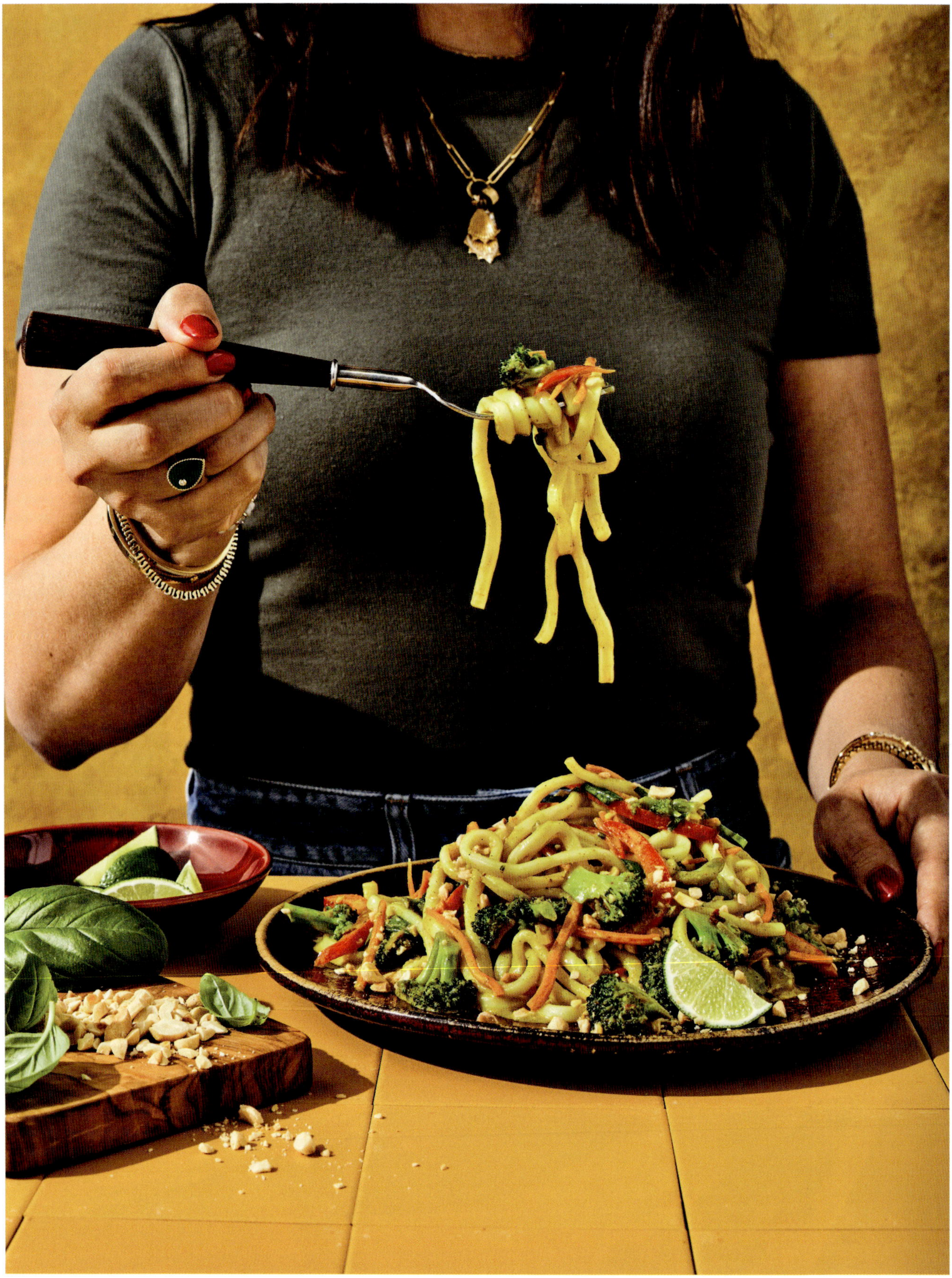

GOLDEN CURRY VEGGIE UDON NOODLES

MAKES 4 SERVINGS | **TOTAL TIME**: 25 MINUTES

DIETARY
DAIRY-FREE
VEGETARIAN
MAKE AHEAD

I love tossing together whatever veggies I have on hand for this curried noodle recipe! The blend of Indian curry powder with Asian-inspired ingredients like fish sauce, coconut aminos, and coconut milk creates a savory, flavor-packed dish. It's the perfect meatless meal—delicious and satisfying!

- 2 tablespoons avocado oil
- 2 cups roughly chopped broccoli florets (about 1 small head)
- 1 medium red bell pepper, seeded and sliced into ¼-inch-wide strips
- 1 cup matchstick carrots
- 4 green onions, thinly sliced, white and green parts kept separate
- 1 teaspoon grated fresh ginger
- 4 garlic cloves, minced
- ½ teaspoon freshly ground black pepper
- 1 teaspoon kosher salt, plus more to taste
- 1 tablespoon curry powder
- 1 teaspoon ground turmeric
- ½ teaspoon crushed red pepper flakes
- ¼ cup coconut aminos
- 2 teaspoons fish sauce
- 1 cup unsweetened full-fat coconut milk
- One 9.5-ounce package udon noodles (3 bundles)
- 2 tablespoons freshly squeezed lime juice (about 1 lime)
- ¼ cup thinly sliced fresh basil leaves
- ¼ cup roughly chopped peanuts, for serving
- Lime wedges, for serving

BRING a medium pot of water to a boil.

MEANWHILE, in a large, deep skillet, heat the oil over medium-high heat. Add the broccoli, bell pepper, carrots, white parts of the green onions, ginger, garlic, black pepper, and salt. Cook, stirring, until the veggies begin to soften, about 4 minutes.

REDUCE the heat to medium and add the curry powder, turmeric, and pepper flakes. Cook, stirring, toasting the spices until fragrant, about 1 minute.

ADD the coconut aminos, fish sauce, and coconut milk. Bring to a rapid simmer, stirring often. Reduce the heat to low, so that the sauce is simmering very lightly, while you cook the noodles.

ADD the udon noodles and plenty of salt (I use about 1 tablespoon) to the boiling water and cook according to the package directions. When the noodles are cooked, reserve ½ cup of the water, then drain the noodles.

ADD the cooked noodles to the sauce along with the green parts of the green onions, the lime juice, and the basil. Toss until the noodles are well coated in the sauce. If the noodles seem dry, add the reserved pasta water ¼ cup at a time until the pasta is coated in the sauce and glossy. Taste and adjust salt as desired.

DIVIDE the noodles among four bowls and top with the peanuts. Serve with a wedge of lime.

STORE leftovers in an airtight container in the fridge for up to 3 days. Reheat in a saucepan or skillet over medium heat with a splash of broth to loosen the sauce, stirring occasionally until warmed through.

ONE-SKILLET BUFFALO CHICKEN PASTA

MAKES 4 SERVINGS | **TOTAL TIME:** 30 MINUTES

DIETARY
GLUTEN-FREE
MAKE AHEAD

This quick and easy Buffalo chicken pasta is the perfect weeknight dinner, loaded with tangy Buffalo sauce, creamy Greek yogurt, and melty cheese. Ready in thirty minutes, it's bold, comforting, and irresistibly satisfying!

FOR THE PASTA

2 tablespoons avocado oil

4 green onions, thinly sliced, white and green parts kept separate

2 garlic cloves, minced

8 ounces gluten-free brown rice bowtie pasta

4 cups low-sodium chicken broth

1½ teaspoons kosher salt

½ teaspoon freshly ground black pepper

1 teaspoon garlic powder

½ teaspoon paprika

½ cup mild or hot Buffalo sauce

¼ cup whole-milk plain Greek yogurt

¾ cup shredded sharp cheddar cheese

2 cups shredded cooked chicken (I use rotisserie)

¼ cup crumbled blue cheese

FOR THE TOPPING

¼ cup gluten-free panko bread crumbs

1 tablespoon avocado oil

¼ teaspoon kosher salt

¼ cup shredded sharp cheddar cheese

1 tablespoon finely chopped fresh parsley leaves, for serving

POSITION a rack in the middle of the oven and preheat the oven to 400°F.

COOK THE PASTA: In a large, deep oven-safe skillet or 3.5-quart braiser, heat the oil over medium-high. Add the white parts of the green onions and the garlic. Cook, stirring, until softened, about 3 minutes.

ADD the pasta, broth, salt, pepper, garlic powder, and paprika. Bring to a rapid simmer, then reduce the heat to medium for a moderate simmer; you want a constant bubble but not a rapid boil. Cook, stirring often, until the pasta is tender and most of the broth is absorbed (it should still have a little excess liquid), 13 to 15 minutes.

REDUCE the heat to low and add the Buffalo sauce, yogurt, and the ¾ cup cheddar. Stir until the mixture is well combined and the cheese has just melted. Remove from the heat.

ADD the chicken, green parts of the green onions, and the blue cheese. Stir once more to combine. Spread into an even layer across the pan.

MAKE THE TOPPING: In a small bowl, combine the panko, oil, and salt. Stir until well combined and the oil coats the bread crumbs.

SPRINKLE the ¼ cup cheddar over the pasta, followed by the panko mixture. Transfer the skillet to the oven and bake until the cheese is bubbly and the bread crumbs are golden brown, 6 to 7 minutes.

REMOVE from the oven and let cool slightly before garnishing with fresh parsley and serving.

STORE leftovers in an airtight container in the fridge for up to 3 days. Reheat in a saucepan or skillet over medium heat with a splash of broth to loosen the sauce, stirring occasionally, or microwave in 1-minute increments, stirring between, until warmed through.

LEFTOVER Buffalo sauce? Try my Roasted Buffalo Chicken Thighs with Brussels Sprouts and Blue Cheese (page 141).

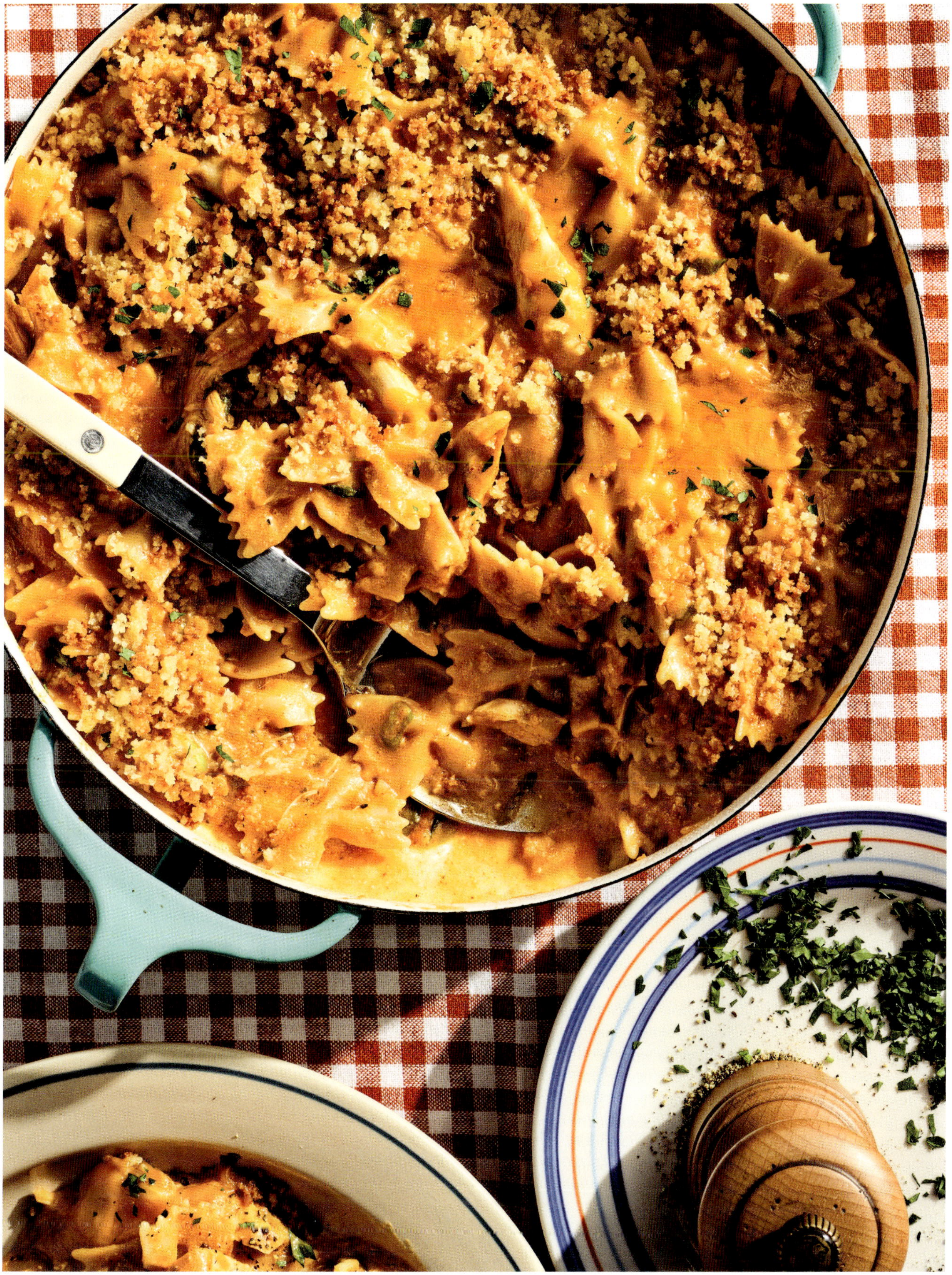

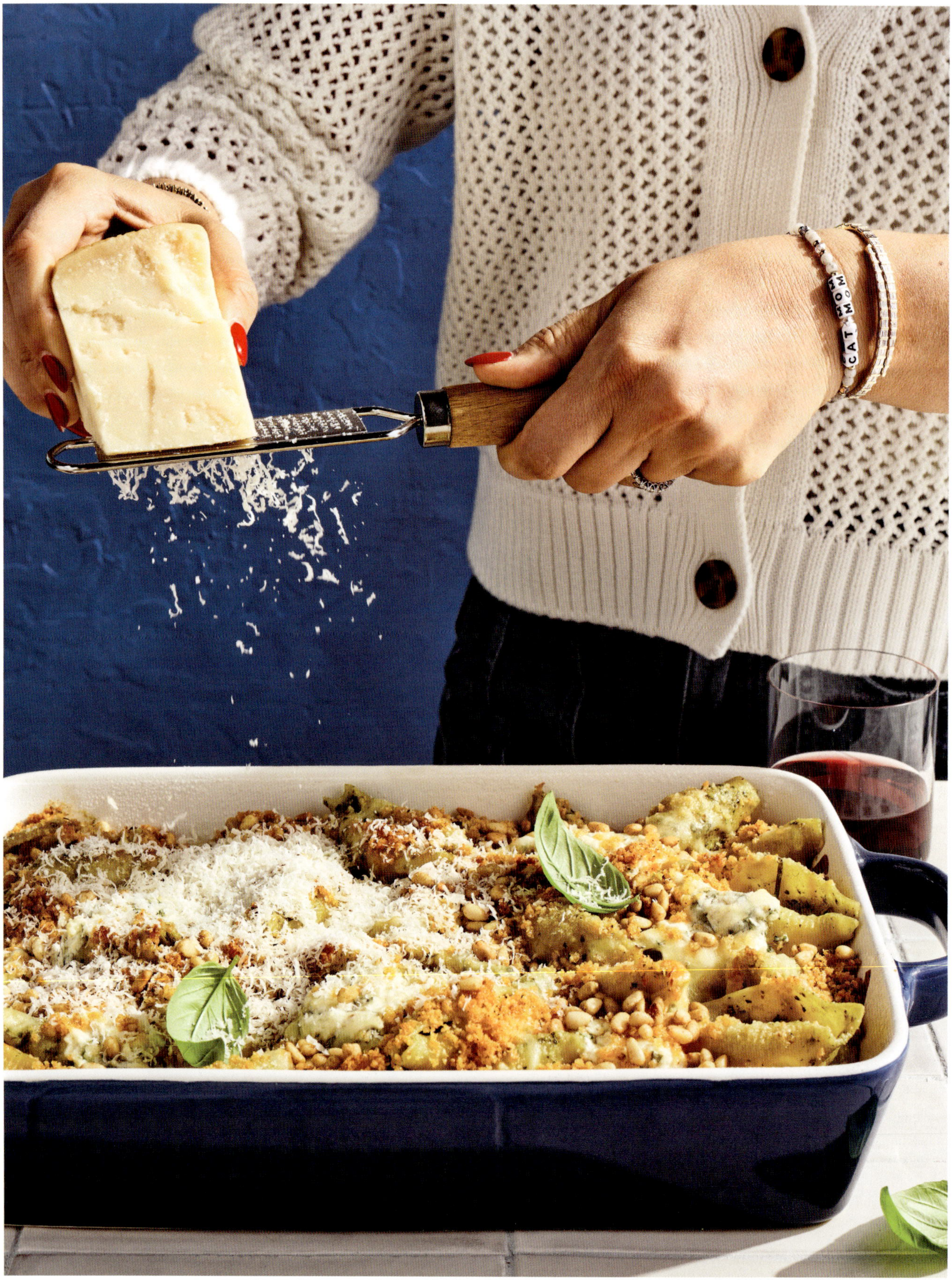
CAT MOM

PESTO UNSTUFFED SHELLS

MAKES 6 SERVINGS | **TOTAL TIME:** 50 MINUTES

DIETARY
VEGETARIAN
GLUTEN-FREE (IF MODIFIED)
MAKE AHEAD

When I ask my daughter Sutton what she wants for dinner, this has been her consistent pick for a few years. This is a less labor-intensive version of the classic with the same results. I use store-bought pesto mixed with creamy ricotta to coat the shells and top the whole thing with lots of parmesan and a crispy, golden panko topping.

Extra-virgin olive oil, for the baking dish

FOR THE RICOTTA MIXTURE

1 cup whole-milk ricotta

3 garlic cloves, minced

½ cup julienned fresh basil leaves, plus more for serving

Grated zest of ½ lemon

2 tablespoons lemon juice (about 1 lemon)

½ teaspoon kosher salt

½ teaspoon freshly ground black pepper

¼ cup freshly grated parmesan

FOR THE BREAD CRUMBS

¾ cup gluten-free panko bread crumbs

2 tablespoons extra-virgin olive oil

¼ teaspoon kosher salt

1 teaspoon dried oregano

1 teaspoon paprika

FOR THE PASTA

Kosher salt

1 pound jumbo shell pasta (sub gluten-free rigatoni)

1 cup store-bought or homemade basil pesto

1 cup grated mozzarella

½ cup freshly grated parmesan

½ cup toasted pine nuts, for garnish (see note)

POSITION a rack in the middle of the oven and preheat the oven to 375°F. Grease a 9 × 13-inch baking dish with oil and set aside.

MAKE THE RICOTTA MIXTURE: In a medium bowl, mix together the ricotta, garlic, basil, lemon zest, lemon juice, salt, pepper, and parmesan. Set aside in the fridge.

MAKE THE BREAD CRUMBS: In a medium bowl, mix together the panko, oil, salt, oregano, and paprika, ensuring the panko is evenly coated in the oil and seasoning. Set aside.

COOK THE PASTA: Bring a large pot of water to a boil. When the water comes to a boil, add plenty of salt (I use about 1 tablespoon) and the pasta. Cook until al dente according to the package directions. When the pasta is cooked, reserve 1 cup of the pasta water, then drain the pasta and transfer it back to the pot.

ADD the pesto, ¼ cup of the reserved pasta water, and half of the ricotta mixture. Stir to combine until the shells are evenly coated and the sauce is smooth and glossy, adding more pasta water ¼ cup at a time as needed.

POUR the pasta and the sauce into the prepared baking dish and smooth it into an even layer. Using a spoon, dollop the remaining ricotta mixture on top of the shells. Top with the mozzarella and parmesan. Evenly distribute the bread crumb topping over the dish.

TRANSFER to the oven and bake for 20 minutes, until bubbly with a golden top. Remove from the oven and let cool for 5 minutes to allow the sauce to settle and thicken a bit more. Top with more basil and the pine nuts.

FROM MY KITCHEN TO YOURS

FOR TOASTED PINE NUTS: To toast pine nuts, place them in a dry (no oil) skillet over medium heat and cook, stirring frequently, until golden and fragrant, 3 to 5 minutes. Keep a close eye on them, as they can burn quickly!

MAKE AHEAD: Bake fully as directed, let cool, and refrigerate, covered, for up to 3 days. To reheat, bake, covered with foil, at 350°F until hot and bubbly, about 30 minutes. To freeze, press plastic wrap directly onto the surface so no air touches it, then wrap tightly in heavy-duty foil and freeze for up to 2 months. Thaw overnight in the refrigerator, remove and discard the wrap and foil, then bake as directed.

TIPSY NOODLES

MAKES 4 SERVINGS | **TOTAL TIME:** 35 MINUTES

DIETARY
GLUTEN-FREE
DAIRY-FREE
MAKE AHEAD

"Drunken noodles" are a favorite across the world. This rendition brings inspiration from the flavors of the popular dish to your weeknight table with a convenient twist. Swapping in ground beef for traditional sliced beef cuts down on prep time, making it perfect for busy evenings. While this recipe packs a punch with a hit of heat from Thai chiles, you can easily dial it down for a milder palate.

½ cup coconut aminos
2 tablespoons rice vinegar
1 tablespoon fish sauce
1 teaspoon toasted sesame oil
2 teaspoons coconut sugar
4 garlic cloves, minced
1 teaspoon grated fresh ginger
1 to 3 Thai chiles, minced (see note)
⅓ cup low-sodium beef broth
1 teaspoon tapioca flour or arrowroot flour
1 tablespoon avocado oil
1 pound ground beef (90/10)
1 small red bell pepper, seeded and thinly sliced
4 green onions, cut into 2-inch pieces
1 cup matchstick carrots
9 ounces wide rice noodles
Kosher salt
2 tablespoons freshly squeezed lime juice (about 1 lime)
1 cup packed fresh Thai or regular basil leaves, plus more for garnish

BRING a large pot of water to a boil.

MEANWHILE, in a small bowl, whisk together the coconut aminos, vinegar, fish sauce, toasted sesame oil, coconut sugar, garlic, ginger, Thai chiles, broth, and flour. Set aside.

IN a large, deep skillet, heat the avocado oil over medium-high heat. Add the beef and cook, breaking up the meat with the edge of a spoon, until cooked through and no longer pink, about 7 minutes. Drain off the excess fat and return the beef to the pan.

ADD the bell pepper, green onions, and carrots and cook, stirring, until the veggies begin to soften, 3 to 4 minutes.

REDUCE the heat to medium and pour in the sauce. Stir to combine and bring to a simmer. Cook, simmering and stirring often, until the sauce reduces slightly and begins to thicken, about 4 minutes. When the sauce is looking thicker, reduce the heat to low to keep warm while you boil the noodles.

ADD the rice noodles and plenty of salt (I use about 1 tablespoon) to the boiling water and cook until al dente according to the package directions. Be mindful that rice noodles typically cook between 2 to 6 minutes, depending on how thick they are. Drain and rinse under cold water.

TRANSFER the cooked noodles to the skillet and toss until they are glossy and well coated in the sauce, about 2 minutes.

ADD the lime juice and basil and toss until the basil is just wilted, 1 more minute.

TO SERVE: Divide the noodles among four bowls and top with additional basil.

STORE leftovers in the fridge in an airtight container for 3 to 4 days without the garnishes. Reheat in a saucepan or skillet over medium heat with a splash of broth to loosen the sauce, stirring occasionally, or microwave in 1-minute increments, stirring between, until warmed through.

FROM MY KITCHEN TO YOURS

Thai chiles are small, but they are mighty. You can make this dish according to your spice preference: 3 for spicy, 2 for medium, 1 for mild. If you can't find Thai chiles, I recommend mincing about ½ serrano pepper.

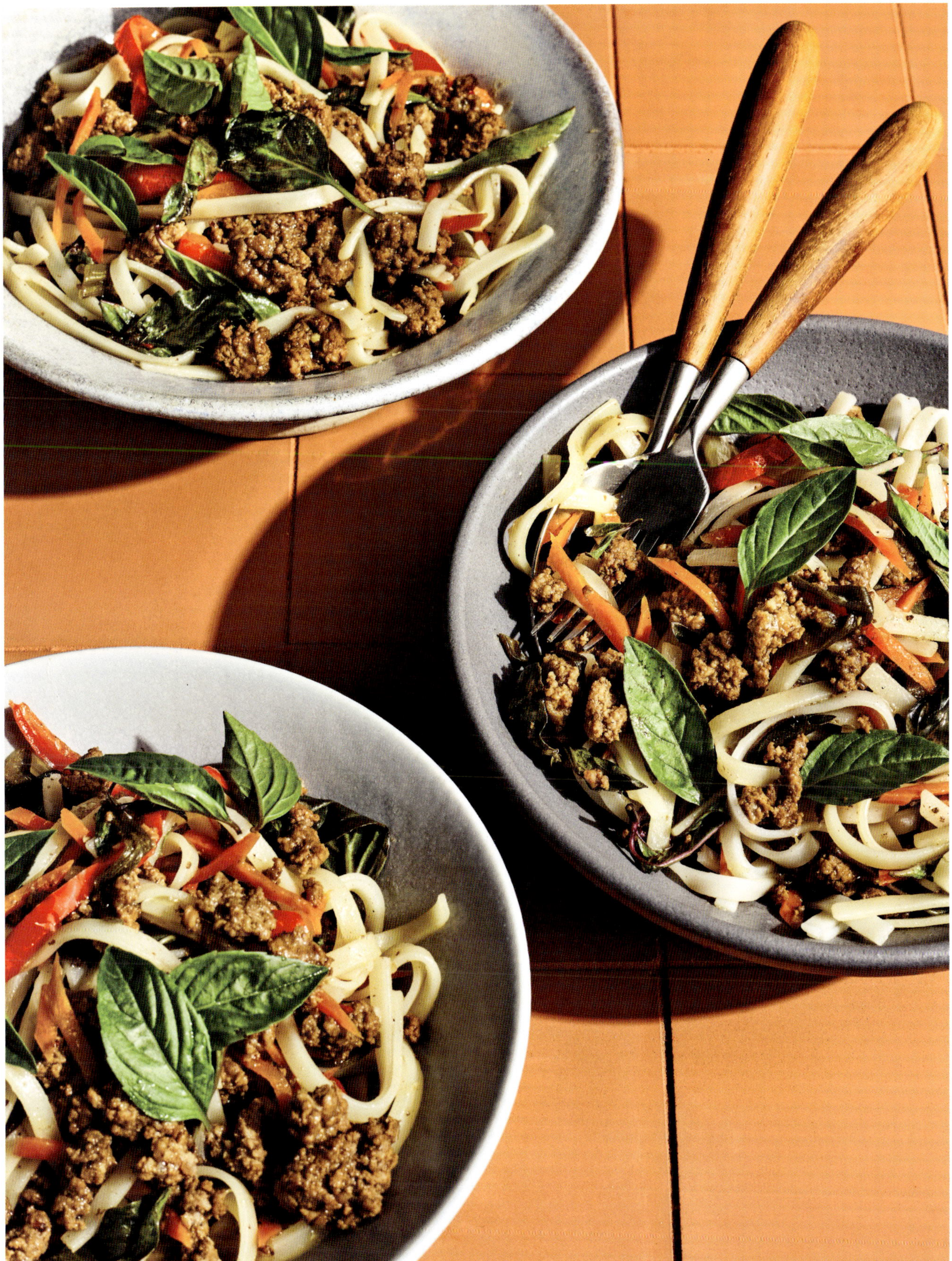

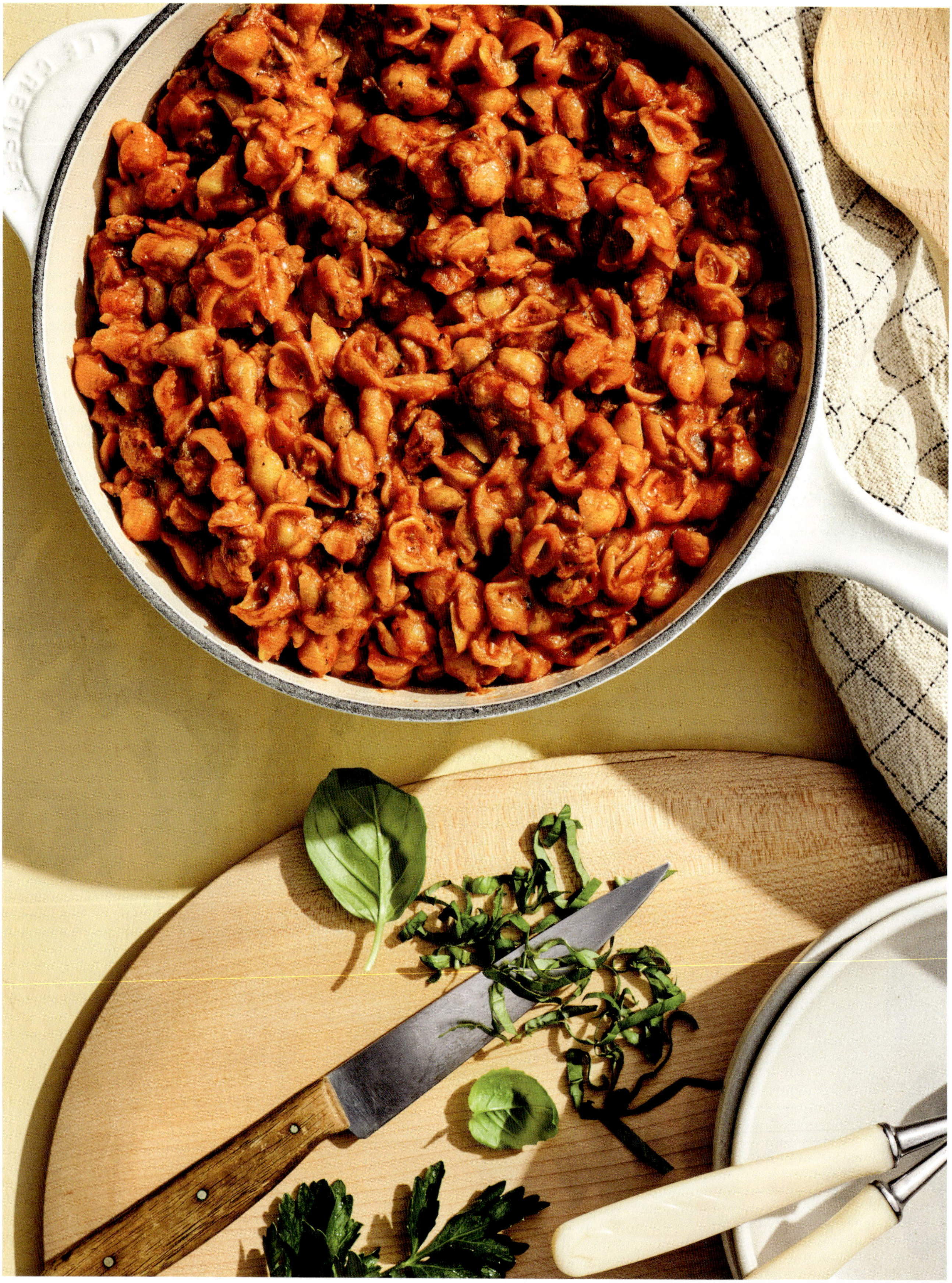

ONE-POT ITALIAN SHELLS AND CHEESE

MAKES 4 SERVINGS | **TOTAL TIME:** 25 MINUTES

DIETARY
GLUTEN-FREE (IF MODIFIED)
MAKE AHEAD

If you know, you know: Cheesy Italian Shells was the elite flavor of Hamburger Helper growing up—and no one can convince me otherwise. This one-pot wonder is my homemade nod to those cozy weeknight dinners of the nineties, but with way better ingredients and a whole lot more flavor. It's saucy, cheesy, herby, and ridiculously easy to throw together—just how I like my comfort food. Whether you're craving something nostalgic or just need a simple dinner win, this cheesy meal totally delivers.

- 1 tablespoon extra-virgin olive oil
- 1 cup finely diced yellow onion (about ½ medium onion)
- 4 garlic cloves, minced
- 1 pound bulk mild or hot Italian sausage
- ½ teaspoon kosher salt, plus more to taste
- ½ teaspoon freshly ground black pepper
- 1½ teaspoons dried oregano
- 2 tablespoons tomato paste
- 12 ounces small pasta shells
- 3 cups low-sodium beef broth
- One 14.5-ounce can tomato sauce
- 2 tablespoons red wine vinegar
- ½ cup shredded mozzarella cheese
- 2 tablespoons thinly sliced fresh basil leaves, for serving
- ½ cup chopped fresh parsley, for serving

IN a large, deep-sided skillet or pot, heat the oil over medium-high heat. When the oil is shimmering, add the onion and garlic and cook, stirring occasionally, until just softened, about 2 minutes.

ADD the sausage and cook, breaking up the meat with the edge of a spoon, until the sausage is cooked through and no longer pink, about 7 minutes. Drain all but 2 tablespoons of fat from the pan and return the sausage to the pan.

REDUCE the heat to medium and add the salt, pepper, and dried oregano. Stir to combine. Add the tomato paste and stir until it is well incorporated with the sausage.

ADD the pasta, broth, tomato sauce, and vinegar and stir to combine. Bring the contents in the pot to a boil. Immediately reduce the heat to a gentle simmer, about medium-low heat, and cook, stirring often, until most of the liquid has absorbed and the pasta is al dente, 13 to 15 minutes.

WHEN the pasta is cooked, reduce the heat to low. Stir in the mozzarella until melted and well combined. Taste and add more salt, if desired.

TO SERVE: Top with fresh basil and parsley.

STORE leftovers in an airtight container in the fridge for up to 3 days. Reheat in a saucepan or skillet over medium heat with a splash of broth to loosen the sauce, stirring occasionally, or microwave in 1-minute increments, stirring between, until warmed through.

OVEN-ROASTED SHRIMP SCAMPI

MAKES 4 SERVINGS | **TOTAL TIME:** 30 MINUTES

DIETARY
GLUTEN-FREE
DAIRY-FREE (IF MODIFIED)
MAKE AHEAD

Shrimp scampi is one of life's simple pleasures: a delightful blend of shrimp, garlic, butter, and white wine that is typically prepared in a skillet. Instead of a skillet, here I let the oven do the work. Relying on the oven for dinner is a favorite trick of mine—it frees up time to set the table, prepare sides, or tackle other tasks while everything roasts to perfection. And let me tell you, this pasta is perfection!

- 6 garlic cloves, minced
- ½ cup halved and thinly sliced shallot (about 1 large shallot)
- 1 teaspoon crushed red pepper flakes
- ¼ cup extra-virgin olive oil
- ½ cup dry white wine
- Grated zest of ½ lemon
- 1 teaspoon kosher salt, plus more to taste
- ½ teaspoon freshly ground black pepper
- 1 pound peeled, deveined, and tail-off shrimp (31/40 count), patted dry
- 8 ounces gluten-free linguine
- ⅓ cup grated parmesan cheese (omit for dairy-free)
- ¼ cup roughly chopped fresh parsley leaves
- Lemon wedges, for serving

PREHEAT the oven to 375°F. Bring a large pot of water to a boil.

MEANWHILE, in a 9 × 13-inch baking dish, combine the garlic, shallot, pepper flakes, oil, wine, lemon zest, salt, black pepper, and shrimp. Toss until well mixed then spread into an even layer.

TRANSFER to the oven and bake until the shrimp is pink and cooked through, about 13 minutes.

MEANWHILE, when the water comes to a boil, add plenty of salt (I use about 1 tablespoon) and the pasta. Cook the pasta according to the package directions.

DRAIN the pasta, add it to the baking dish with the cooked shrimp, and gently toss until coated. Add the parmesan (if using) and parsley and toss once more. Taste and add more salt, if desired.

TO SERVE: Divide the pasta and shrimp among four bowls. Serve with lemon wedges.

STORE leftovers in an airtight container in the fridge for up to 3 days. Reheat in a saucepan or skillet over medium heat with a splash of broth to loosen the sauce, stirring occasionally, or microwave in 1-minute increments, stirring between, until warmed through.

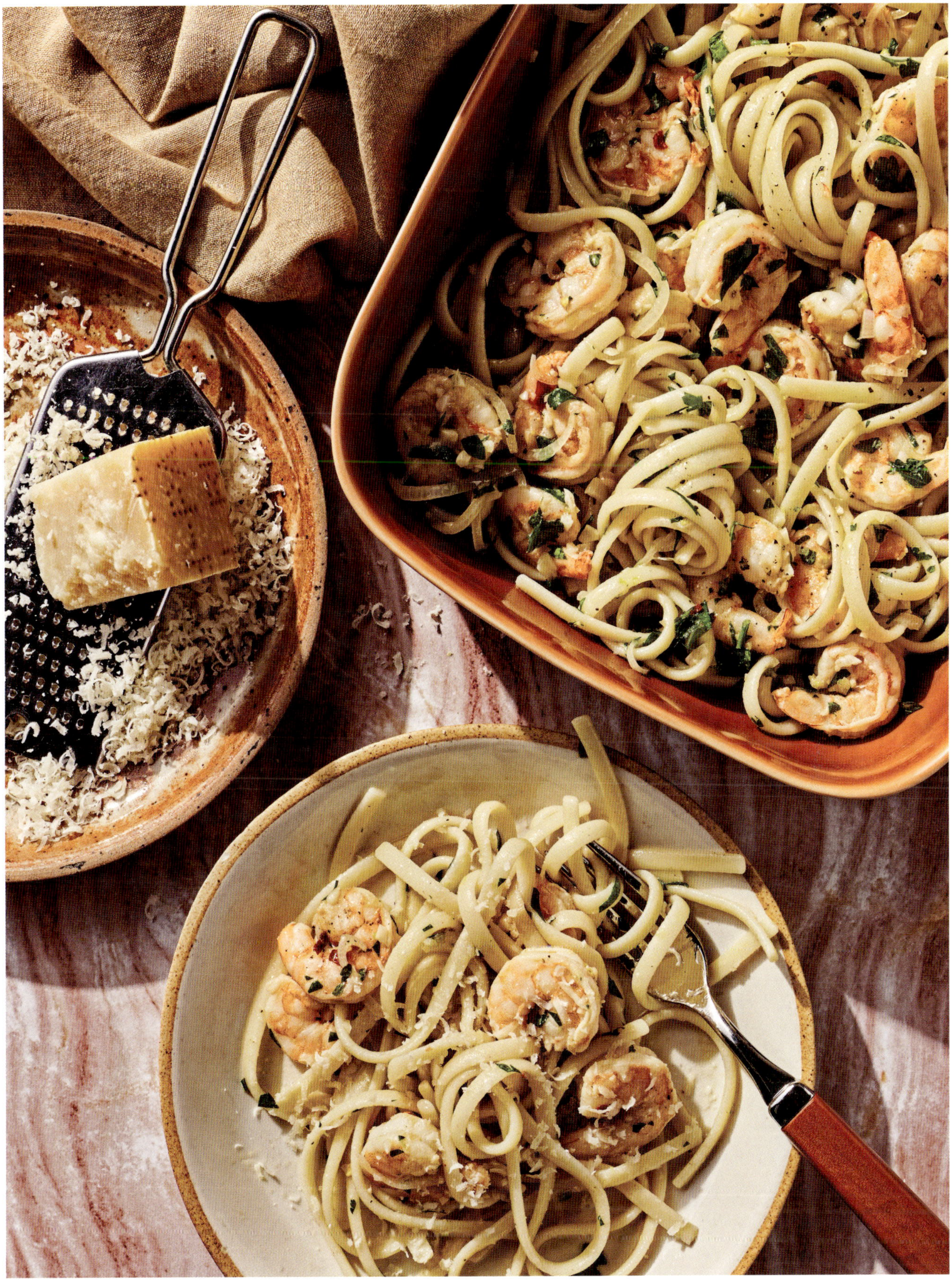

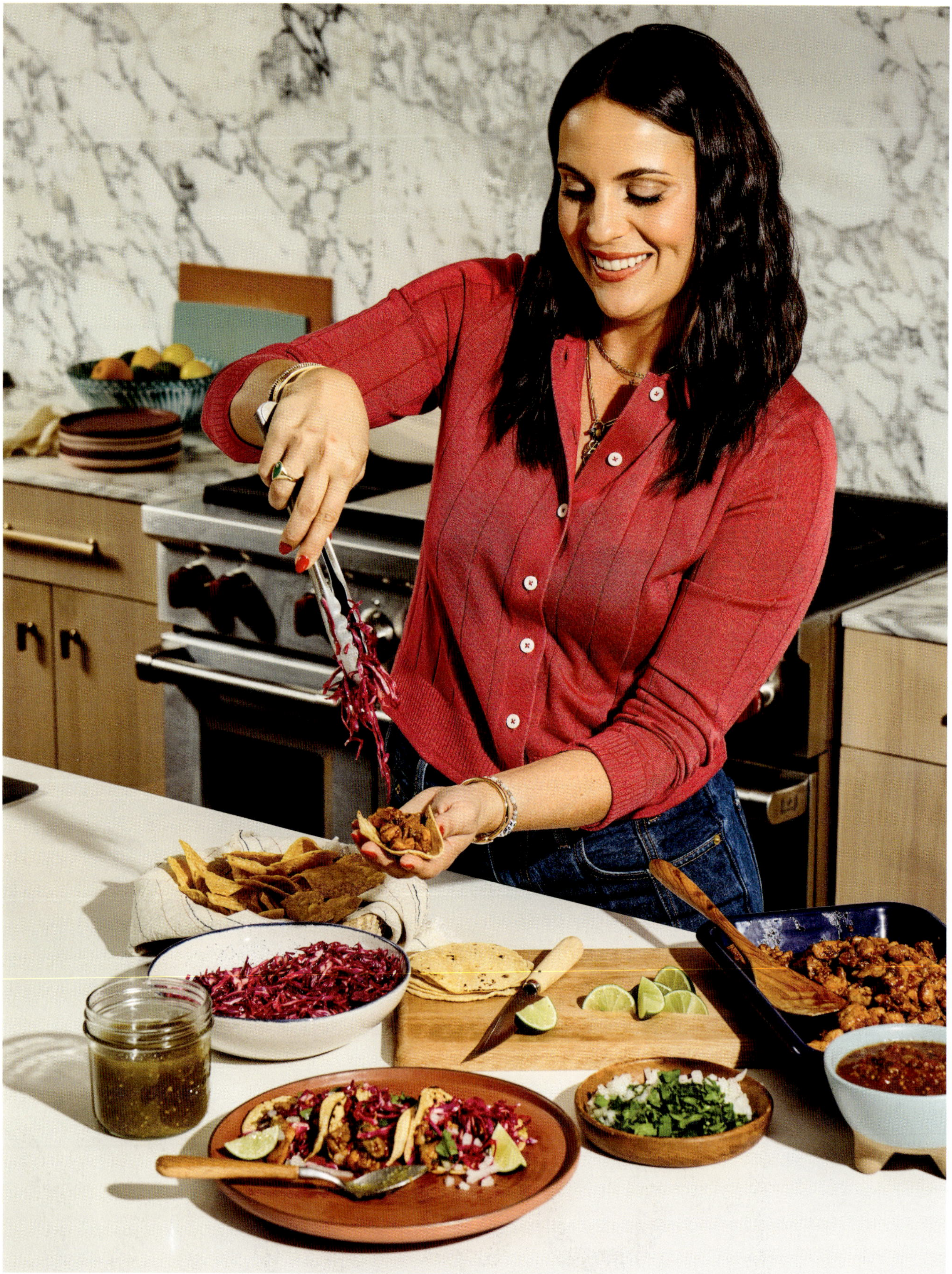

POULTRY

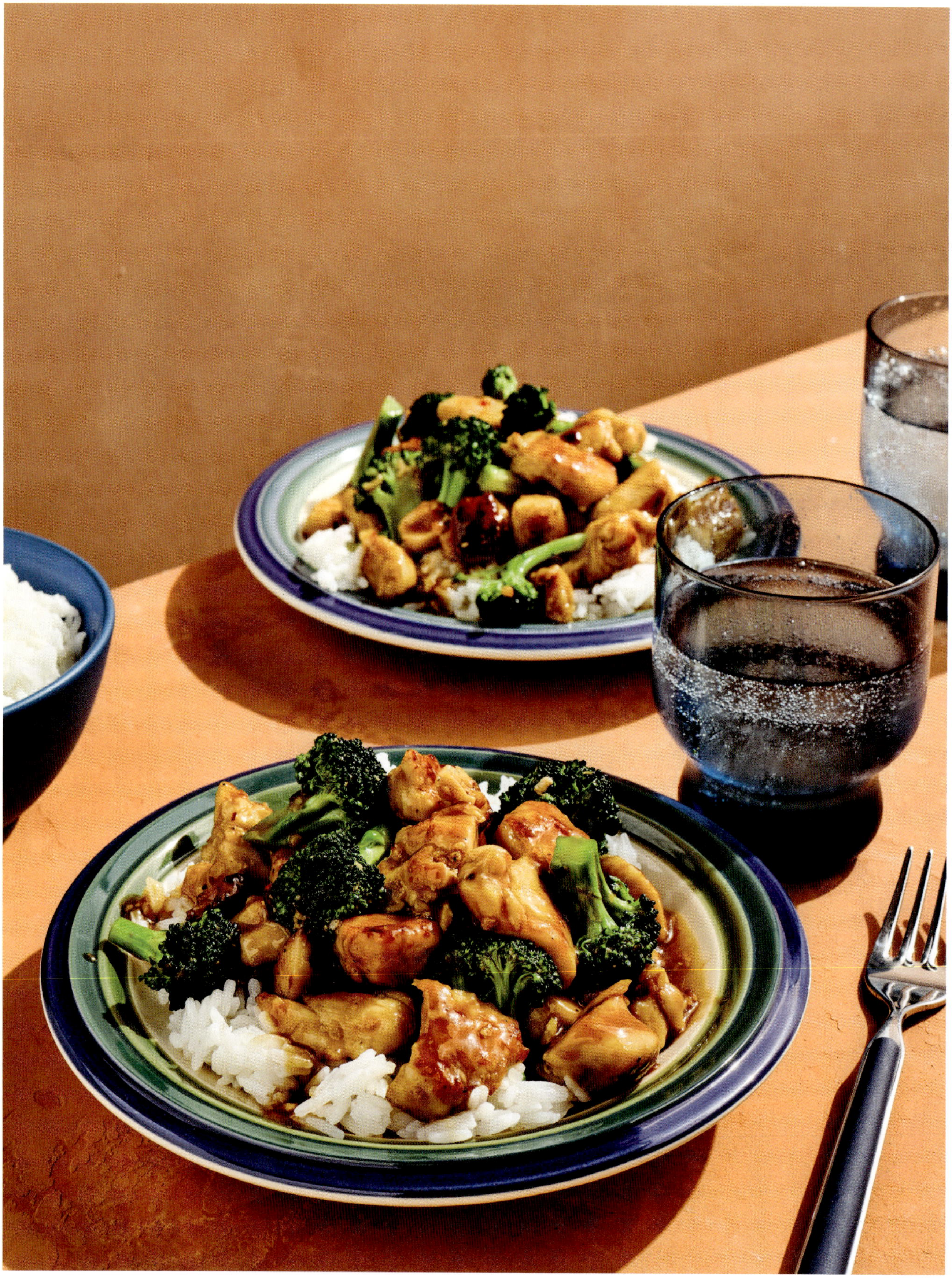

CHICKEN AND BROCCOLI STIR-FRY

MAKES 4 SERVINGS | **TOTAL TIME:** 30 MINUTES

DIETARY
- GLUTEN-FREE
- GRAIN-FREE
- DAIRY-FREE
- PALEO
- **MAKE AHEAD**

Growing up in a small town with few dining options, my best friends and I would happily drive forty-five minutes to our favorite Chinese restaurant just to satisfy our cravings. My order was always the chicken and broccoli—it's a dish that's forever etched in my heart as a comforting classic. With tender chicken and crisp broccoli smothered in a savory brown sauce, this version captures those nostalgic flavors while being a healthier, family-approved favorite.

FOR THE CHICKEN

2 pounds boneless, skinless chicken breasts, trimmed of excess fat and patted dry

2 teaspoons kosher salt

1 teaspoon freshly ground black pepper

2 tablespoons tapioca flour

1 tablespoon coconut aminos

½ teaspoon baking soda

FOR THE STIR-FRY

⅓ cup coconut aminos

1 teaspoon toasted sesame oil

1 teaspoon fish sauce

¾ cup low-sodium chicken broth

4 garlic cloves, minced

1 teaspoon grated fresh ginger

½ teaspoon crushed red pepper flakes, optional

1 tablespoon tapioca flour

2 tablespoons avocado oil

4 cups roughly chopped broccoli florets (about 1 large head)

Prepared cauliflower rice or steamed rice

PREPARE THE CHICKEN: Place the chicken breasts on a cutting board and cover with parchment paper or plastic wrap. Using a meat mallet or the bottom of a heavy skillet, pound the chicken to a uniform ½-inch thickness and cut into 1-inch pieces.

IN a medium bowl, toss together the chicken, salt, black pepper, flour, coconut aminos, and baking soda until well combined. Set aside.

MAKE THE SAUCE: In a small bowl, whisk together the coconut aminos, toasted sesame oil, fish sauce, broth, garlic, ginger, pepper flakes (if using), and flour until well combined. Set aside.

COOK THE STIR-FRY: In a large, deep nonstick skillet, heat the avocado oil over medium-high heat. Working in batches as necessary so as not to overcrowd the pan, add the chicken in a single layer and cook, undisturbed, until a golden-brown crust forms, about 3 minutes. Flip the chicken and continue to cook until both sides are golden brown, about 3 minutes more. Transfer the cooked chicken to a clean plate and set aside.

REDUCE the heat to medium and add the broccoli to the pan along with ¼ cup water. Cook, scraping up any browned bits off the bottom of the pan, until broccoli is bright green and the water has evaporated, about 3 minutes.

ADD the cooked chicken and any of its juices back to the skillet and pour in the sauce. Cook, simmering and stirring occasionally, until the sauce thickens and coats the chicken, about 3 more minutes.

REMOVE from the heat and let cool slightly. Serve over prepared rice.

STORE in an airtight container for 3 to 4 days. Reheat gently in a skillet over medium heat with a splash of broth to loosen the sauce, stirring occasionally, or microwave in 1-minute increments, stirring between, until warmed through.

SHEET PAN CHICKEN WITH SOPPRESSATA AND PEPPERS

MAKES 4 SERVINGS | **TOTAL TIME:** 50 MINUTES

DIETARY
GLUTEN-FREE
GRAIN-FREE
DAIRY-FREE (IF MODIFIED)
PALEO (IF MODIFIED)
MAKE AHEAD

This sheet pan chicken dinner is an easy, flavorful meal packed with zesty lemon, savory soppressata, and roasted veggies. Topped with goat cheese, fresh mint, and fresh oregano, it's a simple dinner with bold Mediterranean flair.

3 tablespoons extra-virgin olive oil
1 teaspoon Dijon mustard
2 garlic cloves, minced
Grated zest of ½ lemon
2 tablespoons freshly squeezed lemon juice (about 1 lemon)
2 tablespoons roughly chopped fresh oregano leaves, divided
2 teaspoons kosher salt
1 teaspoon freshly ground black pepper
1 teaspoon smoked paprika
½ teaspoon crushed red pepper flakes
3 pounds bone-in, skin-on chicken thighs, trimmed of excess fat and patted dry
1 pound mini bell peppers, halved and seeded
½ cup halved and thinly sliced red onion (about ½ small onion)
3 ounces hard soppressata or salami, casings removed, cut into small dice (about ¾ cup)
½ cup torn pitted Castelvetrano olives
½ cup crumbled goat cheese (omit for dairy-free and paleo)
2 tablespoons roughly torn fresh mint leaves

PREHEAT the oven to 425°F. Line a sheet pan with parchment paper and set aside.

IN a small bowl, whisk together the oil, mustard, garlic, lemon zest, lemon juice, 1 tablespoon of the oregano, the salt, black pepper, paprika, and pepper flakes until well combined. Set aside.

PLACE the chicken thighs on the prepared sheet pan. Scatter the bell peppers, onion, and soppressata around the chicken. Pour the mustard mixture over the ingredients on the sheet pan and toss until well combined, massaging the mixture into the chicken thighs. Spread the ingredients into a single layer with the chicken thighs skin side up.

TRANSFER to the oven and bake until the chicken is cooked through and golden brown, 30 to 40 minutes. Toss the veggies halfway through the cook time.

REMOVE from the oven and let cool slightly. Top with the olives. To serve, divide the chicken and veggies among four plates and finish by topping with the crumbled goat cheese (if using), the remaining 1 tablespoon oregano, and the mint.

STORE the chicken and veggies in an airtight container in the fridge for up to 3 days separate from the goat cheese and herbs. Reheat in a 350°F oven or air fryer for 8 to 10 minutes to keep the chicken skin crisp. Alternatively, microwave in 1-minute increments, tossing after each, until warmed through. The skin won't stay as crisp in the microwave. Finish with the crumbled goat cheese (if using) and herbs.

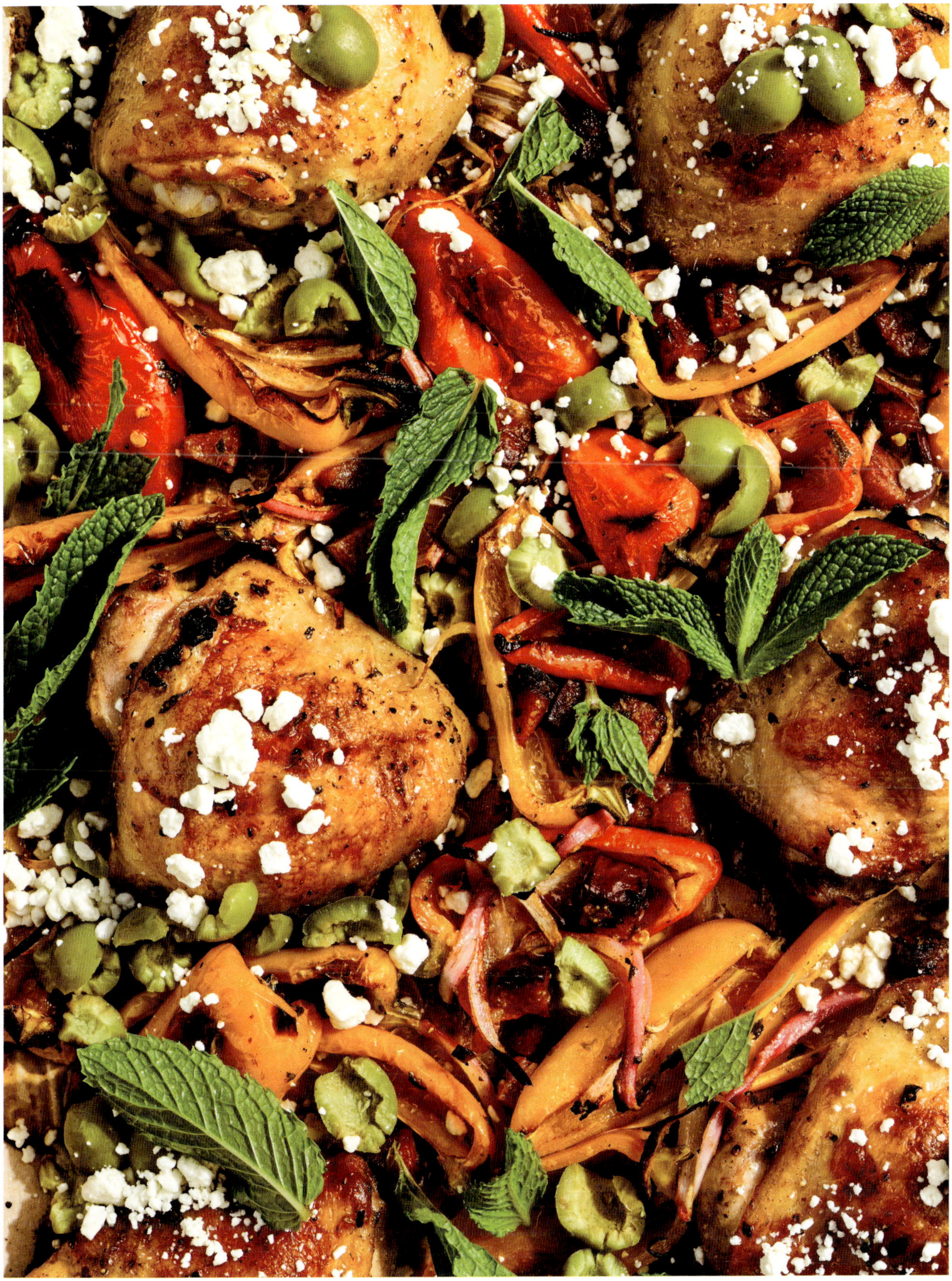

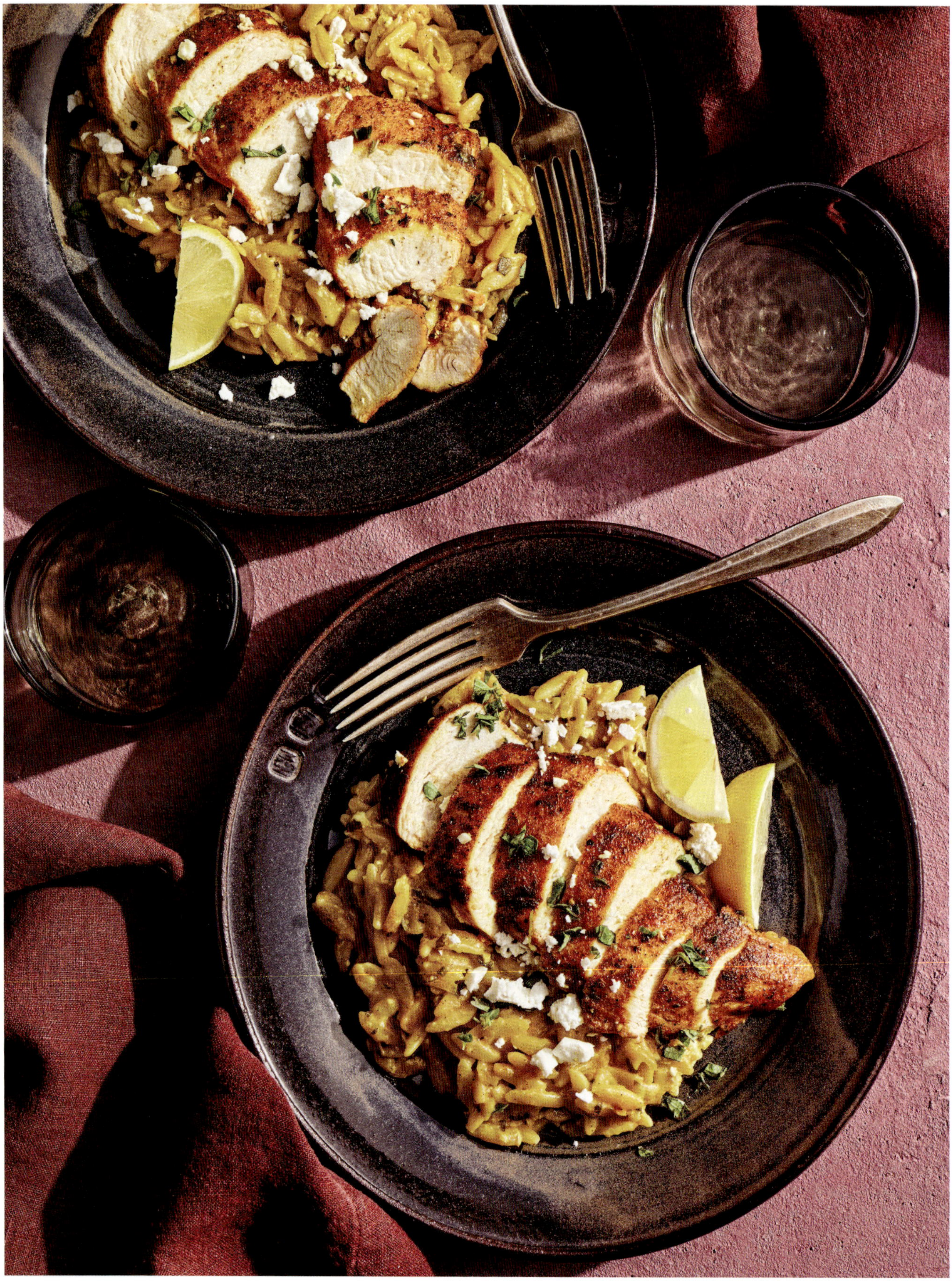

CREAMY ONE-POT LEMON FETA CHICKEN WITH ORZO

MAKES 4 SERVINGS | **TOTAL TIME:** 40 MINUTES

DIETARY
GLUTEN-FREE (IF MODIFIED)
MAKE AHEAD

You will soon discover why this dish is a favorite on my blog! Tender, spiced chicken meets creamy feta orzo in a one-pot meal that's as easy to make as it is delicious. With its simple yet elegant flavors, it's sure to become a recipe ready for any occasion.

FOR THE CHICKEN

1 teaspoon kosher salt

½ teaspoon freshly ground black pepper

1 teaspoon ground turmeric

1 teaspoon smoked paprika

¼ teaspoon cayenne pepper

1½ pounds boneless, skinless chicken breasts, trimmed of excess fat and patted dry

2 tablespoons extra-virgin olive oil

FOR THE ORZO

1 large shallot, halved lengthwise and thinly sliced (about ½ cup)

3 garlic cloves, minced

½ teaspoon crushed red pepper flakes

1 teaspoon Dijon mustard

½ cup dry white wine

1 cup orzo (sub gluten-free brown rice orzo for gluten-free)

2 cups low-sodium chicken broth

Grated zest of ½ lemon

2 tablespoons freshly squeezed lemon juice (about 1 lemon)

½ teaspoon kosher salt

1 tablespoon chopped fresh oregano leaves, plus more for serving

1 tablespoon chopped fresh parsley leaves

¾ cup feta crumbles, divided

Lemon wedges, for serving

PREHEAT the oven to 375°F.

PREPARE THE CHICKEN: In a small bowl, combine the salt, black pepper, turmeric, paprika, and cayenne.

SEASON both sides of the chicken breasts generously with the spice blend. In a large, deep oven-safe skillet or 3.5-quart braiser, heat the oil over medium-high heat. Add the chicken in a single layer and cook until browned on both sides, about 3 minutes per side. The chicken will not be fully cooked through, as it will continue to cook in the oven. Transfer to a clean plate and set aside.

PREPARE THE ORZO: Using the same skillet, reduce the heat to medium and sauté the shallot, garlic, and pepper flakes for 2 minutes. Add the mustard and wine, stirring and scraping up any browned bits off the bottom of the pan. Continue to cook until the wine has reduced by half, about 2 more minutes.

ADD the orzo, broth, lemon zest, lemon juice, salt, oregano, parsley, and ½ cup of the feta. Stir to combine, then nestle the chicken into the skillet, along with any juices from the plate.

TRANSFER to the oven and bake, uncovered, until chicken is cooked through and the orzo is almost cooked through, about 15 minutes.

REMOVE from the oven and top with the remaining ¼ cup feta. Return to the oven and continue to bake until the orzo is cooked through and the feta has softened, about 5 more minutes.

REMOVE from the oven and garnish with more oregano. Serve with lemon wedges.

STORE in an airtight container in the fridge for up to 3 days. Reheat gently in a skillet over medium heat with a splash of broth until warmed through, or microwave in 1-minute increments, stirring after each, until warmed through.

LARB GAI–INSPIRED LETTUCE WRAPS

MAKES 4 SERVINGS | **TOTAL TIME:** 25 MINUTES

DIETARY
GLUTEN-FREE
GRAIN-FREE
DAIRY-FREE
PALEO
MAKE AHEAD

When it comes to Thai food, the bold and fresh flavors of larb make it one of my favorite dishes. My twist on the classic is effortlessly delicious and healthy. Plus, I've given it a modern twist by swapping traditional toasted rice for crunchy cashews, adding a delightful nutty flavor while keeping it grain-free.

½ cup raw, unsalted cashews, roughly chopped

1 tablespoon white sesame seeds

2 tablespoons avocado oil

1 cup halved and thinly sliced shallot (about 2 large shallots)

2 pounds ground chicken or turkey, preferably dark meat

1 teaspoon kosher salt

½ teaspoon freshly ground black pepper

4 garlic cloves, minced

1 to 3 Thai chiles, minced (see note, page 122)

2 tablespoons coconut aminos

¼ cup freshly squeezed lime juice (about 2 limes)

1 tablespoon coconut sugar

2 tablespoons fish sauce

½ cup finely chopped fresh cilantro leaves, plus more for garnish

¼ cup finely chopped fresh mint leaves, plus more for garnish

FOR SERVING

2 heads butter lettuce, separated into individual lettuce leaves

2 Persian (mini) cucumbers, thinly sliced on the diagonal (about 2 cups)

Lime wedges

IN a large, dry (no oil) skillet, toast the cashews and the sesame seeds over medium heat until golden and fragrant, being careful not to burn them, about 2 minutes. Transfer to a clean bowl and set aside.

INCREASE the heat beneath the skillet to medium-high and add the oil. Add the shallot and sauté until slightly tender, about 2 minutes.

ADD the ground chicken, salt, black pepper, garlic, and Thai chiles. Cook, breaking up the meat with the edge of a spoon, until cooked through and no longer pink, about 7 minutes.

REDUCE the heat to medium-low and add the coconut aminos, lime juice, coconut sugar, fish sauce, and three-quarters of the cashew-sesame mixture, reserving the rest for serving. Cook, stirring, until the ingredients are well combined and the flavors have melded, about 4 minutes. Remove from the heat. Add the cilantro and mint and stir to combine.

TO SERVE: Spoon the larb mix into lettuce cups and top with sliced cucumbers. Top with more of the cashew-sesame mixture and garnish with more cilantro and mint. Serve with lime wedges.

STORE the chicken mixture in an airtight container in the fridge for up to 3 days, keeping the lettuce, cucumbers, and cashew-sesame topping separate. Reheat the chicken in a skillet over medium heat, or microwave in 1-minute increments, stirring after each, until warmed through. Assemble with fresh lettuce, cucumbers, and cashew-sesame topping. Garnish with fresh herbs and serve with lime wedges.

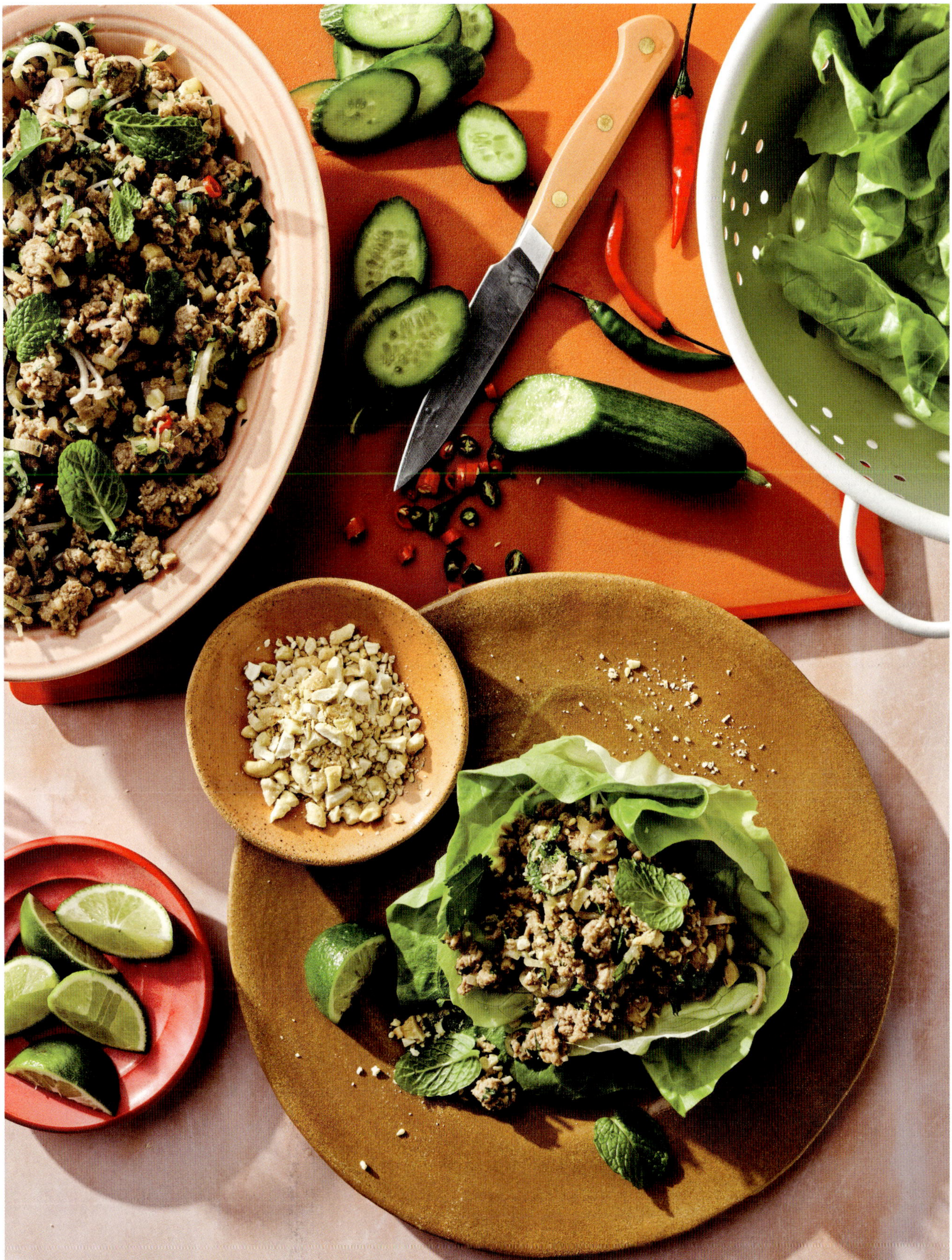

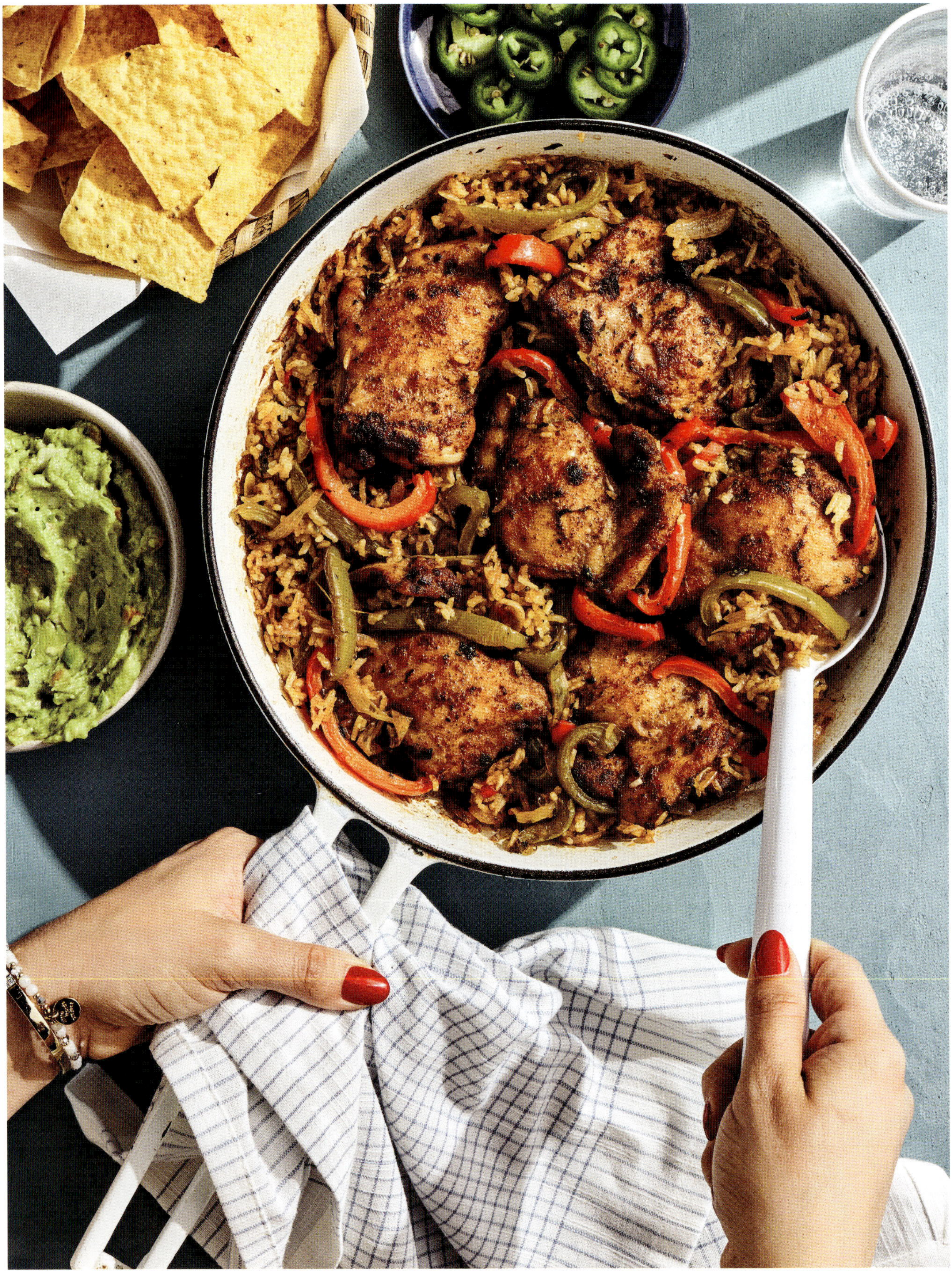

CHICKEN AND RICE TACO SKILLET

MAKES 4 SERVINGS | **TOTAL TIME:** 45 MINUTES

DIETARY
GLUTEN-FREE
DAIRY-FREE
MAKE AHEAD

This easy, family-friendly skillet is the perfect way to use up a packet of taco seasoning—and the one you choose will really shape the flavor. I go with a mild blend so it's not too spicy for the kids, then add sliced jalapeños to mine for a little kick. Once it's in the oven, you've got time to tidy up, make some guacamole if you want, and get the table set—just how weeknight dinners should be.

FOR THE CHICKEN

2 pounds boneless, skinless chicken thighs, trimmed of excess fat and patted dry

1 teaspoon kosher salt

2 tablespoons taco seasoning

3 tablespoons avocado oil

FOR THE VEGGIES AND RICE

1 small red bell pepper, seeded and thinly sliced

1 small green bell pepper, seeded and thinly sliced

½ yellow onion, thinly sliced (about 1 cup)

2 garlic cloves, minced

1 cup white jasmine rice, rinsed well and drained

¼ teaspoon kosher salt

1 tablespoon taco seasoning

1½ cups low-sodium chicken broth

Grated zest of ½ lime

2 tablespoons freshly squeezed lime juice (about 1 lime)

¼ cup finely chopped cilantro leaves, plus more for garnish

OPTIONAL FOR SERVING

Sliced pickled jalapeños

Guacamole

Corn tortilla chips

PREHEAT the oven to 350°F.

PREPARE THE CHICKEN: Season both sides of the chicken evenly with the salt and taco seasoning.

IN a large, oven-safe skillet or 3.5-quart braiser with a fitted lid, heat the oil over medium-high heat. Add the chicken in a single layer and cook until golden brown on both sides, about 3 minutes per side. The chicken does not need to be fully cooked through, as it will continue to cook in the oven. Transfer to a clean plate and set aside.

PREPARE THE VEGGIES AND RICE: Using the same skillet, reduce the heat to medium and add the bell peppers, onion, and garlic. Cook, stirring, until the veggies are tender, about 4 minutes.

ADD the rice, salt, and taco seasoning and continue to cook, stirring, toasting the rice until fragrant and lightly browned, about 2 minutes.

ADD the broth, lime zest, lime juice, and cilantro. Stir to combine and bring to a simmer. Nestle the chicken back into the skillet along with any of its juices. Cover and transfer to the oven and bake for 25 minutes. Carefully uncover the skillet and continue baking until the rice is tender and the chicken is cooked through, 8 to 10 more minutes.

REMOVE from the oven and fluff the rice with a fork. Garnish with more cilantro.

TO SERVE: Spoon the chicken and rice onto plates and garnish as desired. I like to top mine with some sliced jalapeños, a dollop of guacamole, and some corn tortilla chips for scooping and crunch!

STORE leftovers in an airtight container in the fridge for up to 3 days. Reheat in a skillet over medium heat with a splash of broth to keep the rice from drying out, or microwave in 1-minute increments, stirring after each, until warmed through.

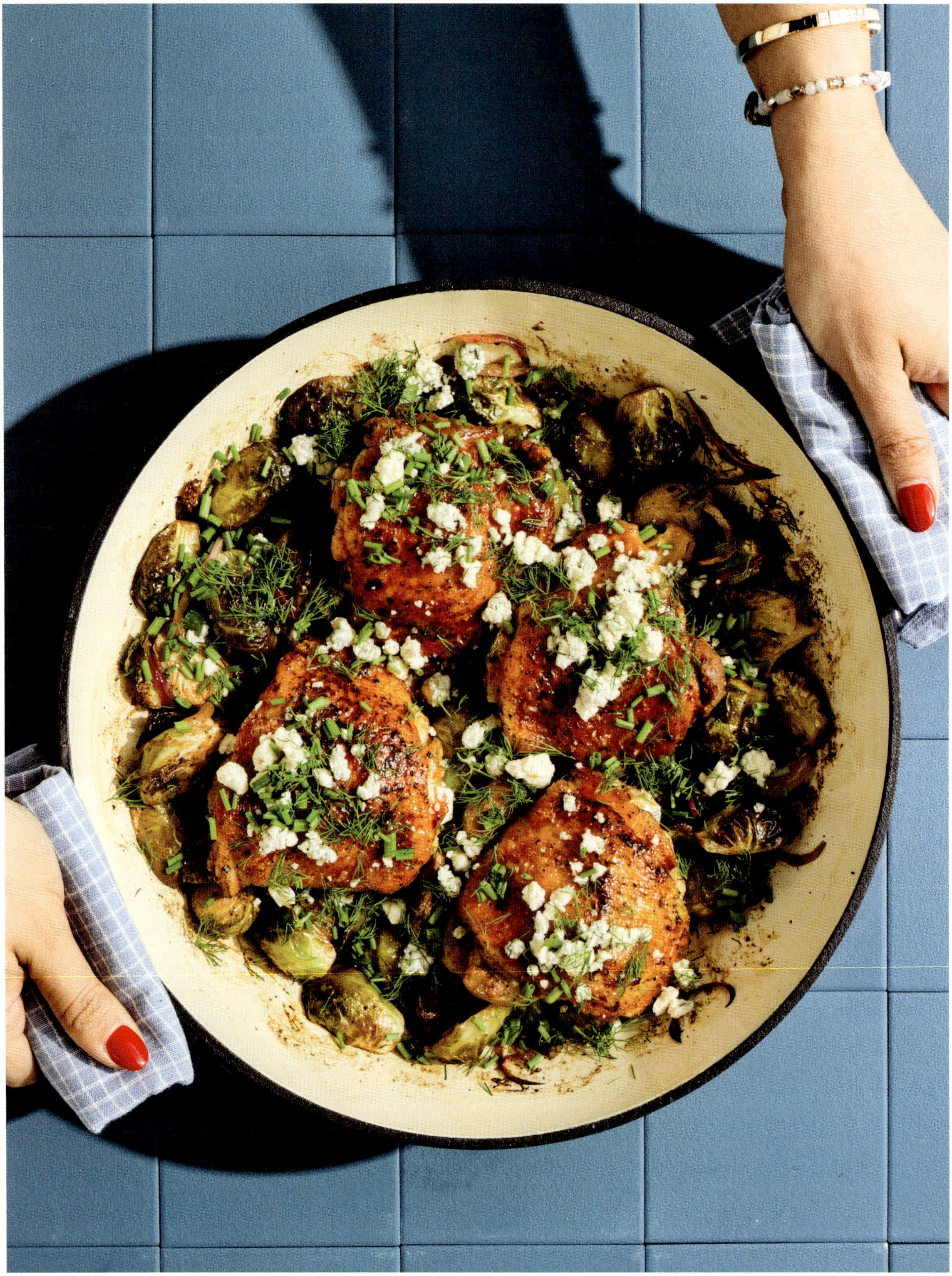

ROASTED BUFFALO CHICKEN THIGHS WITH BRUSSELS SPROUTS AND BLUE CHEESE

MAKES 4 SERVINGS | **TOTAL TIME:** 50 MINUTES

DIETARY
GLUTEN-FREE
GRAIN-FREE
DAIRY-FREE (IF MODIFIED)
PALEO (IF MODIFIED)
MAKE AHEAD

When in doubt, add Buffalo sauce! It's in my regular rotation for quick weeknight dinners because it instantly amps up the flavor. Here, juicy chicken thighs and tender Brussels sprouts are roasted, then tossed in a tangy Buffalo wing sauce. Topped with creamy blue cheese and fresh herbs, this dish is bold, comforting, and incredibly easy to throw together.

4 large bone-in, skin-on chicken thighs, trimmed of excess fat and patted dry

1½ teaspoons kosher salt, divided

½ teaspoon freshly ground black pepper

1 teaspoon onion powder

1 teaspoon garlic powder

2 tablespoons avocado oil

1 pound Brussels sprouts, trimmed and halved lengthwise

1 cup halved and thinly sliced red onion (about 1 small onion)

2 tablespoons freshly squeezed lemon juice (about 1 lemon)

¼ cup mild or hot Buffalo sauce

⅓ cup crumbled blue cheese (omit for dairy-free and paleo)

¼ cup chopped fresh dill

2 tablespoons finely chopped fresh chives

PREHEAT the oven to 400°F.

SEASON both sides of the chicken evenly with 1 teaspoon of the salt, the pepper, onion powder, and garlic powder.

IN a large, deep oven-safe skillet or a 3.5-quart braiser, heat the oil over medium-high heat. Add the chicken thighs, skin-side down, and cook, undisturbed, until a golden-brown crust forms and the chicken lifts easily from the pan, about 4 minutes. The chicken does not need to be fully cooked through, as it will continue to cook in the oven. Transfer to a clean plate and set aside.

REDUCE the heat to medium-low and add the Brussels sprouts, onion, the remaining ½ teaspoon of salt, and the lemon juice to the pan. Cook, deglazing the pan, scraping up any browned bits off the bottom of the pan, until the lemon juice has reduced by half, 1 to 2 minutes. Spread the Brussels sprouts into an even layer.

REMOVE from the heat. Arrange the browned chicken thighs skin side up on top of the Brussels sprouts. Place in the oven, uncovered, and roast until the chicken is almost cooked all the way through and the edges of the Brussels sprouts are lightly browned, about 25 minutes.

CAREFULLY remove the skillet from the oven and gently toss the Brussels sprouts. Spoon 1 tablespoon of the Buffalo sauce over each chicken thigh and spread so that it evenly coats the tops of the chicken. Return to the oven and continue roasting until the sauce has caramelized and the chicken is cooked through, 5 to 8 more minutes, taking care not to let it burn.

REMOVE from the oven and finish with the blue cheese (if using), dill, and chives.

STORE in an airtight container in the fridge for up to 3 days. Reheat in a 350°F oven or air fryer for 8 to 10 minutes to keep the chicken skin crisp. Alternatively, microwave in 1-minute increments, tossing after each, until warmed through. The skin won't stay as crisp in the microwave.

LEFTOVER Buffalo sauce? Try my One-Skillet Buffalo Chicken Pasta (page 118).

SAUCY CHIPOTLE CHICKEN TACOS

MAKES 4 SERVINGS | **TOTAL TIME:** 30 MINUTES

DIETARY
GLUTEN-FREE
DAIRY-FREE
GRAIN-FREE (IF MODIFIED)
MAKE AHEAD

There's nothing like a saucy taco after a hectic day—it's an instant mood booster. This recipe is one of my favorites, featuring quick and delicious flavor from a chipotle pepper in adobo sauce for smoky, saucy chicken served in flavorful corn tortillas. Topped with a fresh slaw, these tacos are sure to become your new favorite in no time!

FOR THE CABBAGE SLAW

3 cups thinly shredded red cabbage (about ½ small head)

1 tablespoon avocado oil

½ teaspoon kosher salt

½ teaspoon ground cumin

2 tablespoons freshly squeezed lime juice (about 1 lime)

FOR THE CHICKEN

2 tablespoons avocado oil

1½ pounds boneless, skinless chicken thighs, trimmed of excess fat, patted dry, and cut into ½-inch pieces

1 teaspoon kosher salt

½ teaspoon freshly ground black pepper

1 teaspoon smoked paprika

1 teaspoon dried oregano

½ teaspoon ground cumin

3 garlic cloves, minced

1 tablespoon tomato paste

1 canned chipotle pepper in adobo sauce, finely minced, plus 1 tablespoon of the sauce

½ cup low-sodium chicken broth

1 tablespoon apple cider vinegar

1 tablespoon honey

MAKE THE SLAW: In a large bowl, combine all the slaw ingredients and toss until well combined. Set aside.

COOK THE CHICKEN: In a large nonstick skillet, heat the oil over medium-high heat. When hot, add the chicken in a single layer and season with the salt, black pepper, paprika, oregano, and cumin. Cook, tossing occasionally, until golden brown on all sides and cooked through, 4 to 5 minutes.

REDUCE the heat to medium and add the garlic, tomato paste, chipotle pepper, and adobo sauce to the skillet with the chicken and stir until well combined. Continue cooking until the garlic is toasted and fragrant, about 2 minutes.

STIR in the broth, vinegar, and honey until well combined, scraping up any browned bits off the bottom of the pan. Bring to a simmer and cook, stirring, until the sauce has reduced slightly, 3 to 4 minutes. Reduce the heat to low while you warm the tortillas.

WARM THE TORTILLAS: In a small skillet, heat ½ teaspoon oil over medium heat. One at a time, place a tortilla into the skillet and warm for 30 seconds on each side. Continue, adding more oil as needed, until all the tortillas are warmed. Alternatively, you can use tongs to char the tortillas directly over a gas flame for a few seconds.

TO ASSEMBLE AND SERVE: Fill the warm tortillas with the chicken. Top with the cabbage slaw, a drizzle of salsa, and a sprinkle of onion and cilantro. Serve with lime wedges.

STORE the saucy chicken in an airtight container in the fridge for up to 3 days, keeping the slaw, tortillas, and toppings separate. Reheat the chicken in a skillet over medium heat, or in the microwave in 1-minute increments, stirring after each, until warmed through. Assemble tacos in warmed tortillas just before serving with fresh slaw and toppings.

FOR ASSEMBLY AND SERVING

Avocado oil

12 corn tortillas (sub almond flour tortillas for grain-free)

Salsa verde

½ cup finely diced white onion (about ½ small onion)

½ cup chopped fresh cilantro leaves

Lime wedges

LEFTOVER chipotles in adobo? Try my Chipotle Chimichurri Steak Bite Bowls (page 166) or Sheet Pan Chipotle-Honey Butter Salmon (page 218).

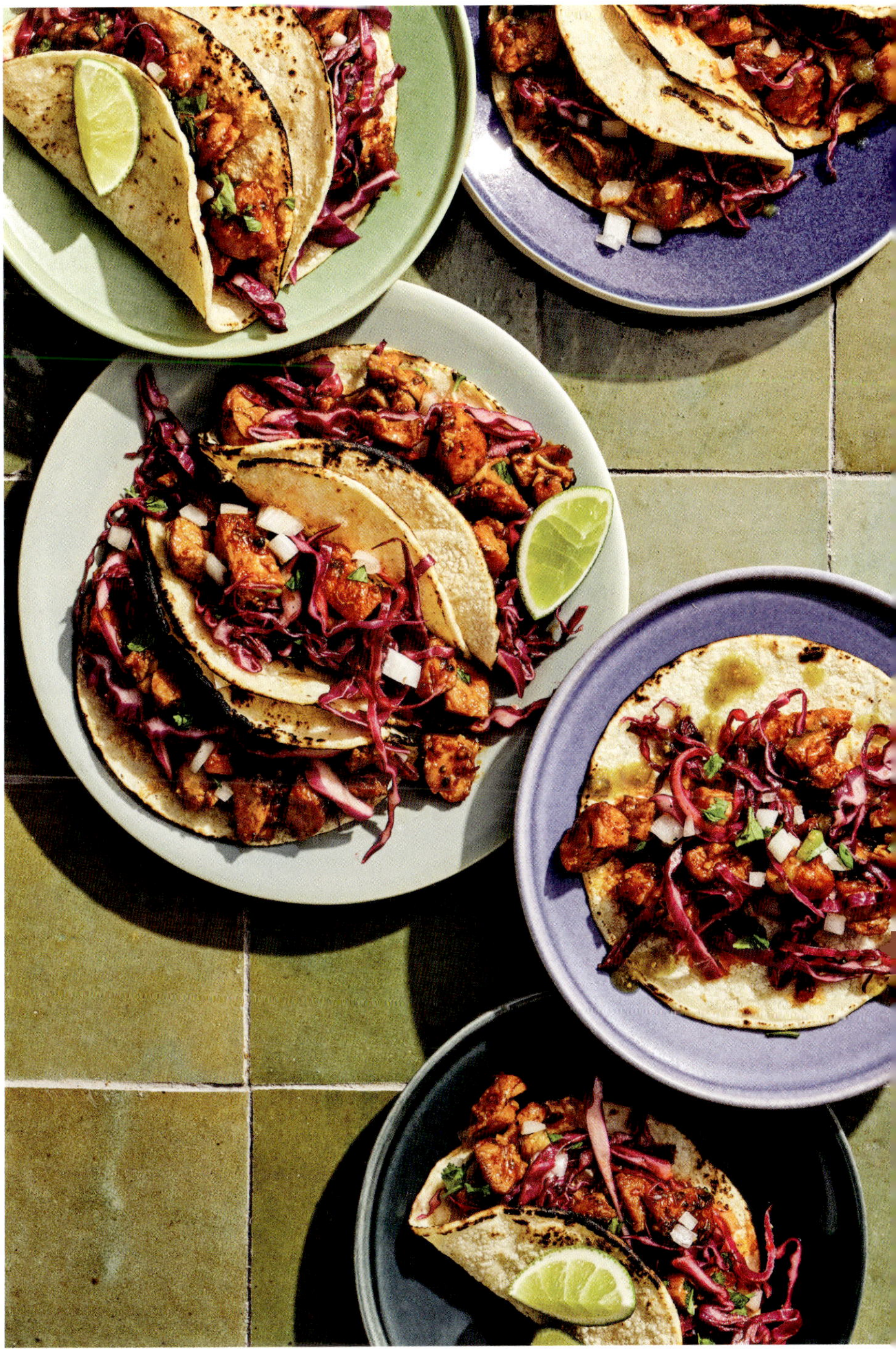

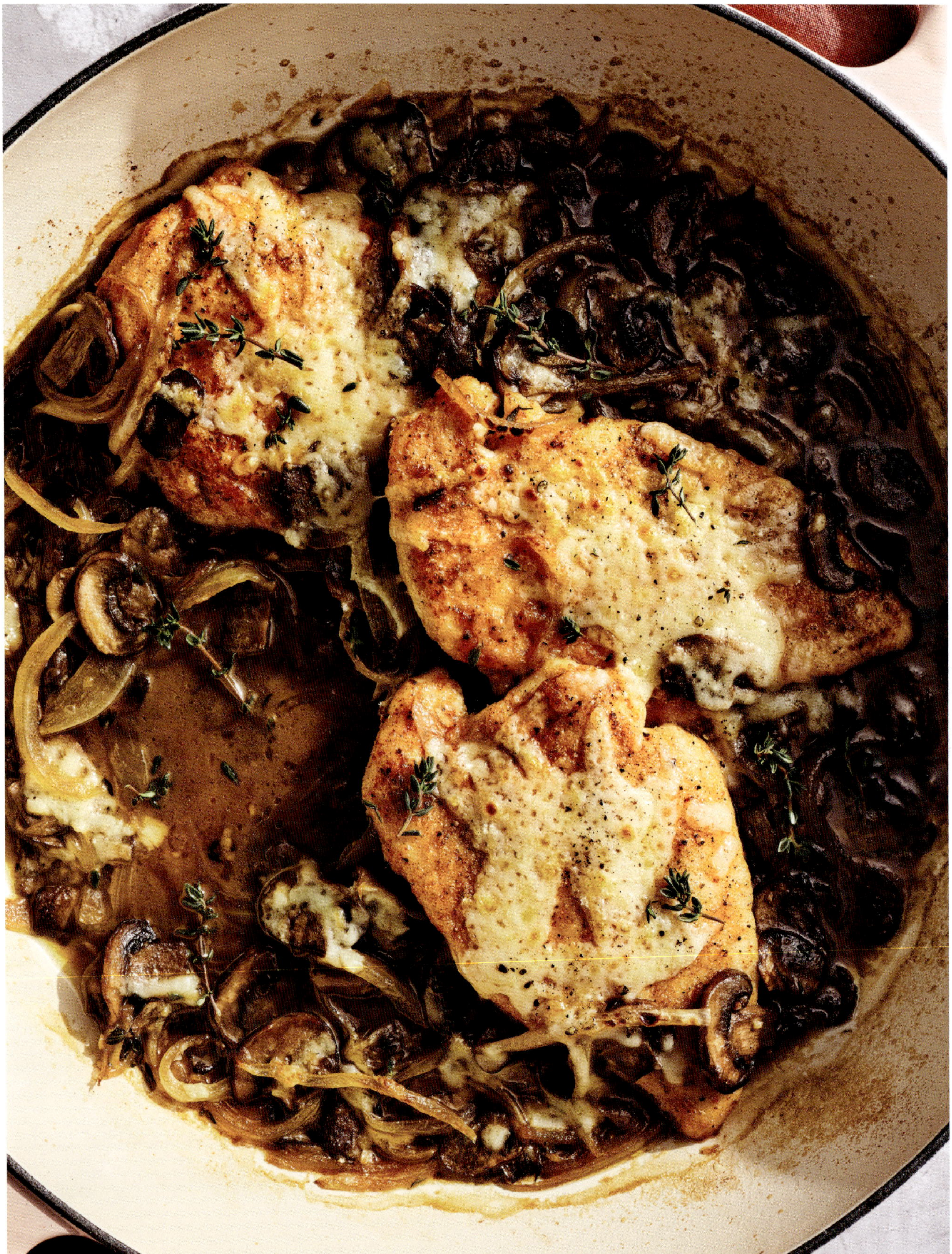

SKILLET FRENCH ONION CHICKEN WITH MUSHROOMS

MAKES 4 SERVINGS | **TOTAL TIME:** 35 MINUTES

DIETARY
GLUTEN-FREE
GRAIN-FREE
MAKE AHEAD

This skillet captures the rich, savory flavors of French onion soup in a hearty, protein-packed dish. Tender chicken breasts are cooked with caramelized onions, earthy mushrooms, and aromatic thyme, then finished in the oven with a layer of melty Gruyère cheese. This dish offers a comforting, flavorful dinner option that's perfect for any night of the week. Pair it with roasted vegetables or a simple side salad for a well-rounded, satisfying meal.

4 small boneless, skinless chicken breasts, trimmed of excess fat and patted dry

1½ teaspoons kosher salt, divided

½ teaspoon freshly ground black pepper

½ teaspoon smoked paprika

3 tablespoons cassava flour

3 tablespoons extra-virgin olive oil, divided

1 small yellow onion, halved and thinly sliced (about 1 cup)

One 8-ounce package thinly sliced baby bella mushrooms

2 garlic cloves, minced

2 teaspoons Dijon mustard

2 tablespoons coconut aminos

2 teaspoons roughly chopped fresh thyme leaves

½ cup dry white wine

¼ cup low-sodium chicken broth

½ cup freshly grated Gruyère cheese

PREHEAT the oven to 375°F.

PLACE the chicken breasts on a cutting board and cover with parchment paper or plastic wrap. Using a meat mallet or the bottom of a heavy skillet, pound the chicken to a uniform ½-inch thickness. Season both sides of the chicken evenly with 1 teaspoon of the salt, the pepper, and the paprika.

PLACE the flour in a large, shallow bowl. Dredge each piece of chicken in the flour until well coated on both sides, shaking off any excess.

IN a large, oven-safe skillet or 3.5-quart braiser, heat 2 tablespoons of the oil over medium-high heat. Working in batches as necessary so as not to overcrowd the pan, add the chicken and cook until golden-brown on both sides, 2 to 3 minutes per side. The chicken doesn't need to be fully cooked through, as it will continue to cook in the oven. Transfer the browned chicken to a clean plate and set aside.

REDUCE the heat to medium. Add the remaining 1 tablespoon oil, the onion, mushrooms, garlic, and the remaining ½ teaspoon salt. Cook, stirring, until the onions and mushrooms are tender, 5 to 7 minutes.

STIR in the mustard, coconut aminos, and thyme until combined. While stirring, add the wine and broth. Stir until well combined.

NESTLE the chicken and any juices back into the skillet and top with the cheese. Transfer to the oven and bake, uncovered, until the chicken is cooked through and the cheese is lightly browned and bubbly, about 12 minutes.

REMOVE from the oven and serve.

STORE leftovers in an airtight container in the fridge for up to 3 days. Reheat gently in a skillet over medium-low heat until warmed through, or microwave in 1-minute increments, stirring after each, until warmed through.

CREAMY PEPERONCINI CHICKEN

MAKES 4 SERVINGS | **TOTAL TIME:** 35 MINUTES

DIETARY
GLUTEN-FREE
GRAIN-FREE
MAKE AHEAD

If you love the briny, tangy bite of peperoncini peppers, this one-skillet meal is for you. Inspired by the bold flavors of a classic deli sandwich, this dish balances creamy richness with a pop of acidity. Tender, golden-seared chicken simmers in a silky sauce made with Dijon mustard, Greek yogurt, and plenty of those punchy little peppers. It's the perfect balance of savory, creamy, and bright—great for a quick weeknight meal that still feels special. Serve it over rice, over egg noodles with crusty bread on the side, or alongside roasted potatoes to soak up every last drop.

FOR THE CHICKEN

4 small boneless, skinless chicken breasts

1 teaspoon kosher salt

½ teaspoon freshly ground black pepper

2 teaspoons Italian seasoning

2 tablespoons cassava flour

2 tablespoons extra-virgin olive oil

FOR THE VEGGIES AND SAUCE

1 tablespoon unsalted butter

½ small yellow onion, thinly sliced (about 1 cup)

1 large red bell pepper, seeded and thinly sliced

4 garlic cloves, minced

3 tablespoons brine from jarred peperoncini

1 tablespoon Dijon mustard

1 tablespoon whole-grain Dijon mustard

¾ cup low-sodium chicken broth

1 tablespoon freshly squeezed lemon juice (about ½ lemon)

½ cup sliced peperoncini peppers, drained

½ cup whole-milk plain Greek yogurt or sour cream

2 tablespoons grated parmesan cheese

2 tablespoons finely chopped fresh Italian parsley

PLACE the chicken breasts on a cutting board and cover with parchment paper or plastic wrap. Using a meat mallet or the bottom of a heavy skillet, pound the chicken to a uniform ½-inch thickness. Season both sides of the chicken evenly with the salt, black pepper, and Italian seasoning. Sprinkle with the flour, ensuring all pieces are evenly coated.

IN a large, deep skillet or 3.5-quart braiser, heat the oil over medium-high heat. Add the chicken and cook until golden brown on both sides, 2 to 3 minutes per side. The chicken does not need to be fully cooked through, as it will continue to cook in the sauce. Transfer to a clean plate and set aside.

REDUCE the heat to medium, add the butter, and let it melt. Add the onion and bell pepper and cook, stirring, until the veggies begin to soften, about 3 minutes.

ADD the garlic and the peperoncini brine. Stir to combine, scraping up any browned bits off the bottom of the pan, and cook until the liquid has reduced by half, 1 to 2 minutes.

ADD the Dijon mustard, whole-grain mustard, broth, lemon juice, and peperoncini peppers. Stir to combine and bring to a rapid simmer. Reduce the heat to a gentle simmer, about medium-low heat. Stir in the yogurt and parmesan until well combined and the sauce is smooth. Be careful not to let the sauce boil, as this will cause the yogurt to curdle.

NESTLE the chicken into the pan along with its juices. Cook, uncovered and gently simmering, until the sauce has thickened and the chicken is fully cooked through, about 5 more minutes.

FINISH with parsley and serve.

STORE leftovers in an airtight container in the fridge for up to 3 days. Reheat gently in a skillet over medium-low heat, adding a splash of broth to loosen the sauce, or microwave in 1-minute increments, stirring after each, until warmed through.

LEFTOVER sliced peperoncini? Try my Italian Deli Chicken Salad (page 46).

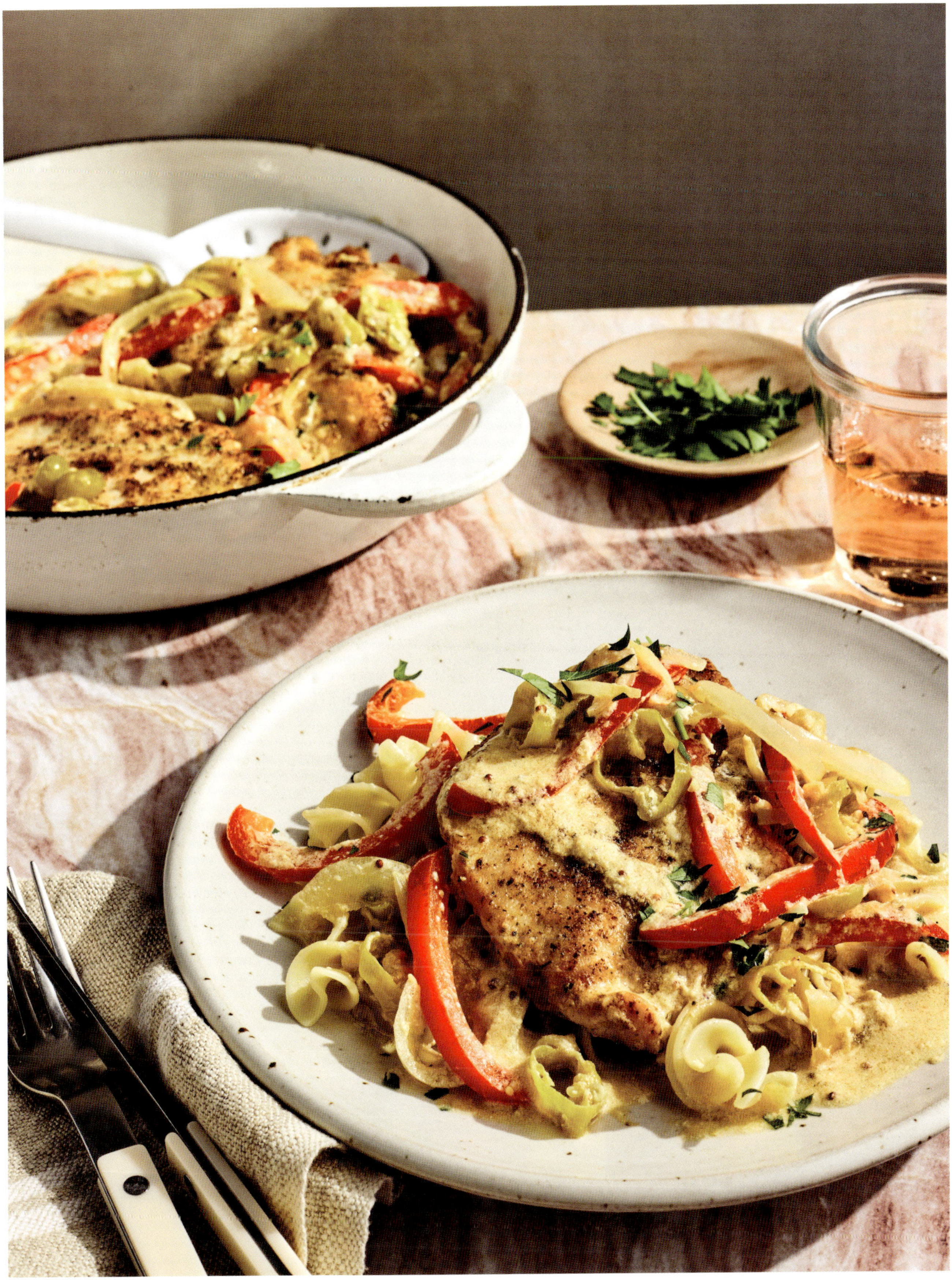

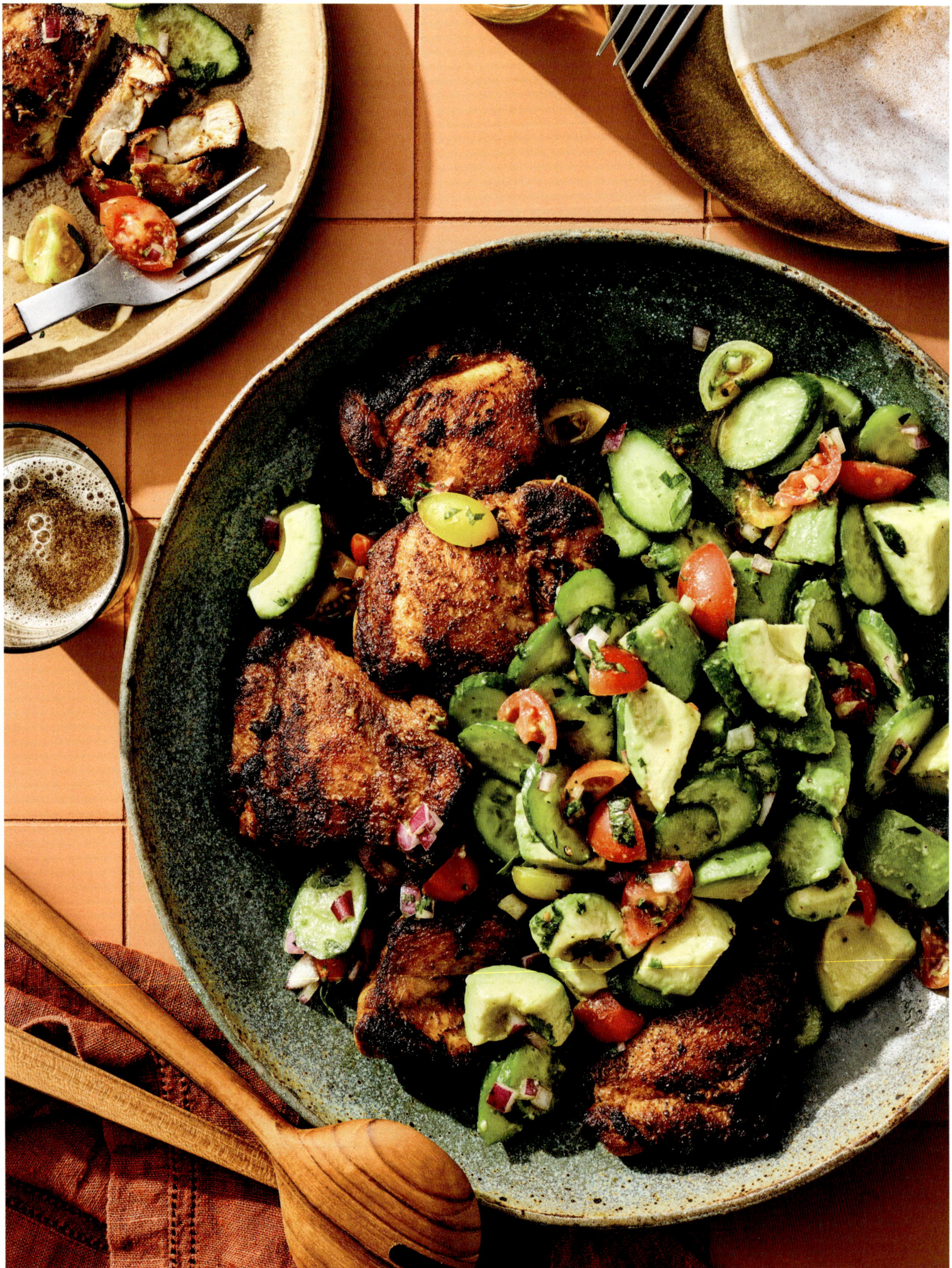

CUMIN-CRUSTED CHICKEN WITH AVOCADO-CUCUMBER SALAD

MAKES 4 SERVINGS | **TOTAL TIME:** 35 MINUTES

DIETARY
GLUTEN-FREE
GRAIN-FREE
DAIRY-FREE
PALEO

This vibrant and flavorful meal comes together quickly and easily. Juicy chicken thighs are seasoned with cumin and paprika, then paired with a refreshing salad of creamy avocado, crisp cucumbers, and tangy citrus. A perfect healthy meal that is ideal for busy weeknights or casual gatherings.

FOR THE CHICKEN

2 pounds boneless, skinless chicken thighs, trimmed of excess fat and patted dry

4 tablespoons extra-virgin olive oil, divided, plus more as needed

1 tablespoon freshly squeezed lime juice (about ½ lime)

2 teaspoons kosher salt

1 teaspoon freshly ground black pepper

2 teaspoons ground cumin

2 teaspoons chili powder

1 teaspoon smoked paprika

¼ teaspoon cayenne pepper

FOR THE SALAD

4 Persian (mini) cucumbers, thinly sliced (about 2 cups)

1 cup quartered grape tomatoes

2 garlic cloves, minced

¼ cup finely diced red onion (about ¼ small onion)

¼ cup finely chopped fresh cilantro leaves

1 tablespoon extra-virgin olive oil

1 teaspoon kosher salt

½ teaspoon freshly ground black pepper

2 tablespoons freshly squeezed lime juice (about 1 lime)

2 tablespoons freshly squeezed lemon juice (about 1 lemon)

2 medium avocados, diced

Lime wedges, for serving

MARINATE THE CHICKEN: In a large bowl, combine the chicken thighs, 2 tablespoons of the oil, the lime juice, salt, black pepper, cumin, chili powder, paprika, and cayenne. Mix until well combined and set aside to marinate at room temperature for 10 minutes while you prepare the salad.

PREPARE THE SALAD: In a large bowl, combine the cucumbers, tomatoes, garlic, onion, cilantro, olive oil, salt, black pepper, lime juice, and lemon juice. Toss until well combined. Add the avocado and gently toss once more until well combined. Cover and set aside while you cook the chicken.

COOK THE CHICKEN: In a large skillet, preferably cast iron, heat the remaining 2 tablespoons of oil over medium-high heat. Working in batches as necessary so as not to overcrowd the pan, add the chicken in a single layer and cook until the chicken is golden brown on both sides and cooked through, 3 to 4 minutes per side. Transfer the cooked chicken to a serving platter and let cool slightly. Repeat with the remaining pieces of chicken as needed, adding more oil to the pan if it becomes dry.

SPOON the avocado-cucumber salad over the chicken. Serve with lime wedges.

FROM MY KITCHEN TO YOURS

Alternatively, to grill the chicken, preheat a grill to medium-high heat and lightly oil the grates to prevent sticking. Place the marinated chicken thighs directly on the grill and cook for about 5 minutes per side, until the internal temperature reaches 165°F and the chicken is nicely charred. Remove the chicken from the grill and transfer to a serving platter. Let cool slightly before serving with the avocado-cucumber salad.

SPICED CHICKEN AND CHICKPEA SKILLET

MAKES 4 SERVINGS | **TOTAL TIME:** 45 MINUTES

DIETARY
GLUTEN-FREE
GRAIN-FREE
DAIRY-FREE (IF MODIFIED)
MAKE AHEAD

Pantry staples like canned chickpeas, crushed tomatoes, and harissa combine with warming spices to make this comforting and quick one-skillet dinner. This skillet comes together in under an hour and is perfect served as is or with warm pita to soak up all the flavorful broth.

- 1½ pounds boneless, skinless chicken thighs, trimmed of excess fat and patted dry
- 1½ teaspoons kosher salt, divided
- 1 teaspoon smoked paprika
- 1 teaspoon ground coriander
- ½ teaspoon ground cumin
- ½ teaspoon ground turmeric
- ½ teaspoon freshly ground black pepper
- 2 tablespoons extra-virgin olive oil, divided
- ½ yellow onion, thinly sliced (about 1 cup)
- 1 large carrot, peeled and thinly sliced (about 1 cup)
- 4 garlic cloves, minced
- 1 tablespoon tomato paste
- 2 tablespoons mild harissa paste
- ½ cup dry white wine
- Grated zest of ½ lemon
- 2 tablespoons freshly squeezed lemon juice (about 1 lemon)
- One 14-ounce can crushed tomatoes
- One 14-ounce can chickpeas, drained and rinsed
- 4 cups de-ribbed and roughly chopped lacinato kale (about 1 bunch)
- 2 tablespoons torn fresh oregano leaves
- ½ cup crumbled feta (omit for dairy-free)

POSITION a rack in the middle of the oven and preheat the oven to 375°F.

SEASON both sides of the chicken evenly with 1 teaspoon of the salt, the paprika, coriander, cumin, turmeric, and pepper, massaging the spices into the chicken.

IN a large, oven-safe skillet, heat 1 tablespoon of the oil over medium-high heat. Working in batches as necessary so as not to overcrowd the pan, add the chicken thighs in a single layer. Cook until golden brown on both sides, about 3 minutes per side. The chicken does not need to be fully cooked through, as it will finish cooking in the oven. Transfer to a clean plate and set aside.

REDUCE the heat to medium and add the remaining 1 tablespoon oil, the onion, and the carrot. Season with the remaining ½ teaspoon of salt and cook, stirring occasionally, until the veggies are tender, about 4 minutes. Add the garlic and cook for 1 minute.

ADD the tomato paste and harissa paste and stir to combine. Cook until the tomato paste begins to soften, about 2 minutes. Add the wine, lemon zest, and lemon juice. Stir to combine, scraping up any browned bits off the bottom of the pan.

BRING to a simmer and cook until the wine has reduced by half, about 3 minutes. Add the tomatoes, chickpeas, and kale and stir to combine. Bring the mixture to a simmer and nestle the chicken back into the skillet along with its juices.

CAREFULLY transfer to the oven, uncovered, and cook for 15 to 17 minutes, until the chicken is cooked through and pieces of the kale have started to crisp.

REMOVE from the oven and allow to cool slightly. Sprinkle the top with oregano and crumbled feta (if using) before serving.

STORE leftovers in an airtight container in the fridge for up to 3 days. Reheat in a skillet over medium heat, or microwave in 1-minute increments, stirring after each, until warmed through.

LEFTOVER harissa? Try my Smashed Lamb Burger Tacos with Harissa-Yogurt Sauce (page 183) or Harissa Salmon Bites with Sesame Cucumber Salad (page 214).

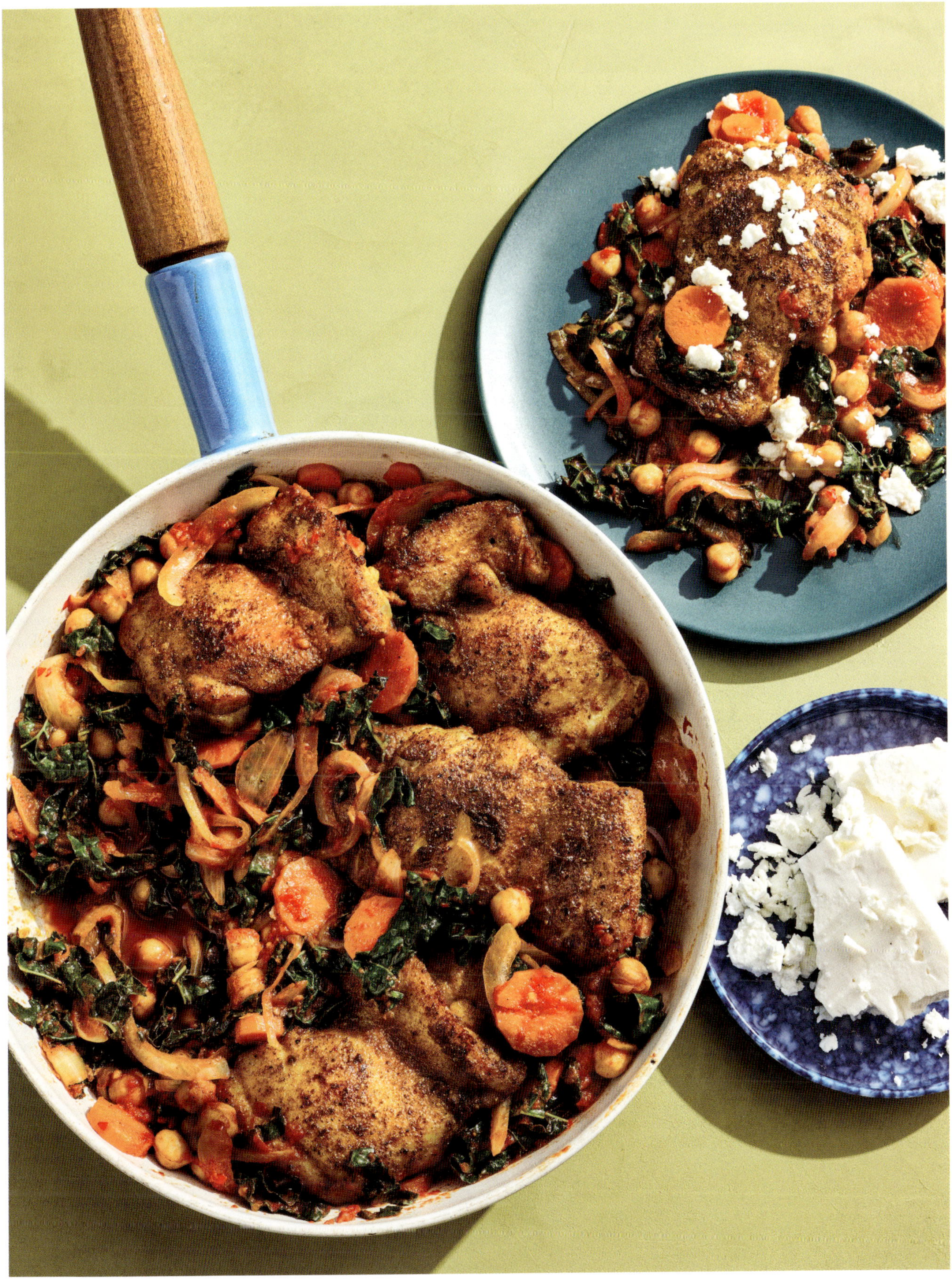

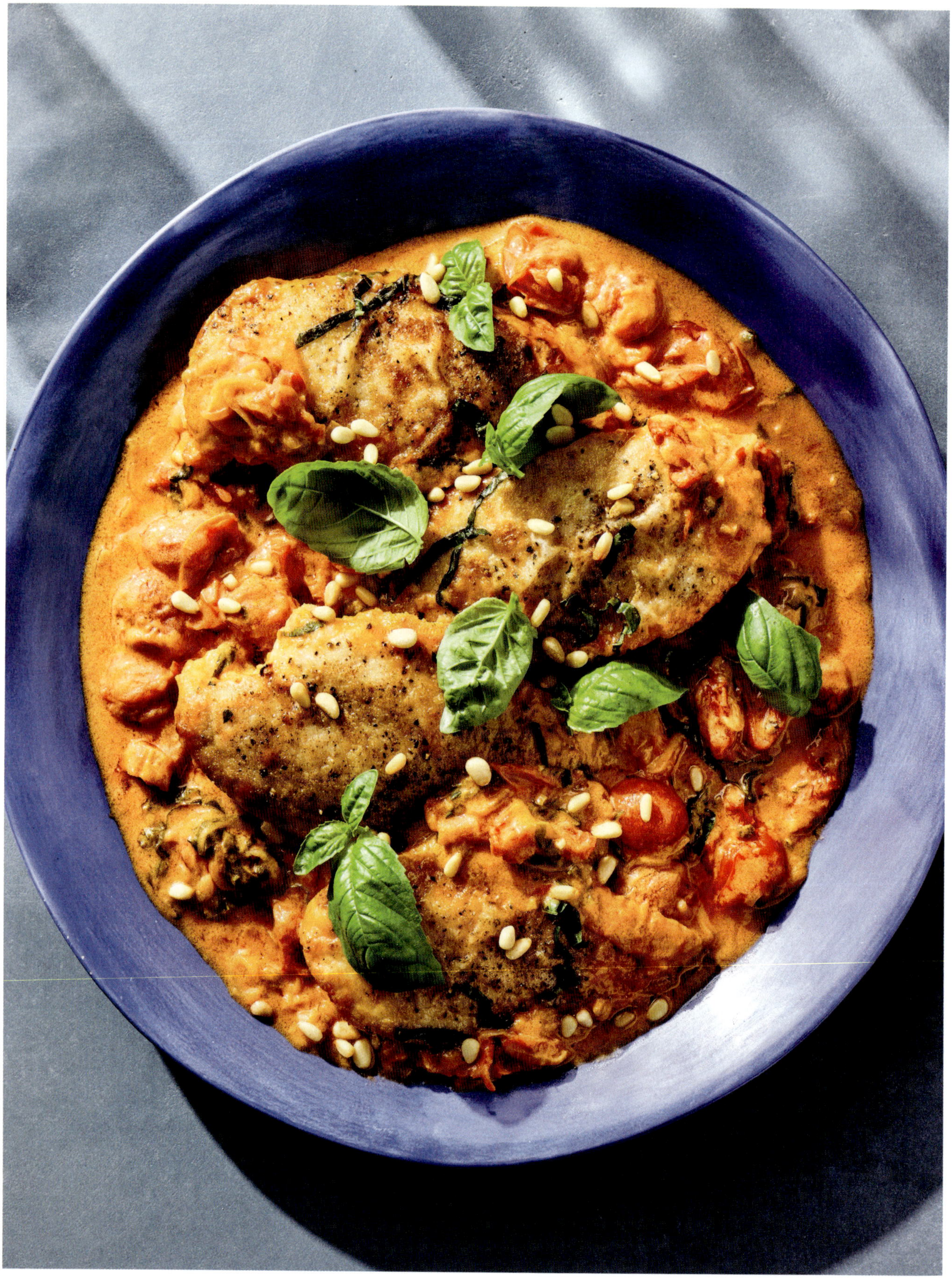

CREAMY SUN-DRIED TOMATO BASIL CHICKEN

MAKES 4 SERVINGS | **TOTAL TIME:** 35 MINUTES

DIETARY
GLUTEN-FREE
GRAIN-FREE
DAIRY-FREE
PALEO
MAKE AHEAD

This creamy, tomato-y chicken dish is a true standout. Bright, juicy tomatoes are combined with rich sun-dried tomatoes to bring a depth of flavor that's both bold and satisfying, while coconut milk adds a velvety finish. It's irresistibly delicious and pairs perfectly with roasted veggies or a fresh side salad, or served over pasta for a hearty, comforting meal.

4 small boneless, skinless chicken breasts, trimmed of excess fat and patted dry

1½ teaspoons kosher salt, divided

1 teaspoon freshly ground black pepper, divided

2 tablespoons cassava flour

2 tablespoons extra-virgin olive oil, plus more if needed

1 pint cherry tomatoes

½ teaspoon crushed red pepper flakes

2 garlic cloves, minced

½ cup halved and thinly sliced shallot (about 1 large shallot)

¾ cup julienne-cut oil-packed sun-dried tomatoes, drained

2 tablespoons tomato paste

1 cup low-sodium chicken broth

1 cup unsweetened full-fat coconut milk

½ cup thinly sliced fresh basil leaves, plus more for garnish

2 tablespoons freshly squeezed lemon juice (1 lemon)

2 tablespoons toasted pine nuts, optional for serving (see note, page 121)

SEASON both sides of the chicken evenly with 1 teaspoon of the salt and ½ teaspoon of the black pepper. Place the flour in a large, shallow bowl. Dredge each piece of chicken in the flour until well coated on both sides, shaking off any excess.

IN a large, deep skillet or 3.5-quart braiser, heat the oil over medium-high heat. Add the chicken and cook until golden brown on both sides, 2 to 3 minutes per side. The chicken does not need to be fully cooked through, as it will finish cooking in the sauce. Transfer to a clean plate and set aside.

REDUCE the heat to medium and add the cherry tomatoes, pepper flakes, garlic, shallot, and sun-dried tomatoes to the skillet. Cook, stirring, until the cherry tomatoes begin to blister and soften, about 4 minutes. It's okay if they begin to burst open.

ADD the tomato paste and broth and stir until well combined. Cook, stirring, until the liquid is reduced by half, about 3 minutes.

STIR in the coconut milk, remaining ½ teaspoon salt, and remaining ½ teaspoon black pepper and bring the sauce to a rapid simmer. Reduce the heat to a gentle simmer, about medium-low heat. Nestle the chicken breasts into the sauce and top with the basil. Simmer, uncovered, until the sauce thickens and the chicken is cooked through, 7 to 10 minutes.

REMOVE from the heat and stir in the lemon juice. Garnish with more basil and top with toasted pine nuts, if desired.

STORE leftovers in an airtight container in the fridge for up to 3 days. Reheat in a skillet over medium heat with a splash of broth to loosen the sauce, or microwave in 1-minute increments, stirring after each, until warmed through.

LEFTOVER sun-dried tomatoes? Try my Freezer-Friendly Mediterranean Breakfast Sandwiches (page 32) or Marry Me White Bean Soup (page 76).

KUNG PAO GROUND CHICKEN

MAKES 4 SERVINGS | **TOTAL TIME:** 30 MINUTES

DIETARY
GLUTEN-FREE
GRAIN-FREE
DAIRY-FREE
PALEO (IF MODIFIED)
MAKE AHEAD

This flavorful high-protein favorite comes together in no time! Ground chicken speeds things up, making it perfect for busy weeknights. Serve this delicious dish over rice, in lettuce wraps, or enjoy it on its own. You will have a versatile, crowd-pleasing option ready to serve!

- 1½ teaspoons toasted sesame oil
- ⅓ cup coconut aminos
- ⅓ cup low-sodium chicken broth
- 2 teaspoons fish sauce
- 1 tablespoon rice vinegar
- 1 tablespoon coconut sugar
- 1 tablespoon tapioca flour
- 3 tablespoons avocado oil, divided
- 1½ pounds ground chicken or turkey, preferably dark meat
- 1 teaspoon kosher salt
- ½ teaspoon freshly ground black pepper
- 1½ cups small-diced red bell pepper (about 1 large bell pepper)
- 1½ cups small-diced zucchini (about 1 small zucchini)
- 4 green onions, thinly sliced, white and green parts kept separate, plus more for garnish
- 4 garlic cloves, minced
- 1 teaspoon grated fresh ginger
- ½ to 1 teaspoon crushed red pepper flakes (depending on your heat preference)
- ½ cup roughly chopped dry roasted peanuts, plus more for garnish (sub cashews for paleo)
- 1 tablespoon freshly squeezed lime juice (about ½ lime)
- Prepared cauliflower rice, steamed rice, or lettuce leaves, optional for serving

IN a small bowl, whisk together the toasted sesame oil, coconut aminos, broth, fish sauce, vinegar, coconut sugar, and flour. Set aside.

IN a large, deep skillet, heat 2 tablespoons of the avocado oil over medium-high heat. Add the ground chicken, salt, and black pepper and spread the chicken into an even layer. Allow the chicken to cook, undisturbed, until a golden crust forms on one side, about 3 minutes. Continue to cook, breaking up the chicken with the edge of a spoon, until it's cooked through and no longer pink, about 4 more minutes. Transfer the chicken to a clean plate and set aside. Drain off any excess fat from the pan.

ADD the remaining 1 tablespoon of avocado oil to the skillet along with the bell pepper, zucchini, and white parts of the green onions. Cook, stirring occasionally, until the veggies begin to soften, about 2 minutes. Add the garlic, ginger, and pepper flakes and cook until the garlic is golden and fragrant, about 2 more minutes.

REDUCE the heat to medium-low and return the chicken along with any of its juices to the skillet. Whisk the sauce once more, then add it to the skillet. Continue to cook, tossing, until the chicken is well coated in the sauce, about 2 minutes.

REDUCE the heat to low and stir in the peanuts, lime juice, and the green parts of the green onions.

SERVE with prepared rice or lettuce leaves and top with more chopped peanuts and green onions, as desired.

STORE leftovers in an airtight container in the fridge for up to 3 days. Reheat in a skillet over medium heat with a splash of broth to loosen the sauce, or microwave in 1-minute increments, stirring after each, until warmed through.

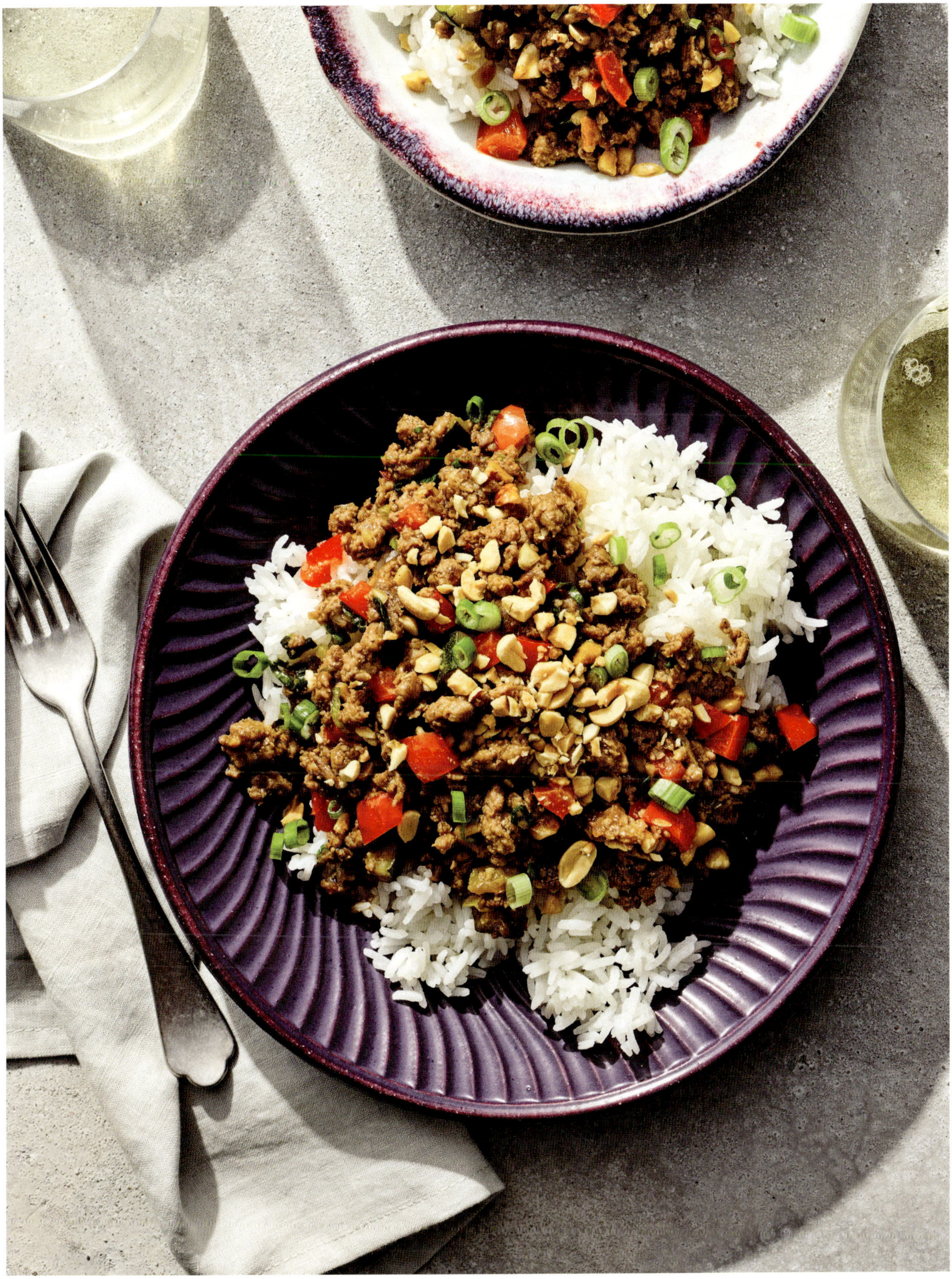

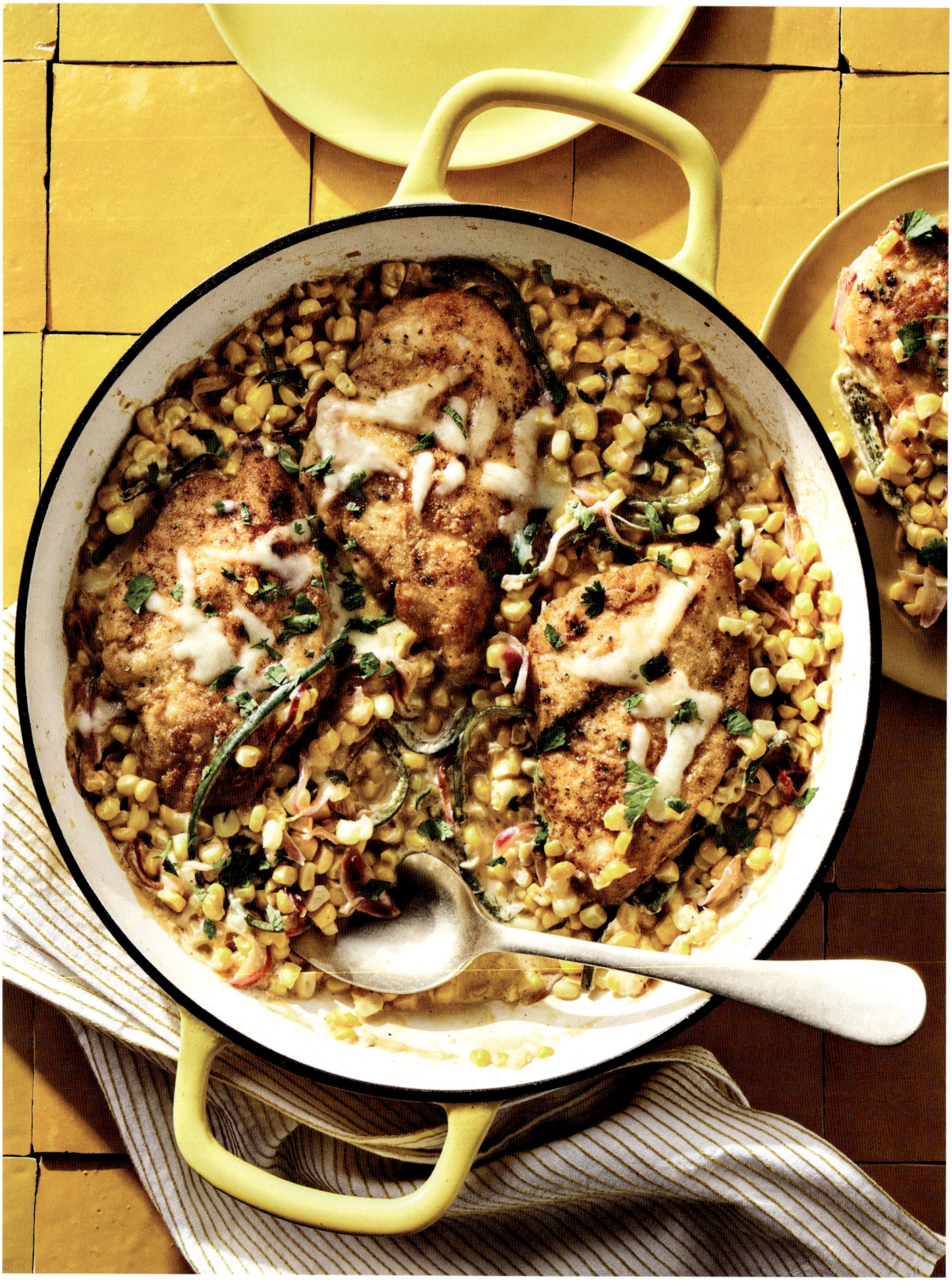

SKILLET CREAMED CORN CHICKEN

MAKES 4 SERVINGS | **TOTAL TIME:** 30 MINUTES

DIETARY
GLUTEN-FREE
DAIRY-FREE (IF MODIFIED)
MAKE AHEAD

This skillet dinner is a tribute to farm days with my grandfather, when picking corn together before dinner was a highlight. The flavors in this dish take me right back to those cherished family moments! Tender chicken simmers in a creamy corn and poblano mix, creating a meal that's both easy to make and absolutely delicious. It's a comforting taste of home that everyone will enjoy.

4 boneless, skinless chicken breasts, trimmed of excess fat and patted dry

2 teaspoons kosher salt, divided

1 teaspoon freshly ground black pepper, divided

1 teaspoon chili powder

2 tablespoons cassava flour

2 tablespoons extra-virgin olive oil

1 large poblano pepper, seeded and sliced into ¼-inch strips

½ cup halved and thinly sliced red onion (about ½ small onion)

2 garlic cloves, minced

4 ears sweet corn, husked and kernels removed

½ cup cream cheese (sub dairy-free cream cheese for dairy-free)

½ cup low-sodium chicken broth

Grated zest of ½ lime

2 tablespoons freshly squeezed lime juice (about 1 lime)

⅓ cup Monterey Jack cheese (omit for dairy-free)

2 tablespoons minced fresh cilantro leaves, for serving

Lime wedges, for serving

PREHEAT the oven to 375°F.

PLACE the chicken breasts on a cutting board and cover them with parchment paper or plastic wrap. Using a meat mallet or the bottom of a heavy skillet, pound the chicken to a uniform ½-inch thickness.

SEASON both sides of the chicken evenly with 1 teaspoon of the salt, ½ teaspoon of the black pepper, and the chili powder.

PLACE the flour in a large, shallow bowl. Dredge each piece of chicken in the flour until well coated on both sides, shaking off any excess.

IN a large, oven-safe skillet or 3.5-quart braiser, heat the oil over medium-high heat. Add the chicken breasts and cook until golden brown on both sides, 2 to 3 minutes per side. The chicken does not need to be cooked through, as it will finish cooking in the oven. Transfer the chicken to a clean plate and set aside.

REDUCE the heat to medium. Add the poblano, onion, and garlic and cook, stirring, until the veggies begin to soften, about 3 minutes.

ADD the corn kernels, the remaining 1 teaspoon salt, and the remaining ½ teaspoon black pepper to the veggies. Cook, stirring, until the corn begins to soften, about 2 more minutes.

REDUCE the heat to medium-low. Stir in the cream cheese, broth, lime zest, and lime juice until well combined.

NESTLE the chicken back into the skillet. Sprinkle the Monterey Jack (if using) evenly over the chicken. Transfer to the oven and bake, uncovered, until the cheese is melted and the chicken is cooked through, 12 to 15 minutes.

REMOVE from the oven and garnish with the cilantro. Serve with lime wedges.

STORE leftovers in an airtight container in the fridge for up to 3 days. Reheat in a skillet over medium heat with a splash of broth to loosen the sauce, or microwave in 1-minute increments, stirring after each, until warmed through.

GROUND TURKEY ENCHILADA SKILLET

MAKES 4 SERVINGS | **TOTAL TIME:** 45 MINUTES

DIETARY
GLUTEN-FREE
MAKE AHEAD

Growing up in small-town Texas, I learned that just about anything can be turned into a casserole—and enchiladas are no exception! This dish takes all the bold, savory flavors of stuffed enchiladas and simplifies them into an easy one-skillet dinner. Sliced tortillas soak up every drop of the zesty sauce, making each bite perfectly comforting. It's basically the best bite of an enchilada—but in one giant skillet. After a busy day, there's nothing better than gathering around this skillet with my family and diving in.

2 tablespoons avocado oil

1 pound ground turkey or chicken, preferably dark meat

1 cup finely diced yellow onion (about ½ medium onion)

1 teaspoon ground cumin

1 teaspoon garlic powder

1 tablespoon chili powder

1 teaspoon kosher salt

½ teaspoon freshly ground black pepper

One 4-ounce can mild diced green chiles

One 15-ounce jar green enchilada sauce

One 15-ounce can pinto beans, drained and rinsed

½ cup low-sodium chicken broth

1 tablespoon freshly squeezed lime juice (about ½ lime)

¼ cup finely chopped fresh cilantro leaves, plus more for garnish

1 cup ¼-inch sliced corn tortillas (see note)

1 cup shredded Monterey Jack cheese

PREHEAT the oven to 400°F.

IN a large, oven-safe skillet or 3.5-quart braiser, heat the oil over medium-high heat. Add the turkey and onion and cook, breaking up the meat with the edge of a spoon, until cooked through and no longer pink, about 7 minutes. Drain off the excess fat and return the turkey and onion to the pan.

REDUCE the heat to medium and add the cumin, garlic powder, chili powder, salt, black pepper, and green chiles. Cook, stirring, to toast the spices, about 2 minutes.

POUR in the enchilada sauce, beans, broth, and lime juice and bring to a simmer. Add the cilantro and sliced tortillas. Gently toss until well combined, then spread the contents of the skillet into a single layer. Sprinkle the cheese evenly over the top.

TRANSFER to the oven and bake, uncovered, until the cheese is golden brown, about 15 minutes. Remove from the oven and let rest for 5 minutes so the sauce can settle and thicken a bit more.

TO SERVE: Place a pile of cabbage in the center of the skillet and scoop the skillet mixture into four shallow bowls. Serve with sliced avocado, sliced jalapeño (if using), and lime wedges.

STORE leftovers in an airtight container in the fridge for up to 3 days, separate of garnishes. Reheat in the oven at 350°F until hot, 15 to 20 minutes, or microwave in 1-minute increments, stirring after each, until warmed through.

FOR SERVING

1 cup shredded green cabbage

1 avocado, sliced

1 jalapeño, thinly sliced, optional

Lime wedges

FROM MY KITCHEN TO YOURS

TORTILLA NOTE: Corn tortillas come in a variety of sizes, so the way you slice them might depend on the type of tortilla you have. If you're using 4-inch round tortillas, simply slice them into ¼-inch strips. For larger tortillas, I recommend slicing them into strips first, then cutting them in half so they aren't such long strips.

FREEZING TIP: After simmering the turkey, beans, sauce, and tortillas together, but before baking, transfer the mixture to an oven-safe, freezer-friendly dish and spread into an even layer. Top with the cheese and let cool completely. Press plastic wrap directly onto the surface so there's no air touching it, then wrap the entire pan tightly in heavy-duty foil. Freeze for up to 2 months. Thaw overnight in the refrigerator. Remove and discard the foil and plastic wrap, then bake at 400°F until hot and bubbly, 20 to 25 minutes.

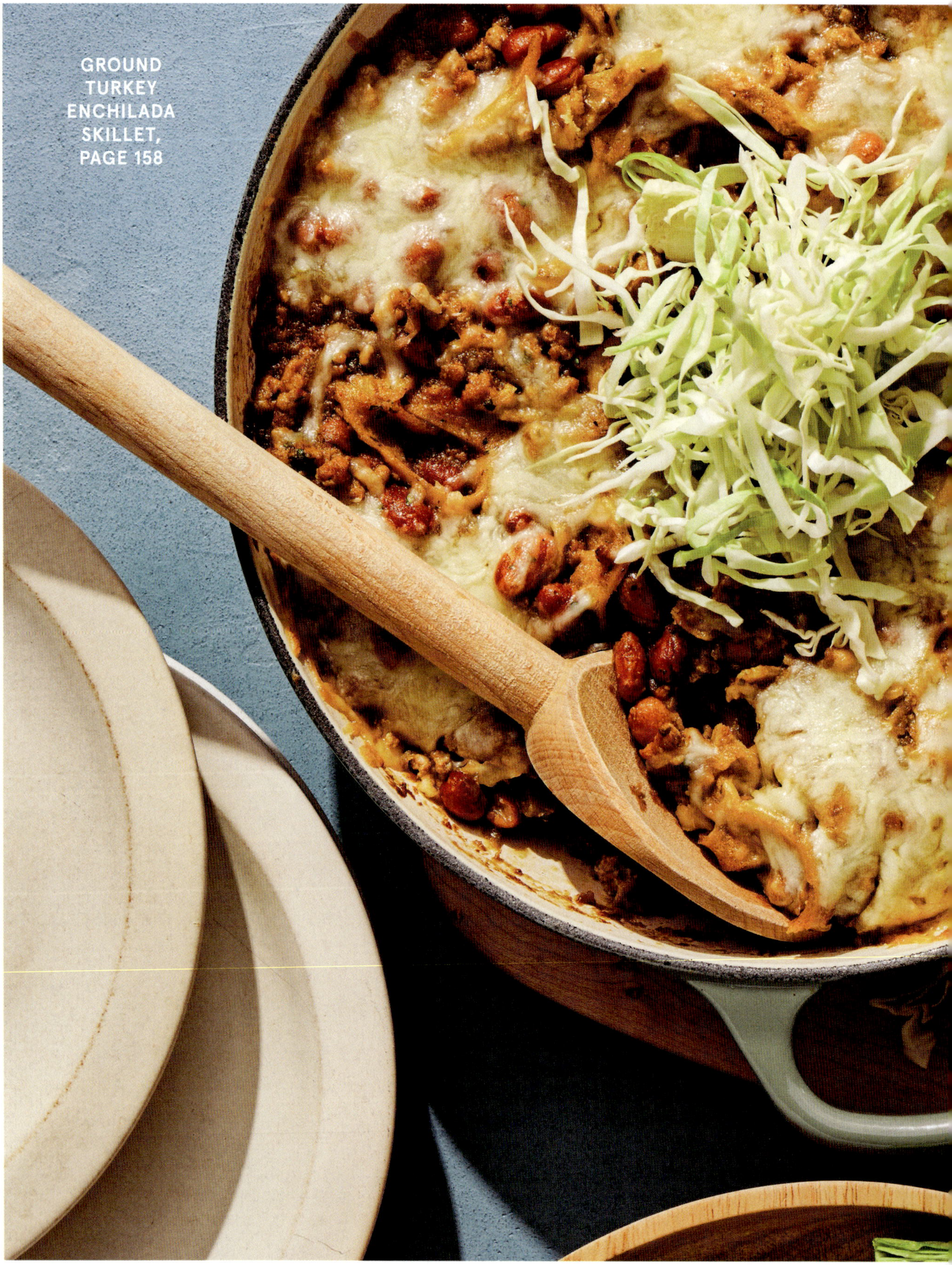

GROUND TURKEY ENCHILADA SKILLET, PAGE 158

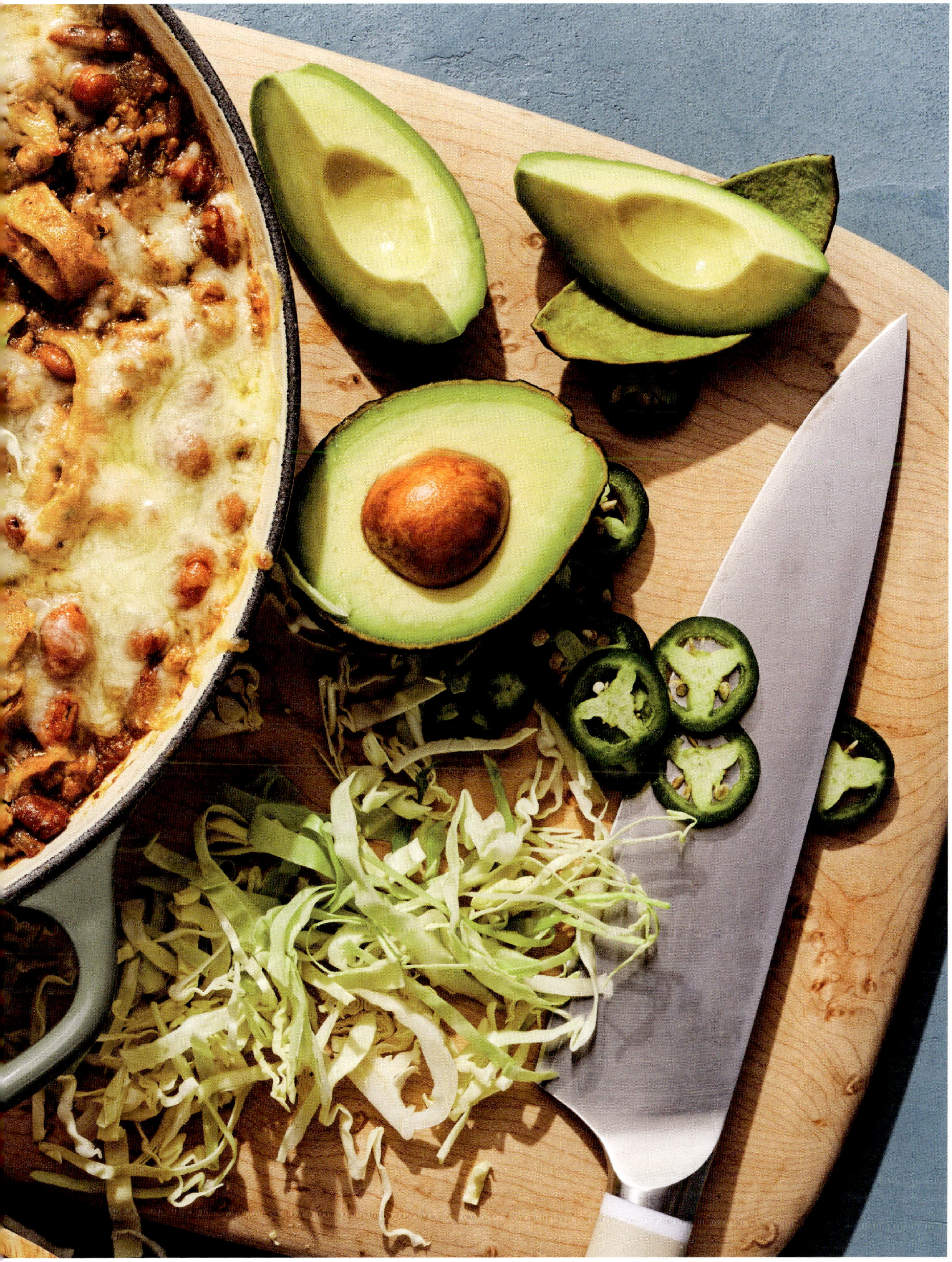

TANGY THAI BRAISED CHICKEN

MAKES 4 SERVINGS | **TOTAL TIME:** 1 HOUR 15 MINUTES

DIETARY
GLUTEN-FREE
GRAIN-FREE
DAIRY-FREE
PALEO
MAKE AHEAD

I do not say this often because I have way too many recipes I love, but this might be one of my favorite recipes—cozy, comforting, and bursting with flavor. The umami flavor from the fish sauce and Thai curry paste, balanced by a hint of sweetness from coconut sugar, makes the braised chicken irresistible. Braising takes a bit of time, but the prep is low effort and the reward is a brothy liquid that's perfect for spooning over rice. It's a meal that feels both indulgent and healthy, ideal for weeknights or relaxed weekends.

FOR THE BRAISING LIQUID

- ⅓ cup coconut aminos
- ½ cup unsweetened full-fat coconut milk
- ½ cup low-sodium chicken broth
- 2 tablespoons Thai red curry paste
- 2 tablespoons fish sauce
- 2 tablespoons coconut sugar
- 3 garlic cloves, minced

FOR THE CHICKEN

- 4 small whole bone-in, skin-on chicken leg quarters or 8 thighs, trimmed of excess fat and patted dry
- 1 teaspoon kosher salt
- ½ teaspoon freshly ground black pepper
- 2 tablespoons avocado oil
- 1 cup halved and thinly sliced shallot (about 2 large shallots)
- 1-inch piece fresh ginger, peeled and cut into thin matchsticks
- 6 green onions, cut into 2-inch pieces
- Fresh Thai or regular basil leaves, for garnish
- Fresh cilantro leaves, for garnish

FOR SERVING

- Prepared cauliflower rice or steamed rice
- Lime wedges

PREHEAT the oven to 375°F.

MAKE THE BRAISING LIQUID: In a medium bowl, combine all the braising liquid ingredients and whisk until very well combined. Set aside.

PREPARE THE CHICKEN: Season both sides of the chicken evenly with the salt and pepper.

IN a large, deep oven-safe skillet or 3.5-quart braiser, heat the oil over medium-high heat. Arrange the chicken, skin side down, in a single layer in the pan and cook until a deep golden-brown crust forms, 6 to 7 minutes. The chicken does not need to be cooked through as it will finish cooking in the oven. Remove from the heat and flip the chicken so that it is skin side up and arrange it in a single layer in the pan. Scatter the shallots, ginger, and green onions over and around the chicken pieces. Pour the braising liquid around and over the chicken.

TRANSFER to the oven, uncovered, and cook until the chicken is cooked through and fork-tender, about 50 minutes.

REMOVE from the oven and let rest for about 5 minutes to allow the juices to settle. Garnish with the Thai basil and cilantro.

TO SERVE: Place prepared rice in four shallow bowls and top with the chicken. Ladle the broth over the top and around the chicken. Serve with lime wedges.

STORE leftovers in an airtight container in the fridge for up to 3 days. Reheat gently in a skillet over medium-low heat, spooning some of the broth over the chicken to keep it moist, or microwave in 1-minute increments, stirring the broth after each, until warmed through.

LEFTOVER red curry paste? Try my Chicken Khao Soi-Inspired Soup (page 87), Thai Red Curry Shrimp Noodles (page 110), or Red Curry Pork Stir-Fry (page 191).

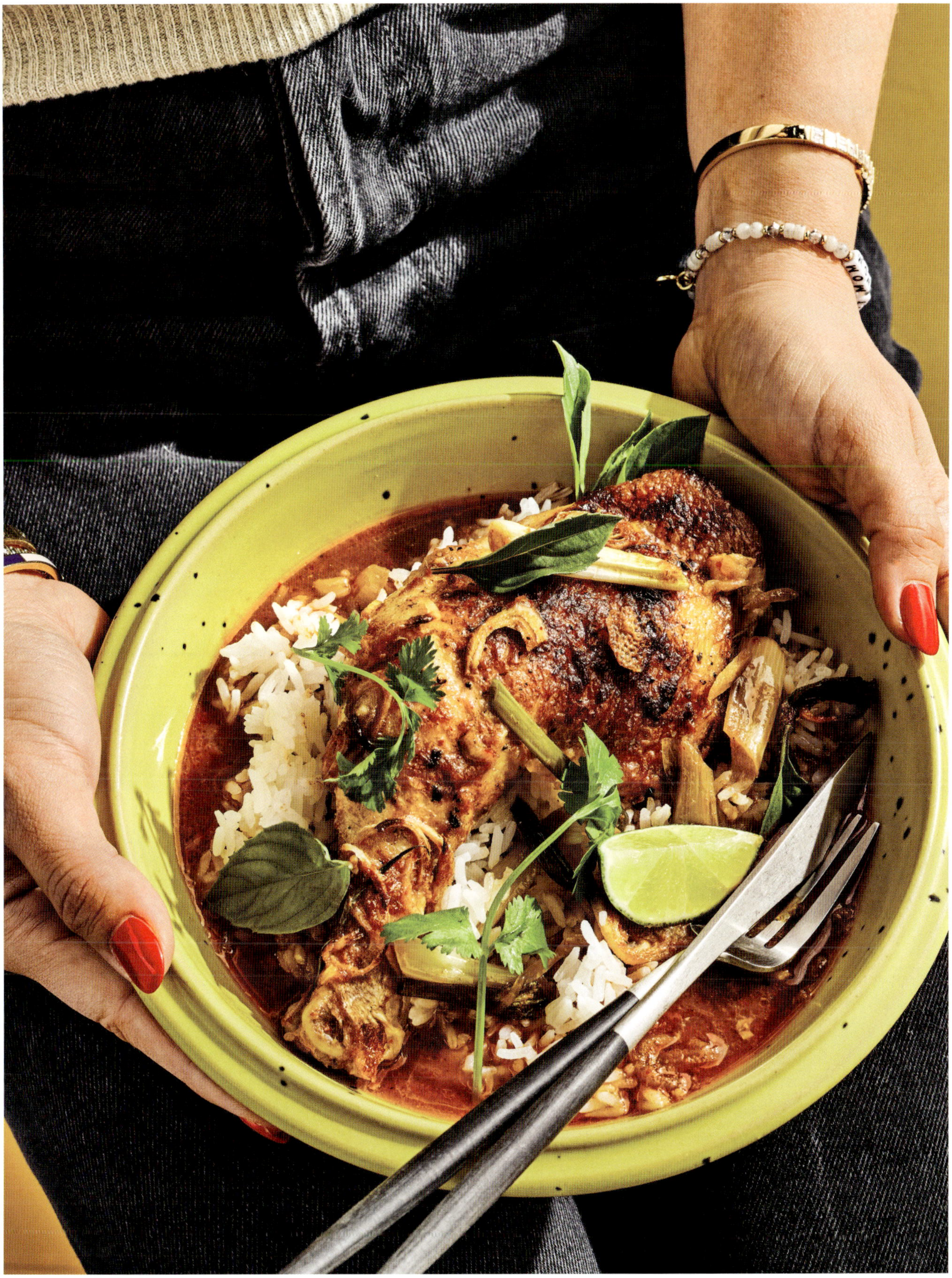

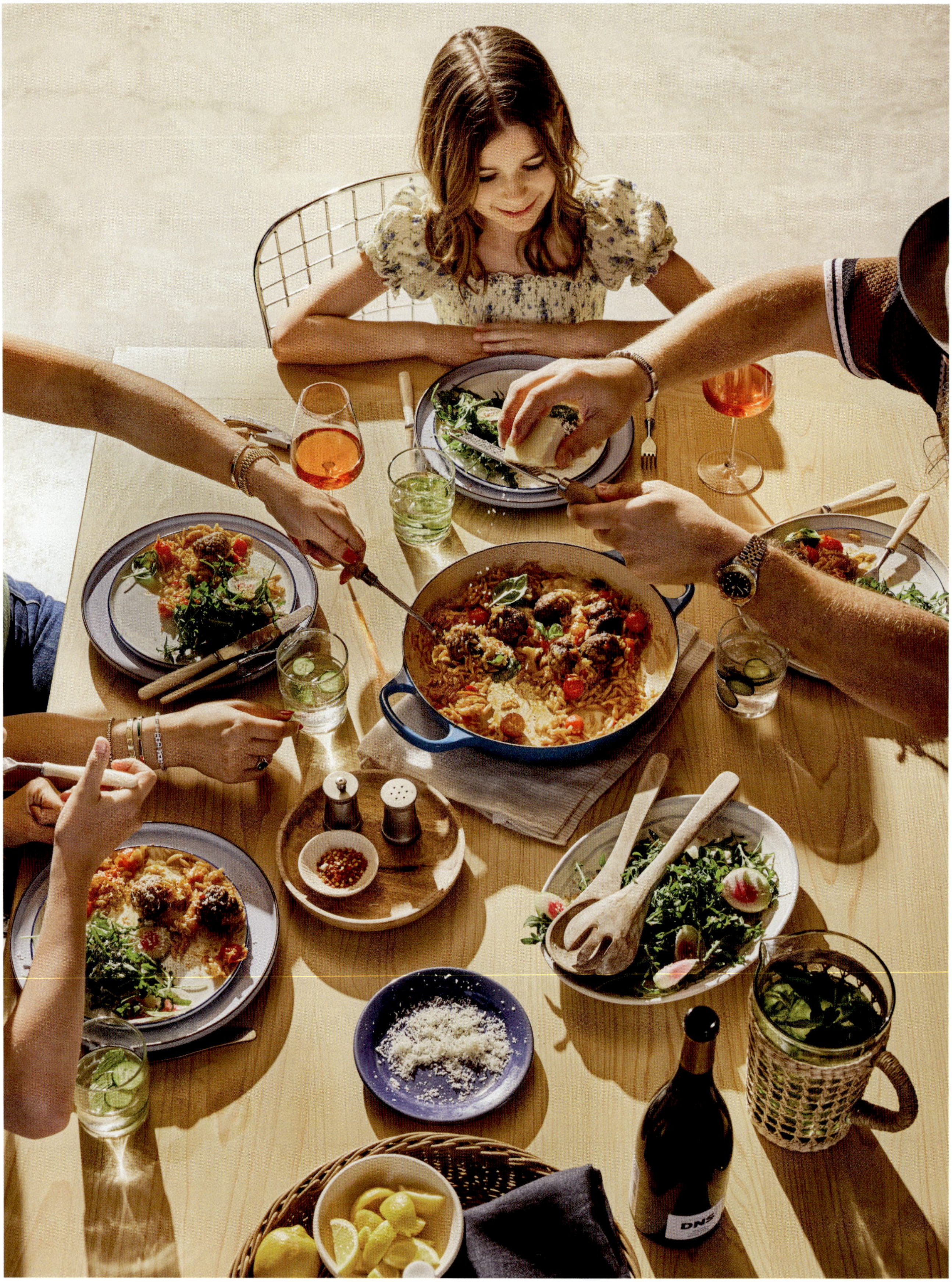
DNS

BEEF, PORK, AND LAMB

CHIPOTLE CHIMICHURRI STEAK BITE BOWLS

MAKES 4 SERVINGS | **TOTAL TIME:** 30 MINUTES

DIETARY
GLUTEN-FREE
DAIRY-FREE
GRAIN-FREE
MAKE AHEAD

If you've ever found yourself with a half-used can of chipotle peppers lingering in the fridge, this bowl is your answer. It's hearty and satisfying thanks to quick-seared steak bites, yet still feels fresh and balanced with a zippy chipotle chimichurri and crisp romaine. Serve it over rice with a scoop of pico de gallo and dinner is served.

FOR THE CHIPOTLE CHIMICHURRI

2 canned chipotle peppers in adobo sauce, minced (about 2 tablespoons)

1 cup roughly chopped fresh cilantro leaves and tender stems

1 cup roughly chopped fresh parsley leaves and tender stems

2 garlic cloves, roughly chopped

½ cup extra-virgin olive oil

2 tablespoons freshly squeezed lime juice (about 1 lime)

2 tablespoons red wine vinegar

½ teaspoon kosher salt

FOR THE STEAK BITES

2 pounds sirloin or flank steak, trimmed of excess fat and patted dry

2 teaspoons kosher salt

1 teaspoon freshly ground black pepper

2 teaspoons ground cumin

2 tablespoons avocado oil

FOR SERVING

Prepared cauliflower rice or steamed rice

Shredded romaine lettuce

Pico de gallo

Chopped fresh cilantro leaves

MAKE THE CHIPOTLE CHIMICHURRI: In a food processor or blender, combine all the chimichurri ingredients and pulse until the mixture is well combined but still slightly chunky with flecks of herbs visible throughout. Set aside. For best results, let it come to room temperature and give it a good stir before serving.

MAKE THE STEAK BITES: Cut the steak into 1-inch cubes, then season generously with the salt, black pepper, and ground cumin. Toss until well combined.

IN a large skillet, preferably cast iron, heat the oil over medium-high heat. Working in batches as necessary so as not to overcrowd the pan, add the steak cubes in a single layer and allow them to sear, undisturbed, for 2 minutes, until a deep golden crust forms on one side. Flip and cook for another 1 to 2 minutes. You're going for a quick sear, not overcooking them. Transfer the steak bites to a clean plate and let them rest for a couple of minutes. This helps keep them juicy.

BUILD THE BOWLS: To serve, divide the prepared rice among four bowls. Add plenty of lettuce, a big scoop of the steak bites, and the pico de gallo. Finish with a generous dollop of the chipotle chimichurri and top with cilantro.

STORE leftovers in an airtight container in the fridge for up to 3 days, keeping the chimichurri separate. Reheat the steak in a skillet over medium-low heat, or microwave just until warmed to avoid overcooking and serve over fresh rice and romaine with chimichurri spooned on top.

LEFTOVER chipotles in adobo? Try my Saucy Chipotle Chicken Tacos (page 142) or Sheet Pan Chipotle-Honey Butter Salmon (page 218).

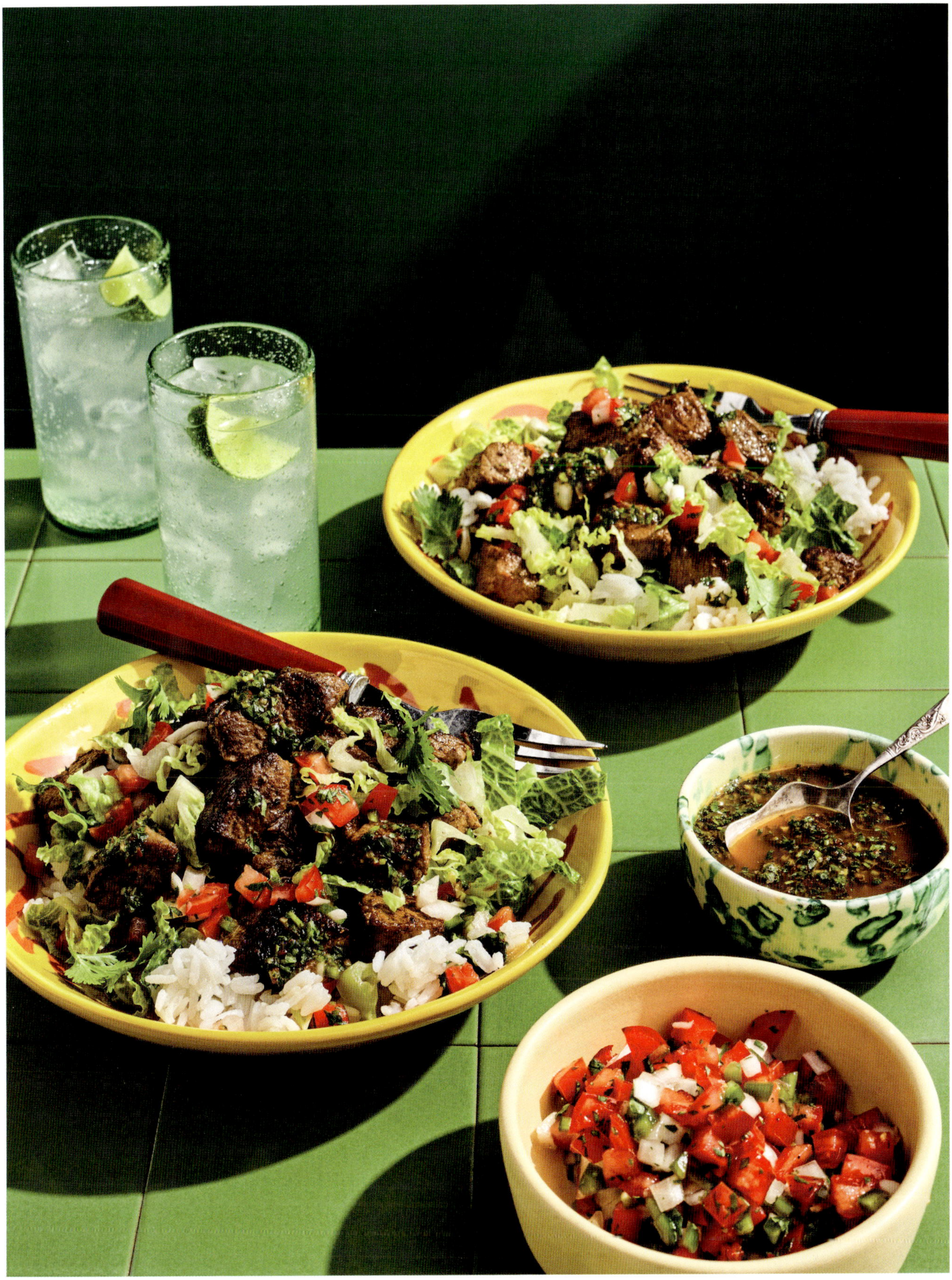

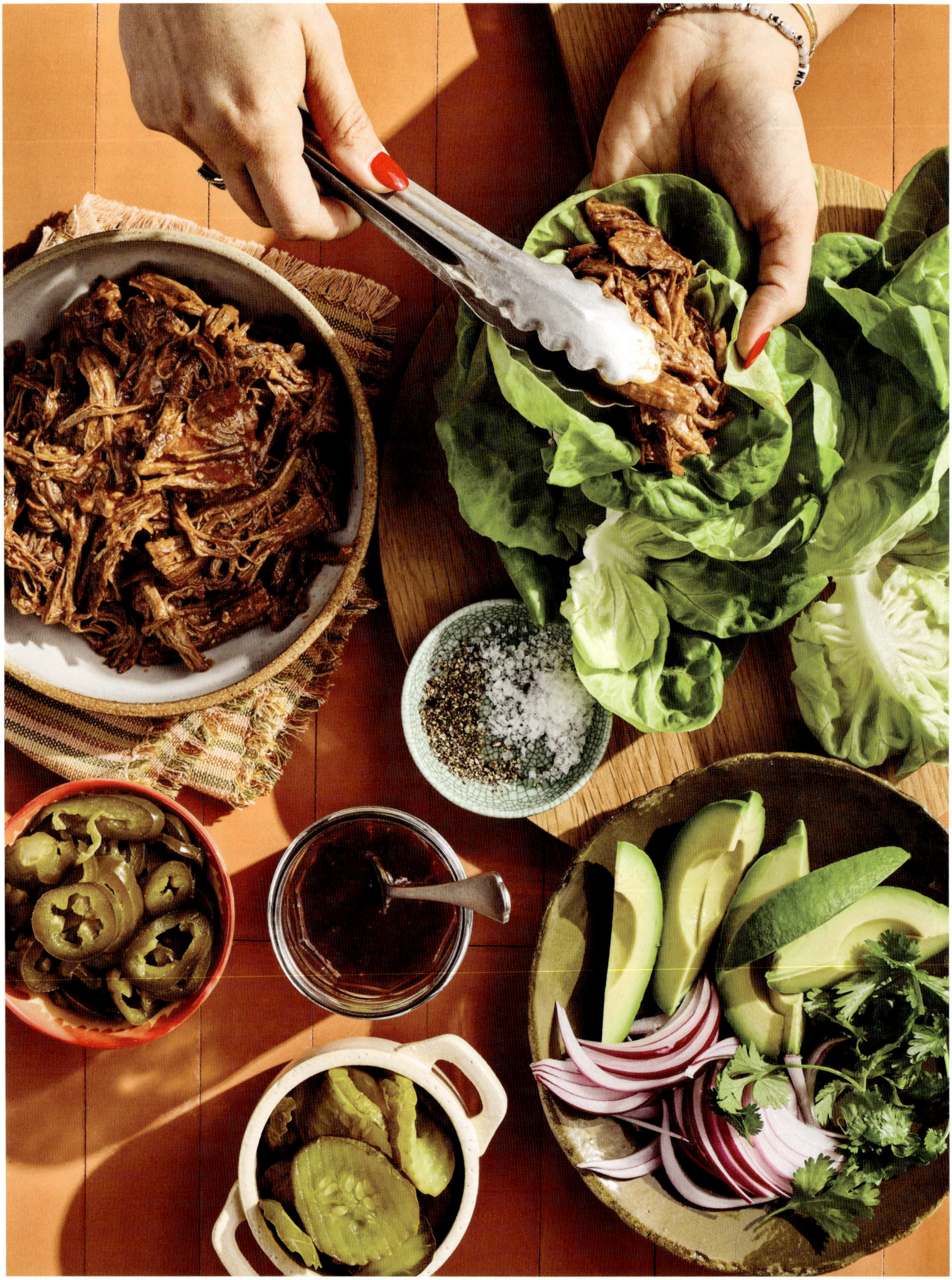

SLOW COOKER OR PRESSURE COOKER BBQ BEEF LETTUCE WRAPS

MAKES 6 SERVINGS | **TOTAL TIME:** 4 TO 8 HOURS (SLOW COOKER) OR 1 HOUR 15 MINUTES (PRESSURE COOKER)

DIETARY
GLUTEN-FREE
GRAIN-FREE
DAIRY-FREE
PALEO
MAKE AHEAD

These wraps have all the smoky, tangy flavors of a classic barbecue sandwich—just in a lighter, fresher form. Let the slow cooker or pressure cooker do the work, then pile on your favorite toppings. The beef is ultra-versatile too—serve it in lettuce wraps (like I did here), pile it over grains or sweet potatoes, or go classic with a BBQ sandwich.

FOR THE BEEF

4 garlic cloves, minced

1 cup halved and thinly sliced red onion (about 1 small onion)

2 tablespoons tomato paste

2 tablespoons brine from jar of pickled jalapeños

¾ cup no-sugar-added barbecue sauce, divided

½ cup low-sodium beef broth

2 tablespoons coconut sugar

2 tablespoons Dijon mustard

2 teaspoons smoked paprika

2 teaspoons garlic powder

2 pounds flank steak, trimmed of excess fat, patted dry, and cut into 4 equal-size pieces

2 teaspoons kosher salt

½ teaspoon freshly ground black pepper

2 tablespoons freshly squeezed lime juice (about 1 lime)

FOR SERVING

2 heads butter lettuce, separated into leaves

1 cup halved and thinly sliced red onion (about 1 small onion)

1 avocado, thinly sliced

Sliced dill pickles

Pickled jalapeño slices

No-sugar-added barbecue sauce

Chopped fresh cilantro leaves

SLOW COOKER METHOD

IN a slow cooker, whisk together the garlic, onion, tomato paste, jalapeño brine, ½ cup of the barbecue sauce, the broth, coconut sugar, mustard, paprika, and garlic powder.

SEASON the steak with the salt and black pepper, then nestle the steak into the sauce. Cover and cook on high for 4 hours or low for 8 hours, until the beef is fall-apart tender.

WHEN the cook time is complete, transfer the steak to a rimmed sheet pan and use two forks to shred the meat. Add the remaining ¼ cup barbecue sauce, the lime juice, and about ½ cup of the cooking liquid. Toss to combine.

TO SERVE: Layer two lettuce leaves on each plate, add the beef, and finish with your desired toppings.

PRESSURE COOKER METHOD

IN a pressure cooker, whisk together the garlic, onion, tomato paste, jalapeño brine, ½ cup of the barbecue sauce, the broth, coconut sugar, mustard, paprika, and garlic powder.

SEASON the steak with the salt and black pepper, then nestle the steak into the sauce. Secure the lid on the pressure cooker and ensure the vent is sealed. Press the "manual" or "pressure cook" button (depending on your model) and set the time to 60 minutes.

WHEN the cook time is complete, release the pressure manually by carefully turning the valve and letting it vent completely. When venting is done, carefully remove the lid. Transfer the steak to a rimmed sheet pan and use two forks to shred the meat. Add the remaining ¼ cup of barbecue sauce, the lime juice, and about ½ cup of the cooking liquid. Toss to combine.

TO SERVE: Layer two lettuce leaves on each plate, add the beef, and finish with your desired toppings.

STORE leftovers in an airtight container in the fridge for up to 4 days, keeping lettuce and toppings separate. Reheat the beef in a skillet over medium heat, or microwave in 1-minute increments, stirring after each, until warmed through. Serve with fresh toppings.

HONEY-ORANGE PORK AND SNAP PEA STIR-FRY

MAKES 4 SERVINGS | **TOTAL TIME:** 30 MINUTES

DIETARY
GLUTEN-FREE
GRAIN-FREE
DAIRY-FREE
PALEO
MAKE AHEAD

This easy pork stir-fry is one of my go-to dinners! Juicy, tender pork bites are stir-fried in a sweet, tangy, and slightly spicy honey-orange glaze that's packed with umami flavors. To keep it fresh and add some crunch, I toss in sugar snap peas—one of my kids' favorite veggies. It's a quick and flavorful way to get a nourishing dinner on the table!

FOR THE HONEY-ORANGE SAUCE

2 tablespoons coconut aminos

1 teaspoon fish sauce

1 teaspoon toasted sesame oil

2 tablespoons no-sugar-added sriracha

1 tablespoon grated orange zest

1 tablespoon freshly squeezed orange juice

2 tablespoons honey

1 teaspoon grated fresh ginger

2 garlic cloves, minced

FOR THE PORK STIR-FRY

1½ pounds pork tenderloin, silver skin removed, patted dry, and cut into 1-inch cubes

1 teaspoon kosher salt

½ teaspoon freshly ground black pepper

2 tablespoons tapioca flour

2 tablespoons avocado oil

½ cup halved and thinly sliced shallot (about 1 large shallot)

8 ounces sugar snap peas

1 tablespoon toasted sesame seeds, for garnish

Prepared cauliflower rice or steamed rice

MAKE THE HONEY-ORANGE SAUCE: In a small bowl, whisk together all the sauce ingredients until well combined. Set aside.

MAKE THE STIR-FRY: In a large bowl, combine the pork, salt, pepper, and flour. Toss until well coated.

IN a large, deep nonstick skillet, heat the avocado oil over medium-high heat. Add the pork in a single layer and let cook, undisturbed, until a golden-brown crust forms on one side, 3 to 4 minutes. Flip and continue to cook, tossing occasionally, until the pork is browned on both sides and cooked through, 3 to 4 more minutes. Using a slotted spoon, transfer the browned pork to a clean plate.

REDUCE the heat to medium. Add the shallot and sauté for 1 minute, until it begins to soften. Add the snap peas and 2 tablespoons water and scrape up any browned bits off the bottom of the pan. Cook, stirring occasionally, until the water has evaporated and the snap peas are bright green and slightly tender but still crunchy, about 4 minutes.

ADD the browned pork back to the pan along with any of its juices and toss until well combined. Pour in the honey-orange sauce and stir once more to combine. Bring to a simmer, then let cook, tossing, until the pork and snap peas are well coated in the sauce, about 2 more minutes.

FINISH with a sprinkle of toasted sesame seeds and serve over prepared rice.

STORE leftovers in an airtight container in the fridge for up to 3 days. Reheat in a skillet over medium heat to keep the pork tender and snap peas crisp, or microwave in 1-minute increments, stirring after each, until warmed through. Garnish with toasted sesame seeds and serve over fresh rice.

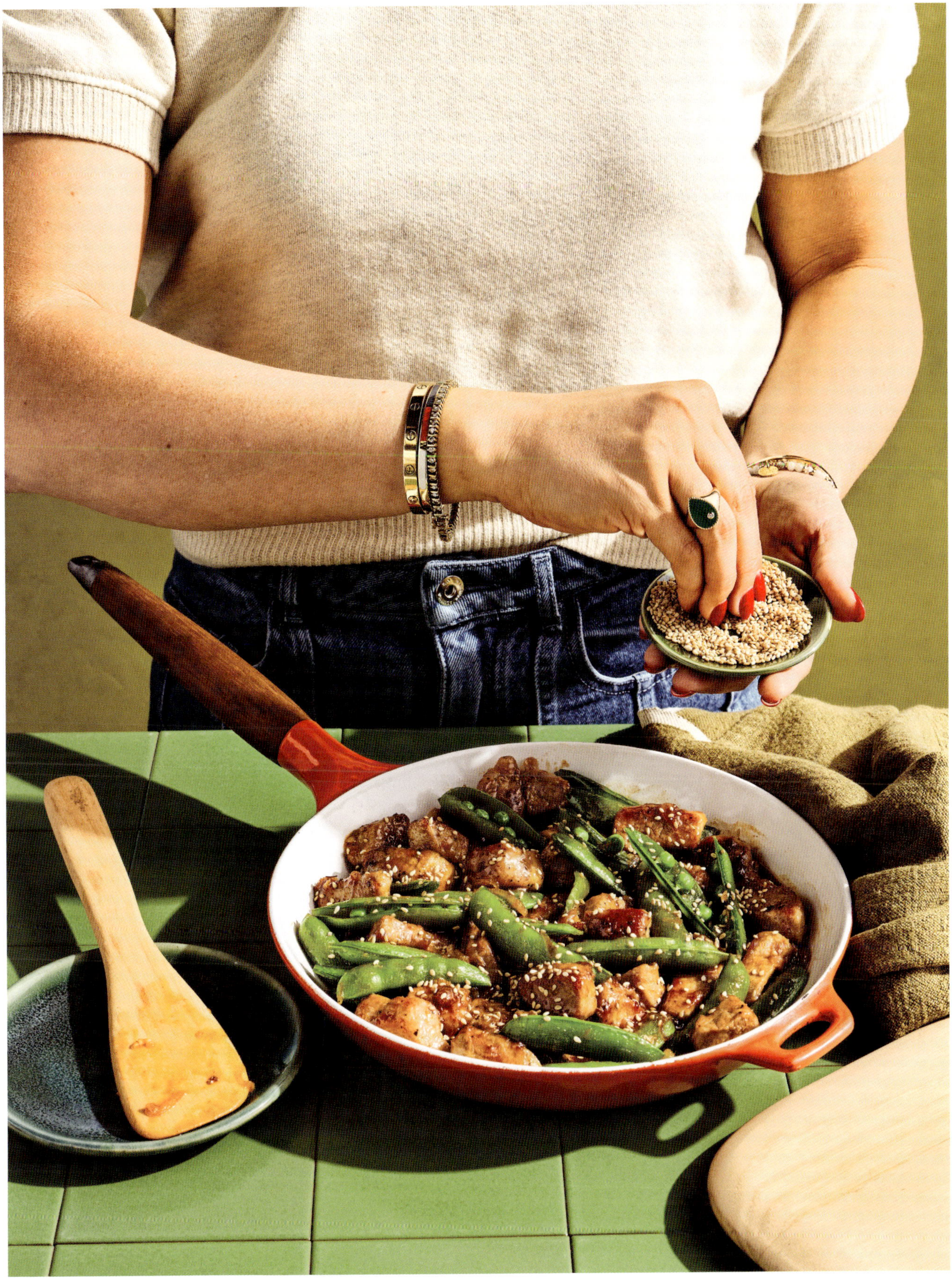

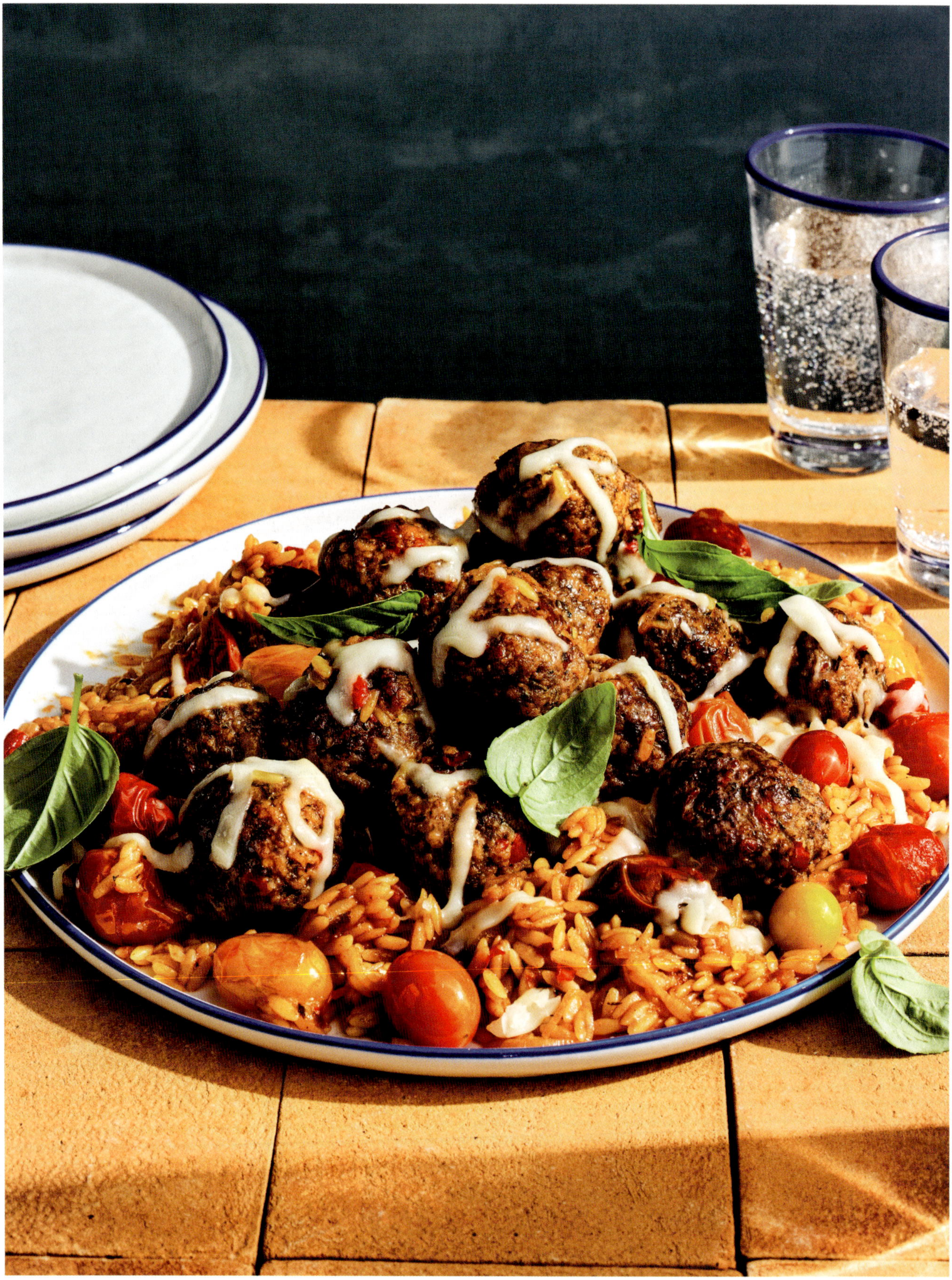

CALABRIAN CHILE MEATBALL ORZO SKILLET

MAKES 4 SERVINGS | **TOTAL TIME:** 45 MINUTES

DIETARY

GLUTEN-FREE (IF MODIFIED)

MAKE AHEAD

Growing up, I was obsessed with SpaghettiOs with meatballs. This recipe is my fun, grown-up take on that nostalgic favorite. Juicy, herb-packed meatballs get a little kick from chopped Calabrian peppers, while a splash of white wine adds brightness to the rich, tomato-y orzo. It all comes together in one skillet—and it's absolutely bursting with flavor.

FOR THE MEATBALLS

1 pound ground beef (90/10)

2 tablespoons chopped Calabrian peppers (see note, page 106)

1 large egg

½ cup gluten-free panko bread crumbs

1 teaspoon kosher salt

1 teaspoon Italian seasoning

½ teaspoon freshly ground black pepper

3 garlic cloves, minced

2 teaspoons finely chopped fresh rosemary leaves

2 tablespoons extra-virgin olive oil

FOR THE ORZO SKILLET

½ cup halved and thinly sliced shallot (about 1 large shallot)

1 pint cherry tomatoes

1 teaspoon kosher salt

1 tablespoon tomato paste

1 tablespoon chopped Calabrian peppers

½ cup dry white wine

1 cup orzo (sub gluten-free orzo for gluten-free)

1½ cups low-sodium beef broth

Grated zest of ½ lemon

½ cup shredded mozzarella cheese

¼ cup torn fresh basil leaves, for serving

MAKE THE MEATBALLS: In a large bowl, add the ground beef, Calabrian peppers, egg, panko, salt, Italian seasoning, black pepper, garlic, and rosemary. Using clean hands, mix together until just combined. Do not overmix or the meatballs will be tough. Form the meat mixture into 16 meatballs, about 1 inch each. Set aside.

IN a large, deep skillet or 3.5-quart braiser with fitted lid, heat the oil over medium-high heat. Add the meatballs in a single layer and cook until golden brown, 2 to 3 minutes per side. The meatballs do not have to be fully cooked through, as they will finish cooking in the orzo. Transfer to a clean plate and set aside.

MAKE THE ORZO: Reduce the heat beneath the skillet to medium, add the shallot and tomatoes to the skillet and cook, stirring, until the tomatoes begin to blister and burst, 3 to 4 minutes.

ADD the salt, tomato paste, and Calabrian peppers and stir to combine. Pour in the wine and continue to cook, stirring, until well combined and the wine is reduced by half, about 2 minutes.

ADD the orzo, broth, and lemon zest and stir to combine. Bring the mixture to a rapid simmer, then reduce the heat to a gentle simmer, about medium-low heat. Nestle the meatballs into the pan, cover, and cook for about 10 minutes, stirring once halfway through to prevent the orzo from sticking to the bottom of the pan. The orzo should be al dente and the meatballs fully cooked through.

REMOVE from the heat and stir once more. Sprinkle the top of the skillet evenly with the mozzarella. Cover to allow the cheese to melt, about 2 more minutes.

TO SERVE: Top with the torn basil leaves. Divide the orzo and meatballs among four shallow bowls.

STORE leftovers in an airtight container in the fridge for up to 3 days. Reheat in a skillet over medium heat with a splash of broth to loosen the orzo, or microwave in 1-minute increments, stirring after each, until warmed through.

LEFTOVER chopped Calabrian peppers? Try my Calabrian Carbonara (page 106).

HIBACHI-INSPIRED STEAK STIR-FRY WITH GINGER SAUCE

MAKES 4 SERVINGS | **TOTAL TIME:** 30 MINUTES

DIETARY
GLUTEN-FREE
GRAIN-FREE
DAIRY-FREE (IF MODIFIED)
PALEO (IF MODIFIED)
MAKE AHEAD

If you have my first cookbook, you likely know and love my recipe for Hibachi-Style Chicken with Magic Mustard Sauce. Let's shake things up with a steak version paired with our other favorite hibachi sauce to dip in: the famous ginger sauce. There is truly nothing like dunking a succulent piece of steak in this zingy ginger sauce on a busy weeknight!

FOR THE GINGER SAUCE

1 cup medium-diced yellow onion (about ½ medium onion)

3 garlic cloves, minced

2 teaspoons grated fresh ginger

2 tablespoons freshly squeezed lemon juice (about 1 lemon)

¼ cup coconut aminos

1 teaspoon fish sauce

2 tablespoons rice vinegar

2 teaspoons toasted sesame oil

1 tablespoon honey

½ teaspoon kosher salt

½ teaspoon freshly ground black pepper

FOR THE STIR-FRY

1½ pounds filet or sirloin steak, patted dry and cut into 1-inch cubes

1 teaspoon kosher salt

½ teaspoon freshly ground black pepper

2 tablespoons avocado oil, plus more as needed

1 cup thinly sliced yellow onion (about ½ medium onion)

2 small zucchini, cut in half crosswise, then each half quartered lengthwise

2 small carrots, cut in half crosswise, then each half quartered lengthwise

2 tablespoons unsalted butter (omit for paleo and dairy-free)

2 tablespoons coconut aminos

1 tablespoon toasted sesame seeds

Prepared cauliflower rice or steamed rice

MAKE THE GINGER SAUCE: In a food processor or blender, combine the sauce ingredients. Blend until just smooth. Set aside. The sauce will keep in an airtight container in the fridge for 3 days.

MAKE THE STIR-FRY: Season the steak with the salt and pepper. Toss to coat.

IN a large skillet, heat the avocado oil over medium-high heat. Working in batches so as not to overcrowd the pan, add the steak in a single layer and sear until a golden-brown crust forms on all sides, about 2 minutes per side. Using a slotted spoon, transfer to a clean plate and set aside.

IF the skillet is dry, add 1 tablespoon more avocado oil. Add the onion, zucchini, carrots, and a pinch of salt. Cook, tossing, until the veggies are slightly tender, about 5 minutes.

REDUCE the heat to medium. Stir in the butter (if using), coconut aminos, and sesame seeds. Return the steak and any of its juices back to the pan. Cook, tossing, until the steak is well coated and the sauce has reduced, about 2 minutes.

SERVE over prepared rice with the ginger sauce on the side for dipping.

STORE the steak stir-fry and ginger dipping sauce in separate airtight containers in the fridge for up to 3 days. Reheat the stir-fry quickly in a skillet over medium heat until warm, or microwave in 1 minute increments, stirring between, until warmed through. Serve with rice and the ginger sauce.

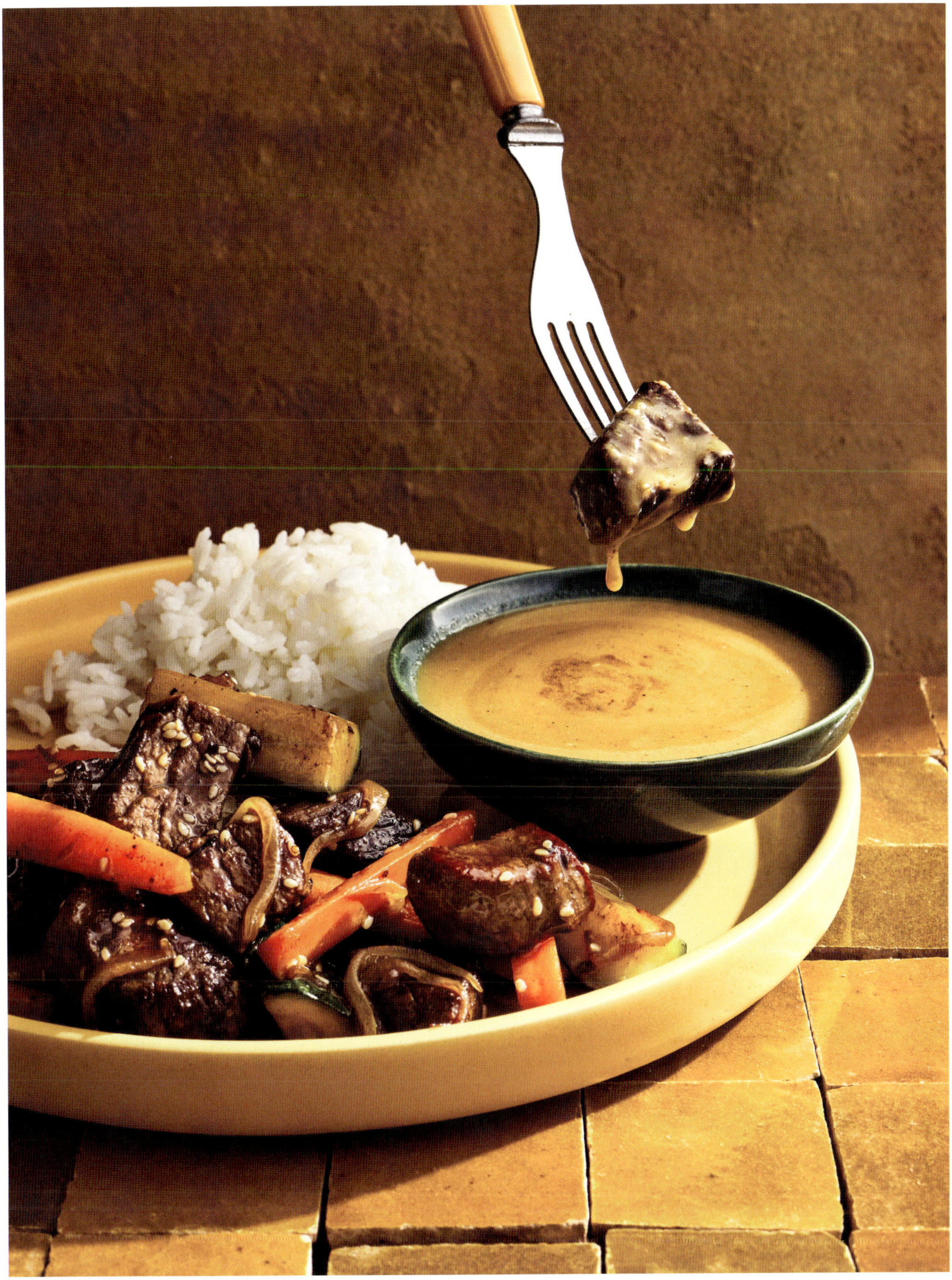

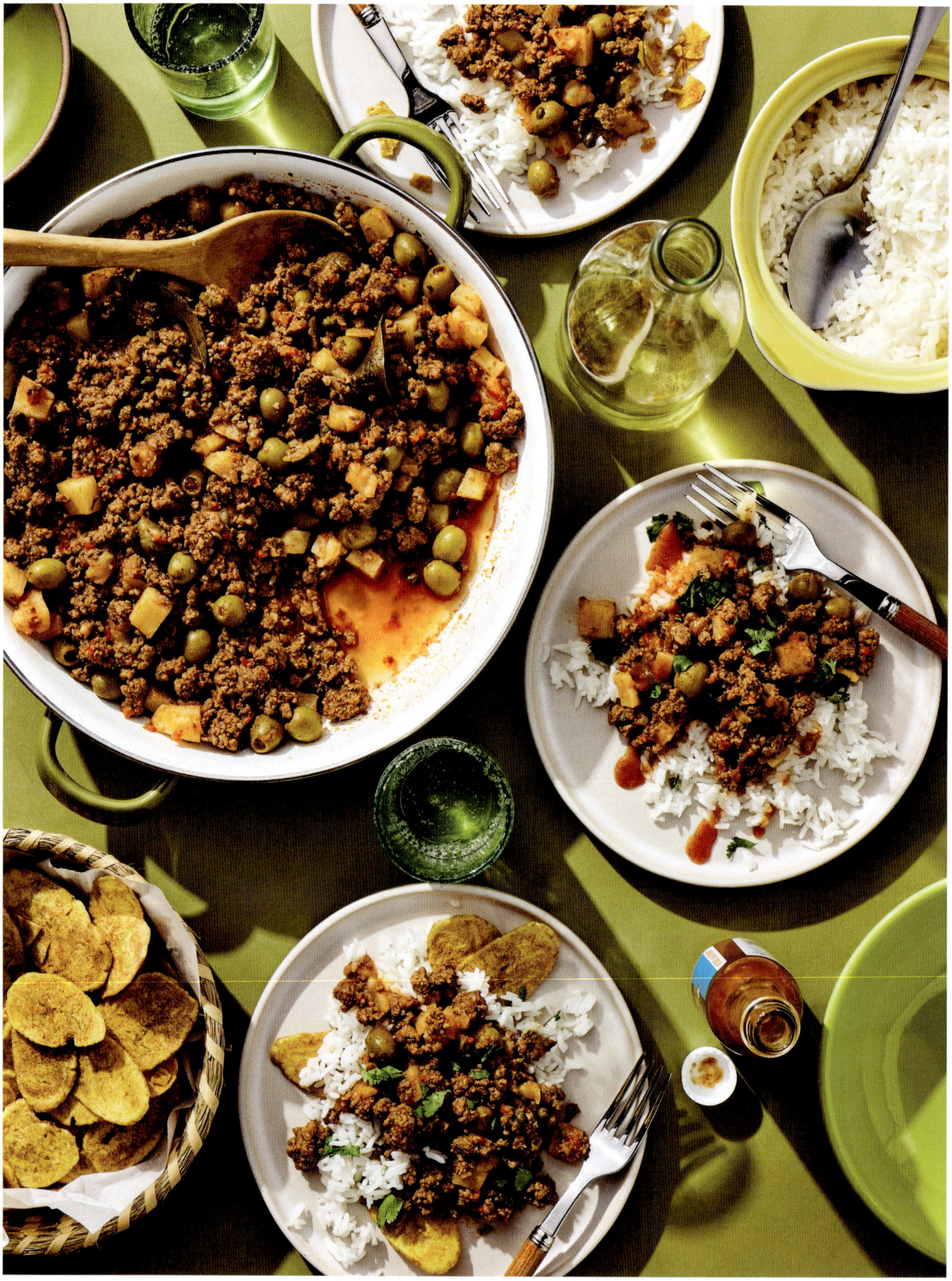

CUBAN-INSPIRED PICADILLO

MAKES 8 SERVINGS | **TOTAL TIME:** 45 MINUTES

DIETARY

GLUTEN-FREE

GRAIN-FREE

DAIRY-FREE

PALEO (IF MODIFIED)

MAKE AHEAD

This hearty, family-friendly dish is sure to become a favorite around the dinner table. It combines ground beef with warming spices, briny olives, capers, and tender potatoes, all simmered together for a deeply satisfying meal. Simple to prepare and full of flavor, it's perfect for a comforting dinner any night of the week, and the leftovers are just as delightful.

2 tablespoons extra-virgin olive oil

1 cup finely diced white onion (about ½ medium onion)

½ cup finely diced red bell pepper (about 1 small bell pepper)

4 garlic cloves, minced

2 pounds ground beef (90/10)

1½ teaspoons kosher salt

½ teaspoon freshly ground black pepper

2 teaspoons garlic powder

1½ teaspoons ground cumin

2 teaspoons dried oregano

2 teaspoons chili powder

2 bay leaves

⅓ cup dry white wine (omit for paleo)

¾ cup low-sodium beef broth

One 8-ounce can tomato sauce

One 5-ounce jar small Manzanilla olives, drained

3 tablespoons capers, drained

1½ cups small-diced peeled russet potato (about 1 large potato)

FOR SERVING

Prepared cauliflower rice or steamed rice

Plantain chips

Chopped fresh cilantro leaves

Your favorite hot sauce, optional

IN a large, deep skillet or 3.5-quart braiser with fitted lid, heat the oil over medium heat. Add the onion, bell pepper, and garlic and cook, stirring, until softened, about 4 minutes.

ADD the ground beef and cook, breaking up the meat with the edge of a spoon, until cooked through and no longer pink, about 7 minutes. Drain off the excess fat and return the beef to the pan.

ADD the salt, black pepper, garlic powder, cumin, oregano, chili powder, and bay leaves and continue to cook, stirring, until the spices are toasted, 2 minutes.

POUR in the wine (if using) and let it reduce by half, about 1 minute. Add the broth, tomato sauce, olives, capers, and potato. Stir to combine and bring to a rapid simmer. Reduce the heat to a gentle simmer, about medium-low heat. Cover and cook, stirring occasionally, until the potato is fork-tender, about 15 minutes. Discard the bay leaves.

TO SERVE: Ladle the picadillo over prepared rice with a side of plantain chips. Garnish with cilantro and top with hot sauce, if desired.

STORE leftovers in an airtight container in the fridge for up to 3 days, separate of garnishes. Reheat in a skillet over medium heat, or microwave in 1-minute increments, stirring after each, until warmed through. Serve over rice and garnish as desired.

ITALIAN SAUSAGE WITH BROTHY WHITE BEANS AND KALE

MAKES 4 SERVINGS | **TOTAL TIME:** 30 MINUTES

DIETARY
GLUTEN-FREE
GRAIN-FREE
DAIRY-FREE (IF MODIFIED)
MAKE AHEAD

This cozy one-pan meal is a perfect balance of hearty and wholesome, featuring juicy Italian sausage, creamy cannellini beans, and tender kale in a garlicky sauce. Keeping the sausage links whole allows them to stay extra juicy while infusing the beans and broth with rich flavor. Serve it with crusty bread for a satisfying, no-fuss dinner that feels both rustic and comforting.

2 tablespoons extra-virgin olive oil

4 mild or hot Italian sausage links

2 large shallots, halved and thinly sliced (about 1 cup)

3 garlic cloves, minced

½ teaspoon crushed red pepper flakes, optional

½ teaspoon kosher salt

½ teaspoon freshly ground black pepper

1 teaspoon Italian seasoning

½ cup dry white wine

1 tablespoon tomato paste

Two 15-ounce cans cannellini beans, drained and rinsed

1 cup low-sodium chicken broth

Grated zest of ½ lemon

1 teaspoon fresh thyme leaves or ½ teaspoon dried

4 cups de-ribbed and roughly chopped lacinato kale (about 1 bunch)

1 tablespoon freshly squeezed lemon juice (about ½ lemon)

Freshly grated parmesan cheese (omit for dairy-free)

Fresh thyme leaves, for garnish

IN a large skillet or 3.5-quart braiser with fitted lid, heat the oil over medium heat. Add the sausage links and sear until browned on both sides, 3 to 4 minutes per side. They don't need to be fully cooked through yet, as they will finish cooking with the beans. Remove from the pan and set aside.

IN the same skillet, add the shallots, garlic, pepper flakes (if using), salt, black pepper, and Italian seasoning. Cook, stirring, until softened, about 2 minutes.

POUR in the wine, scraping up any browned bits off the bottom of the pan. Let it simmer for 2 minutes to reduce slightly.

STIR in the tomato paste until well combined. Add the cannellini beans, broth, lemon zest, and thyme. Bring to a rapid simmer, then reduce the heat to a gentle simmer, about medium-low heat. Nestle the browned sausages back into the pan, cover, and cook for 10 minutes to allow the flavors to meld and sausage to finish cooking.

STIR in the kale and lemon juice and let the kale wilt into the broth, 2 to 3 minutes. Remove from the heat.

TO SERVE: Divide the brothy beans among four shallow bowls and top each with a sausage link. Garnish with grated parmesan (if using) and some fresh thyme.

STORE leftovers in an airtight container in the fridge for up to 3 days. Reheat in a skillet over medium heat, or microwave in 1-minute increments, stirring after each, until warmed through.

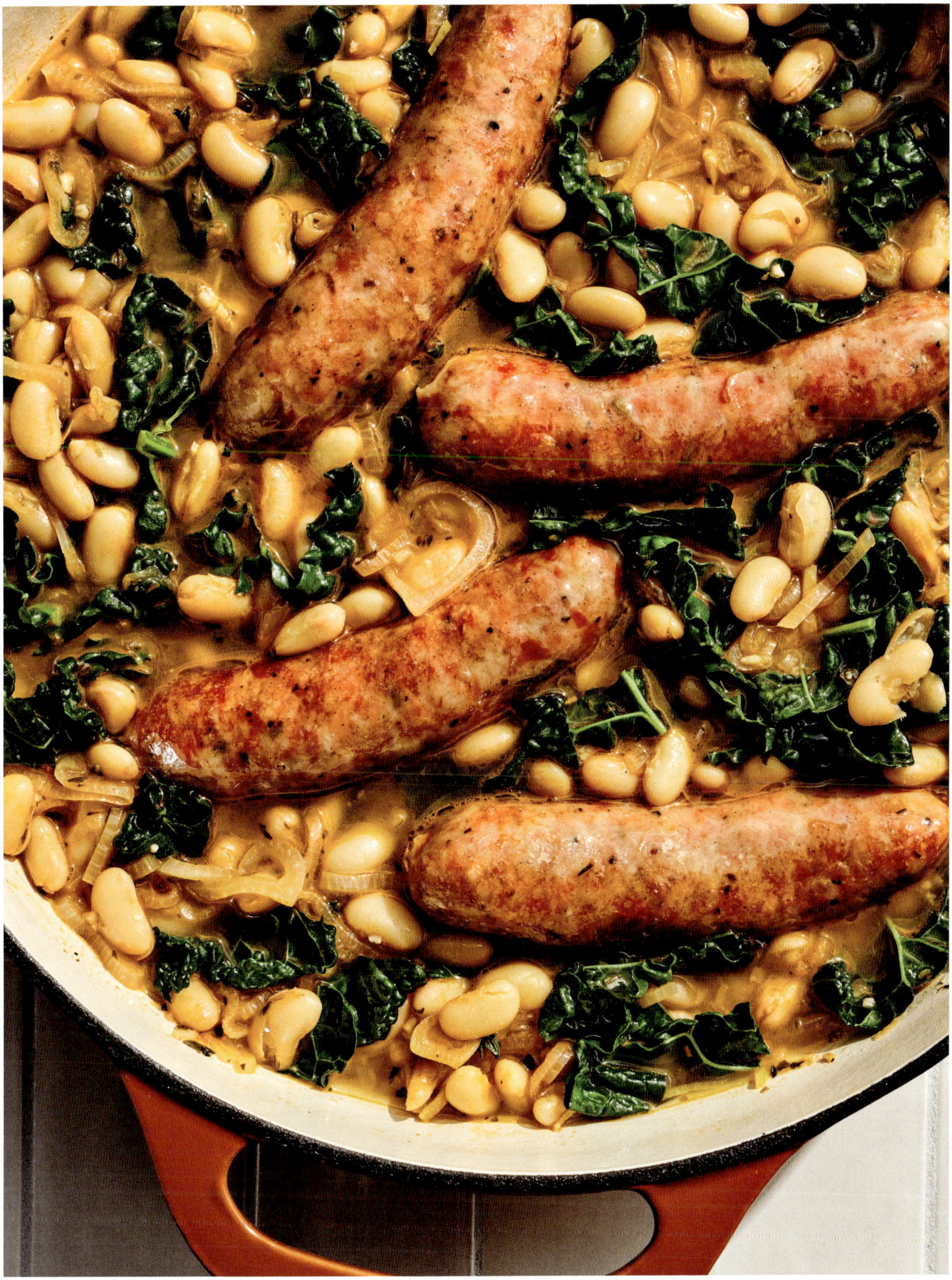

CHORIZO AND SWEET POTATO STREET TACOS

MAKES 6 SERVINGS | **TOTAL TIME:** 30 MINUTES

DIETARY
GLUTEN-FREE (IF MODIFIED)
GRAIN-FREE (IF MODIFIED)
DAIRY-FREE (IF MODIFIED)
MAKE AHEAD

These street tacos are my fresh take on the classic chorizo con papas, swapping out yellow potatoes for sweet potatoes to create an irresistible sweet-and-savory combination. Topped with a creamy, zesty avocado salsa—made by blending salsa verde and avocado—these tacos are as easy to make as they are delicious. They're perfect for a quick weeknight meal, and any leftover chorizo filling transforms into the ultimate breakfast taco when paired with scrambled eggs the next morning. Simple, flavorful, and downright satisfying!

FOR THE CHORIZO MIXTURE

1 pound fresh Mexican chorizo sausage (see note)

1 tablespoon avocado oil, if needed

1 cup finely diced white onion (about ½ medium onion)

1 cup finely diced poblano pepper (about 1 large poblano)

1 cup peeled and small-diced sweet potato (about 1 small sweet potato)

1 teaspoon kosher salt

FOR THE AVOCADO SALSA

½ large avocado, cubed

1 cup salsa verde

1 tablespoon freshly squeezed lime juice (about ½ lime)

Kosher salt, to taste

FOR ASSEMBLY AND SERVING

Twelve 4-inch flour tortillas (sub corn tortillas for gluten-free and sub grain-free tortillas for grain-free)

½ large avocado, cubed

4 ounces queso fresco, crumbled (omit for dairy-free)

¼ cup finely diced white onion (about ¼ small onion)

Finely chopped fresh cilantro

Lime wedges

MAKE THE CHORIZO MIXTURE: Line a plate with paper towels. In a large skillet over medium-high heat, cook the chorizo, breaking up the meat with the edge of a spoon, until the chorizo is browned, crumbly, and fully cooked through with no pink remaining, 7 to 9 minutes. Using a slotted spoon, transfer the cooked chorizo to the prepared plate and set aside.

REDUCE the heat to medium, and if the skillet seems dry, add the avocado oil. Add the onion, poblano, sweet potato, and salt. Cook, stirring frequently, until the potatoes are tender, about 8 minutes.

RETURN the chorizo to the skillet and toss until well combined with the sweet potato mixture and the chorizo is warmed through, 2 to 3 minutes. Reduce the heat to low and keep warm.

MAKE THE AVOCADO SALSA: In a small blender or using an immersion blender in a wide-mouth jar, combine the avocado, salsa verde, and lime juice. Blend until smooth. Taste and add salt as desired. This keeps well in an airtight container in the fridge for up to 3 days.

ASSEMBLE AND SERVE THE TACOS: One at a time, place the tortillas in a dry (no oil) skillet over medium heat and cook for about 30 seconds on each side. Alternatively, you can use tongs to char the tortillas directly over a gas flame for a few seconds.

FILL the tortillas with the chorizo and sweet potato mixture. Top with a dollop of the avocado salsa and cubed avocado. Finish with a sprinkle of the queso fresco (if using), onion, and cilantro. Serve with lime wedges.

STORE leftovers in an airtight container in the fridge for up to 3 days, keeping the tortillas, avocado salsa, and toppings separate. Reheat the filling in a skillet over medium heat, or microwave in 1-minute increments, stirring after each, until warmed through. Assemble tacos with avocado salsa and fresh toppings.

FROM MY KITCHEN TO YOURS

Fresh Mexican chorizo is a flavorful, uncooked sausage made with ground pork and a blend of chili spices, garlic, and vinegar. You can often find it in the refrigerated meat section at your local grocery store, butcher shop, or specialty Latin markets. It's sometimes sold in bulk, but if it comes in casing, simply remove it before cooking. Be sure not to confuse it with cured Spanish chorizo, which is dried and ready to eat, as fresh chorizo must be cooked thoroughly.

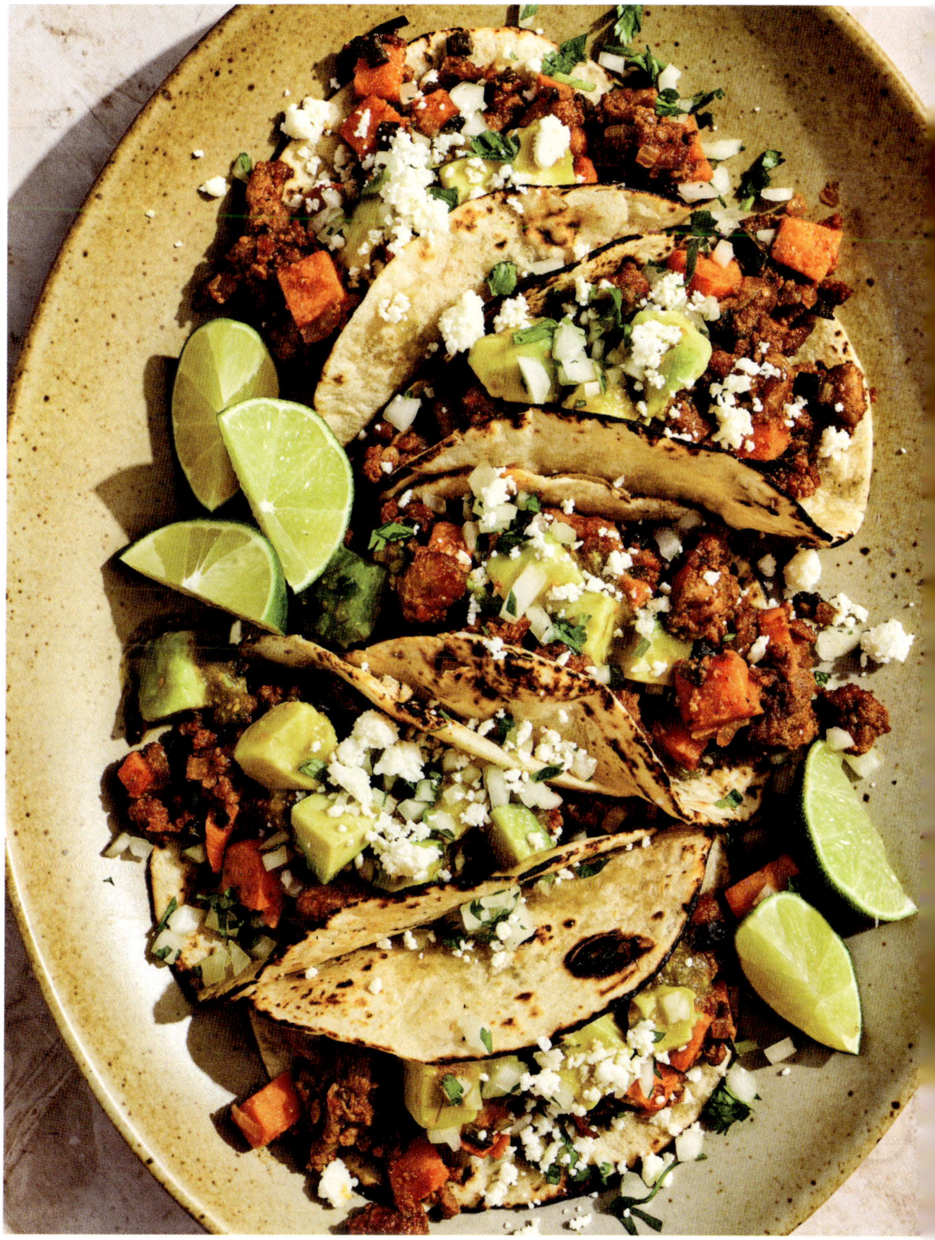

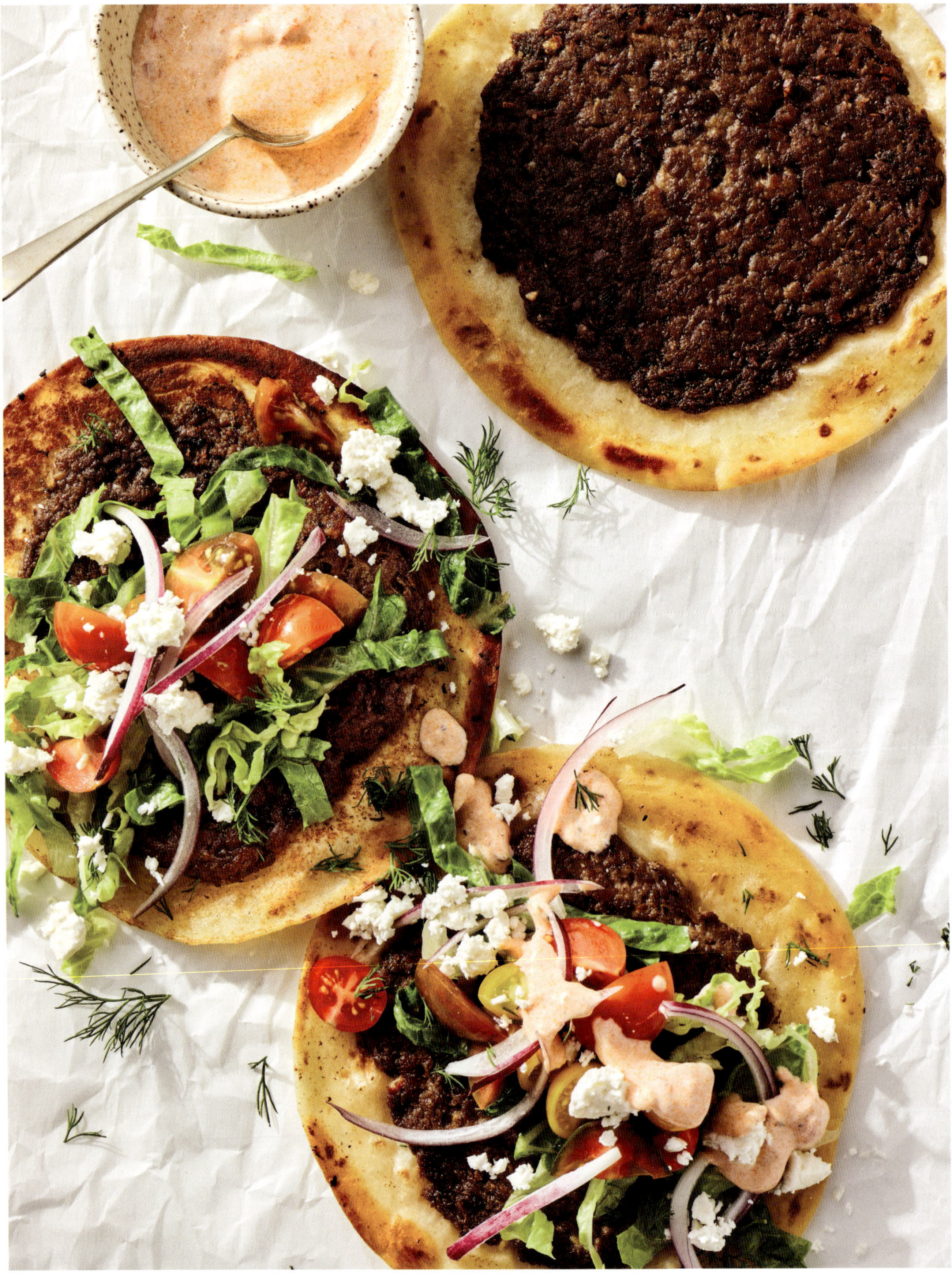

SMASHED LAMB BURGER TACOS WITH HARISSA-YOGURT SAUCE

MAKES 4 SERVINGS | **TOTAL TIME:** 30 MINUTES

DIETARY

GLUTEN-FREE (IF MODIFIED)

GRAIN-FREE (IF MODIFIED)

Get ready to elevate your taco game! This recipe takes inspiration from the classic flavors of a gyro and combines them with the playful trend of smashed burger tacos. Juicy lamb is pressed into tortillas and seared until golden, then topped with creamy feta and a drizzle of tangy, slightly spicy, harissa yogurt sauce that's sure to impress!

FOR THE HARISSA-YOGURT SAUCE

½ cup whole-milk plain Greek yogurt

2 tablespoons mild harissa paste

2 tablespoons freshly squeezed lemon juice (about 1 lemon)

¼ teaspoon kosher salt

¼ teaspoon freshly ground black pepper

FOR THE LAMB BURGERS

1½ pounds ground lamb

4 garlic cloves, minced

1 teaspoon ground cumin

1 teaspoon ground coriander

1 teaspoon dried oregano

½ teaspoon allspice

1½ teaspoons kosher salt

½ teaspoon freshly ground black pepper

Avocado oil

Eight 6-inch flour tortillas (sub almond-flour tortillas for gluten-free and grain-free)

FOR SERVING

2 cups thinly sliced romaine lettuce

¾ cup quartered cherry tomatoes

1 cup halved and thinly sliced red onion (about 1 small onion)

½ cup roughly chopped fresh dill

½ cup crumbled feta

MAKE THE HARISSA-YOGURT SAUCE: In a small bowl, whisk together all the sauce ingredients. Transfer to the fridge until you're ready to serve. The sauce stores well in an airtight container in the fridge for 5 days.

MAKE THE BURGERS: In a medium bowl, combine the lamb, garlic, cumin, coriander, oregano, allspice, salt, and pepper. Using clean hands, mix until just combined and the seasoning is evenly distributed. Do not overwork the meat. Roll the lamb mixture into 8 equal-size meatballs, each about 2 inches.

IN a large skillet or a griddle, heat 1 tablespoon of the oil over medium-high heat. Place 1 or 2 lamb balls in the skillet (don't overcrowd the pan). Place a tortilla on top of each lamb ball. Using a grilling press or sturdy spatula, press down and smash the lamb balls into the skillet, creating a thin patty. Cook, undisturbed, for 3 to 4 minutes, or until the meat is browned and totally cooked through.

USE a stiff spatula to scrape underneath each burger and flip it so that the tortilla is on the bottom. Continue to cook so that the tortilla can warm and slightly crisp on the other side, 1 to 2 more minutes. Transfer to a serving platter or sheet pan. Repeat with the remaining meat and tortillas, adding more oil to the skillet for each batch as needed. Do not stack the tacos as you cook them or the tortillas will get soggy.

TO SERVE: For each taco, add a handful of romaine, tomatoes, onion, dill, and feta. Generously drizzle the top with the harissa-yogurt sauce. Serve immediately.

LEFTOVER harissa? Try my Spiced Chicken and Chickpea Skillet (page 150) or Harissa Salmon Bites with Sesame Cucumber Salad (page 214).

PERFECT OVEN-ROASTED OR SLOW COOKER POT ROAST

MAKES 6 SERVINGS | **TOTAL TIME:** 4 HOURS 30 MINUTES (OVEN-ROASTED) OR 8 TO 10 HOURS (SLOW COOKER)

DIETARY
GLUTEN-FREE
GRAIN-FREE
DAIRY-FREE
PALEO
MAKE AHEAD

There's nothing quite like a pot roast to bring comfort to the dinner table and satisfy a hungry family. This childhood favorite has always been one of my most-loved hearty meals. I love tossing it into the oven or slow cooker on a Sunday to fill the house with cozy aromas then gather everyone for a good old-fashioned Sunday supper. And the best part? Leftovers—if there are any—make for the easiest, most delicious meals throughout the week!

3½ pounds boneless chuck roast, patted dry

2½ teaspoons kosher salt, divided

1½ teaspoons freshly ground black pepper, divided

2 tablespoons tapioca flour or all-purpose flour

2 tablespoons avocado oil

1 large yellow onion, halved and sliced into ¼-inch-wide strips

3 medium carrots, cut into 2-inch pieces

4 celery stalks, cut into 2-inch pieces

3 garlic cloves, smashed

2 teaspoons Dijon mustard

1 tablespoon tomato paste

½ teaspoon smoked paprika

2 tablespoons apple cider vinegar

1 cup low-sodium beef broth

1 teaspoon roughly chopped fresh thyme leaves, plus more for serving

2 bay leaves

1½ pounds medium yellow potatoes, quartered

OVEN-ROASTED METHOD

PREHEAT the oven to 275°F.

SEASON the roast generously with 2 teaspoons of the salt and 1 teaspoon of the pepper. Sprinkle the flour over the meat and rub it in so that the roast is evenly coated.

IN a large Dutch oven, heat the oil over medium-high heat. Sear the beef until a golden-brown crust has formed on both sides, about 4 minutes per side. The beef does not need to be fully cooked through, as it will finish cooking in the oven. Transfer to a clean plate and set aside.

REDUCE the heat to medium and add the onion, carrots, celery, garlic, and the remaining ½ teaspoon salt and ½ teaspoon pepper. Cook, stirring, until the onion begins to soften, about 4 minutes.

ADD the mustard, tomato paste, and paprika and stir until well combined. Pour in the vinegar and continue to cook, stirring and scraping up any browned bits off the bottom, until the vinegar has reduced by half, about 2 minutes.

POUR in the broth and stir until well combined and the contents come to a boil then reduce the heat to a gentle simmer, about medium-low heat. Add the thyme and bay leaves, then nestle the roast and any of its juices back into the center of the pot with the veggies. Add the potatoes all around the roast.

COVER with a fitted lid and transfer to the oven. Roast until the beef is fall-apart tender, about 4 hours.

REMOVE from the oven and let cool for 10 minutes prior to serving to allow the sauce to settle. Discard the bay leaves. Shred the meat into large chunks before serving.

TO SERVE: Divide the shredded roast, onions, carrots, celery, and potatoes among shallow bowls. Ladle the sauce over the top and finish with fresh thyme, if desired.

SLOW COOKER METHOD

SEASON the roast generously with 2 teaspoons of the salt and 1 teaspoon of the pepper. Sprinkle the flour over the meat and rub it in so that the roast is evenly coated.

IN a large skillet, heat the oil over medium-high heat. Sear the beef until a golden-brown crust has formed on both sides, about 4 minutes per side. The beef does not need to be fully cooked through, as it will finish cooking in the slow cooker. Transfer to a clean plate and set aside.

IN a slow cooker, add the onion, carrots, celery, garlic, and the remaining ½ teaspoon salt and ½ teaspoon pepper. Toss to combine. Add the mustard, tomato paste, paprika, vinegar, and broth and stir until well combined with the veggies.

TRANSFER the roast and any of its juices into the slow cooker and nestle it into the center of the veggies. Add the thyme, bay leaves, and potatoes around the roast. Cover and cook on low for 8 to 10 hours, until the beef is fall-apart tender. Discard the bay leaves. Shred the meat into large chunks before serving.

TO SERVE: Divide the shredded roast, onions, carrots, celery, and potatoes among shallow bowls. Ladle the sauce over the top and finish with fresh thyme, if desired.

FROM MY KITCHEN TO YOURS

STORAGE NOTE: Store in an airtight container in the fridge for up to 4 days. Reheat gently in a saucepan over medium-low heat, or microwave in 1-minute increments, stirring after each, until warmed through.

FREEZER NOTE: Allow the roast to cool completely, then transfer it to a freezer-safe container with some of the cooking liquid. Freeze for up to 3 months. Thaw overnight in the refrigerator and reheat as directed.

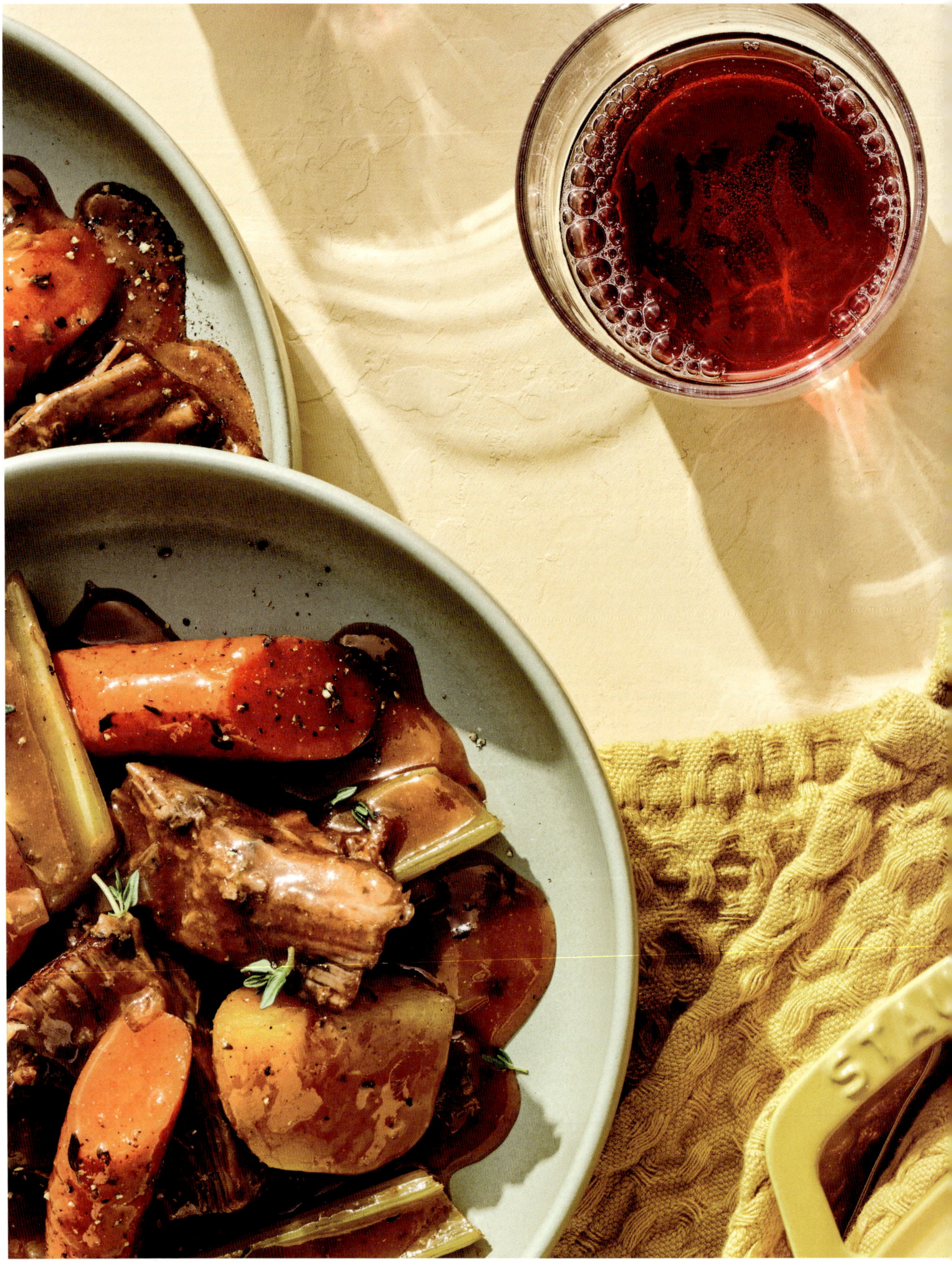

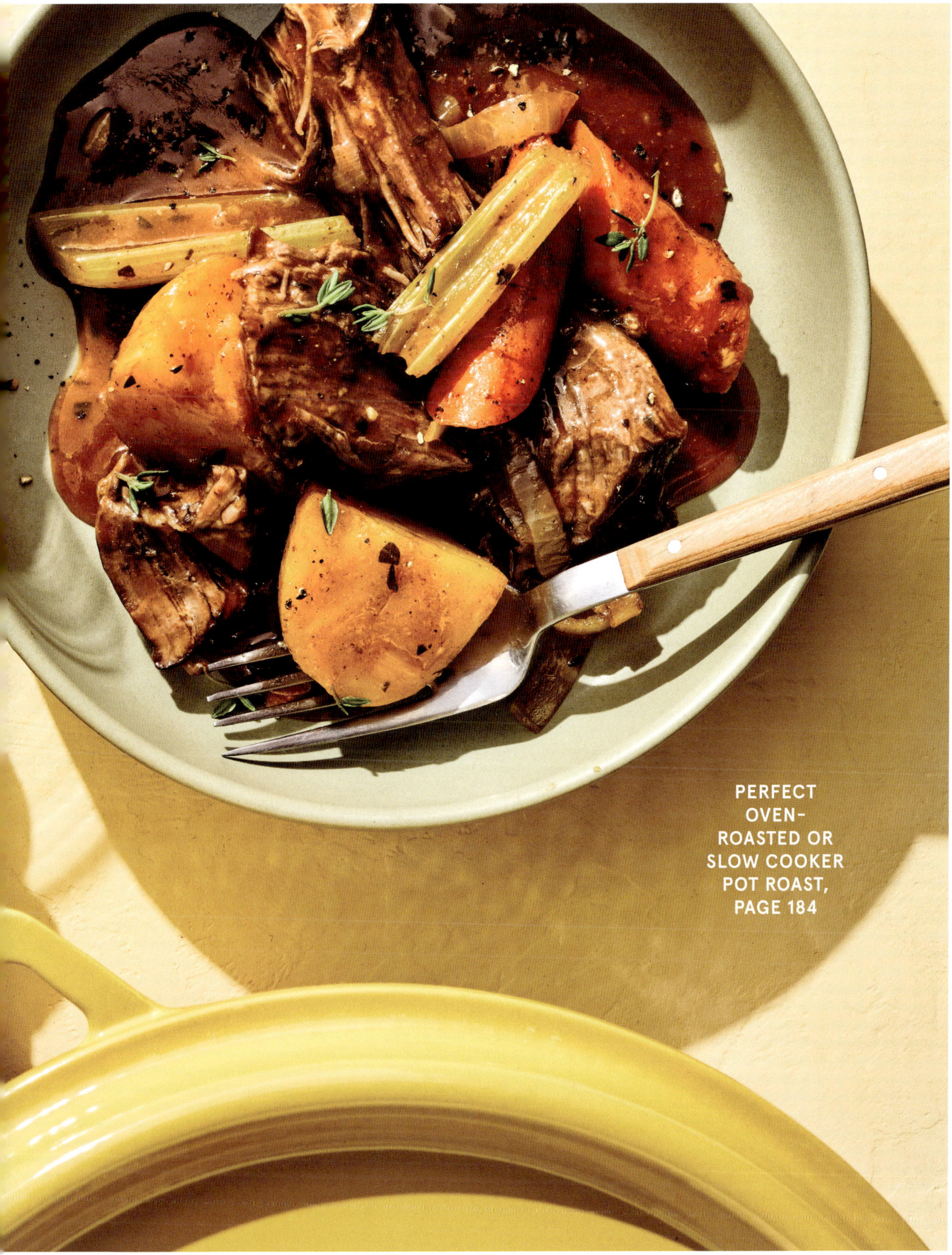
PERFECT OVEN-ROASTED OR SLOW COOKER POT ROAST, PAGE 184

SLOPPY JANES

MAKES 4 SERVINGS | **TOTAL TIME:** 1 HOUR

DIETARY
GLUTEN-FREE
GRAIN-FREE
DAIRY-FREE
PALEO
MAKE AHEAD

Meet the Sloppy Jane—a lighter, nutrient-packed twist on the classic Sloppy Joe! This version keeps all the hearty, comforting flavors but swaps the bun for a baked sweet potato, adding a touch of natural sweetness. Juicy ground beef simmered in a rich, savory sauce makes for a satisfying, family-friendly meal that's just as delicious as the original.

FOR THE SWEET POTATOES

4 medium sweet potatoes

2 tablespoons avocado oil

½ teaspoon kosher salt

FOR THE SLOPPY JANE MIXTURE

2 tablespoons avocado oil

1 cup finely diced yellow onion (about ½ medium onion)

1 cup finely diced green bell pepper (about 1 large bell pepper)

2 garlic cloves, minced

1 pound ground beef (90/10)

1 teaspoon kosher salt

½ teaspoon freshly ground black pepper

2 teaspoons chili powder

2 tablespoons tomato paste

1 tablespoon yellow mustard

¼ cup coconut aminos

Finely chopped fresh parsley leaves, optional for garnish

PREHEAT the oven to 400°F. Line a sheet pan with parchment paper.

PREPARE THE SWEET POTATOES: Scrub and pat dry the sweet potatoes and set them on the prepared sheet pan. Using a fork, pierce each potato about six times all over. Drizzle the potatoes with the oil and, using clean hands, rub the oil into the potatoes evenly. Sprinkle evenly with the salt.

TRANSFER to the oven and bake until the potatoes are tender, about 40 minutes.

MEANWHILE, MAKE THE SLOPPY JANE MIXTURE: In a large skillet, heat the oil over medium heat. Add the onion, bell pepper, and garlic. Cook, stirring, until tender, about 4 minutes.

ADD the ground beef and cook, breaking up the meat with the edge of a spoon, until the meat is cooked through and no longer pink, about 7 minutes. Drain off the excess fat and return the beef to the pan.

ADD the salt, black pepper, chili powder, tomato paste, mustard, and coconut aminos and stir until well combined and the meat is coated in the sauce, 3 to 4 more minutes. Turn the heat to low, cover, and keep warm until the potatoes are ready.

ASSEMBLE THE SLOPPY JANES: When the potatoes are done, remove them from the oven and let cool enough to handle. Carve a slit at the top of each potato and, using a fork, fluff the inside of the potato. Spoon the Sloppy Jane mixture into the center of the sweet potato to stuff it. Garnish with parsley, if desired.

STORE leftovers in an airtight container in the fridge for up to 3 days. Reheat in the microwave in 1-minute increments, stirring the filling after each, until warmed through. Garnish with parsley, if desired.

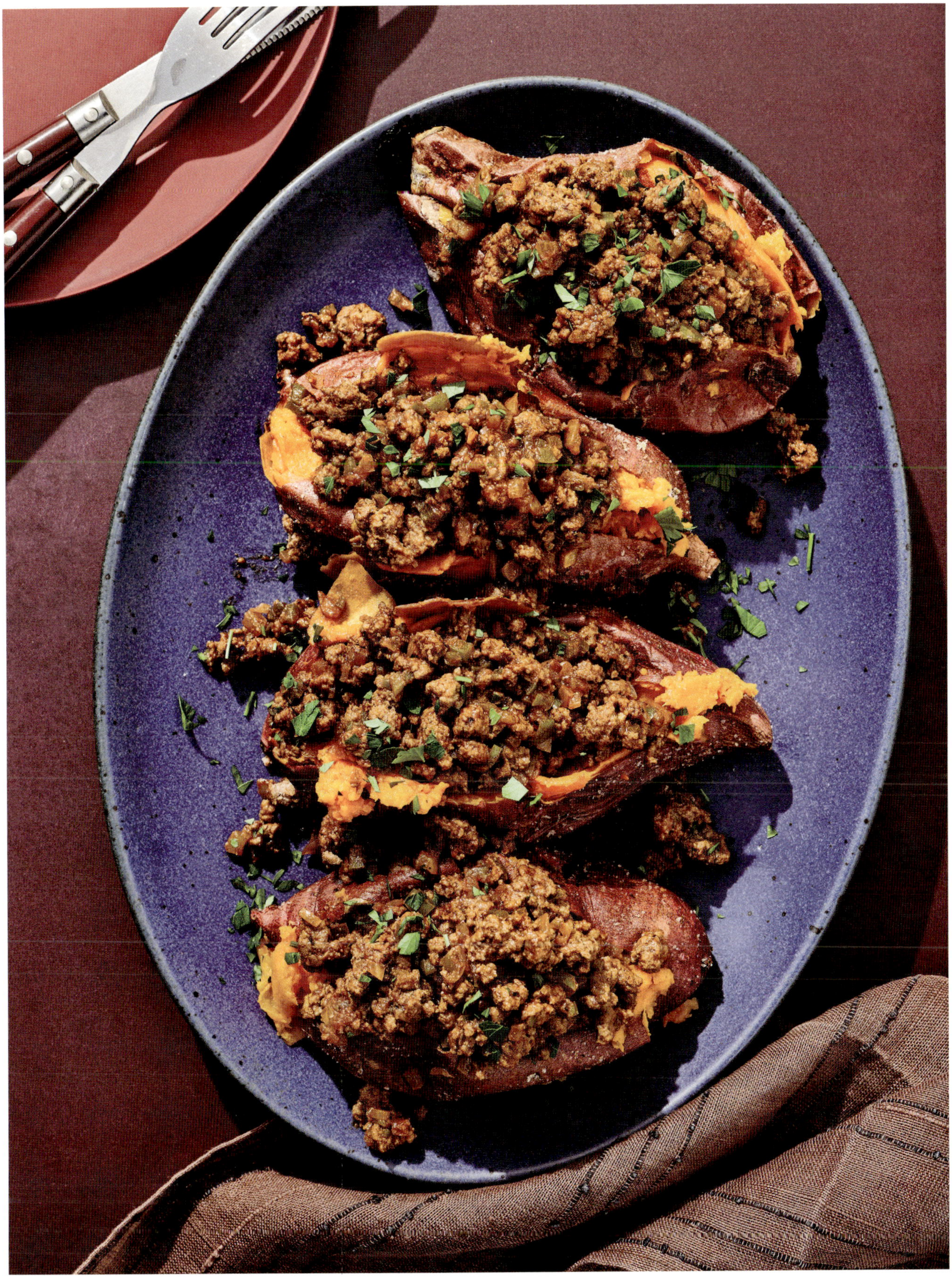

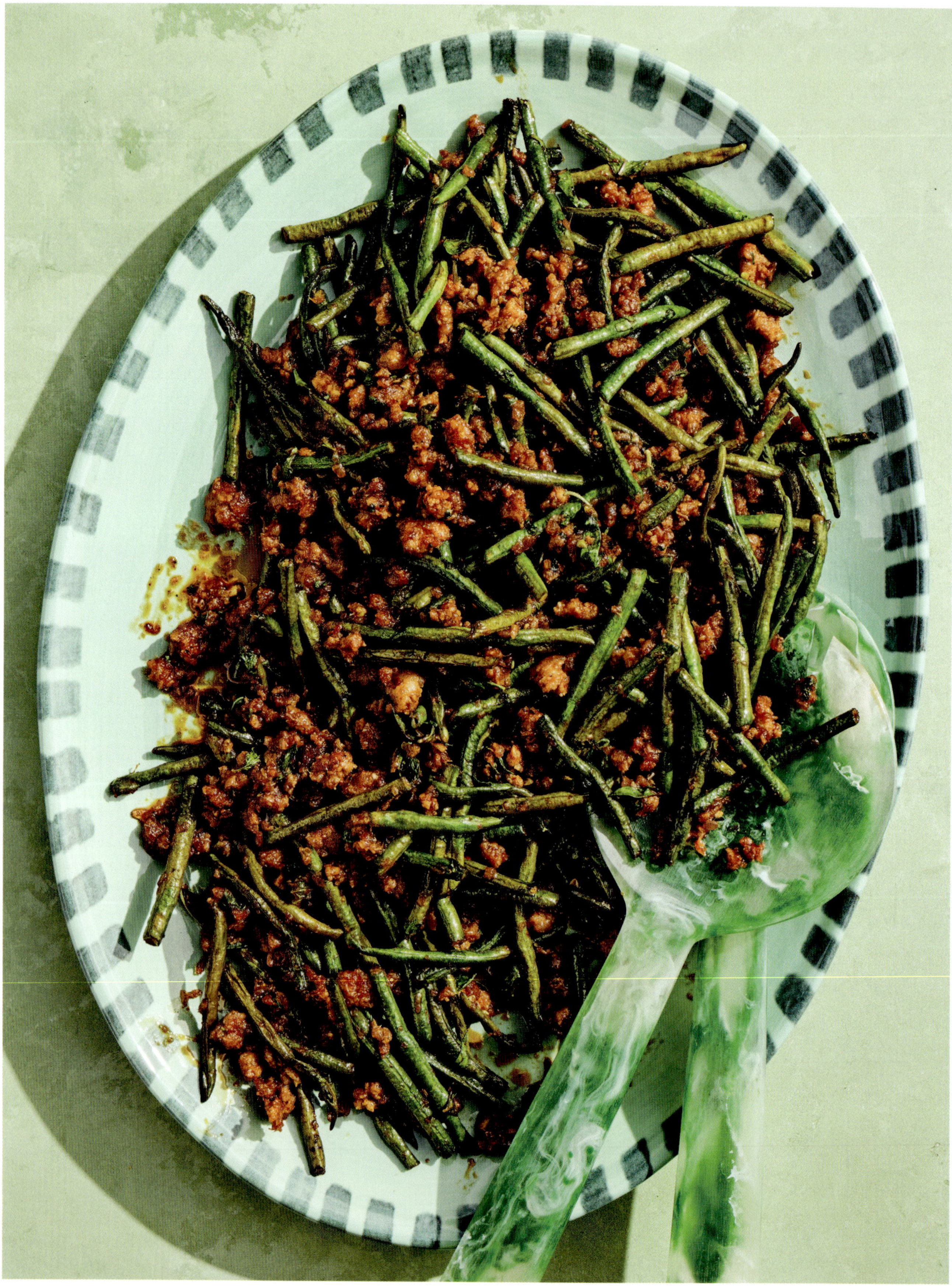

RED CURRY PORK STIR-FRY

MAKES 4 SERVINGS | **TOTAL TIME:** 20 MINUTES

DIETARY
GLUTEN-FREE
GRAIN-FREE
DAIRY-FREE
PALEO
MAKE AHEAD

While on vacation, my mother-in-law, GoGo, taught me how to make pad prik king, her favorite Thai vegetarian dish. Pad prik king is a spicy stir-fry typically made with green beans and red curry paste, but here I've added ground pork to boost the protein and make it even heartier. This recipe is simple yet incredibly flavorful and truly a dish that I can't get enough of.

- 2 tablespoons avocado oil
- 1 pound ground pork
- 1½ teaspoons kosher salt, divided
- 2 teaspoons toasted sesame oil
- ¾ cup minced shallot (about 2 large shallots)
- 2 tablespoons Thai red curry paste
- 1 pound yardlong beans, trimmed into 2-inch pieces (see note)
- ½ teaspoon freshly ground black pepper
- 3 garlic cloves, minced
- ¼ cup coconut aminos
- 2 tablespoons fish sauce
- 1 tablespoon coconut sugar
- 1 tablespoon freshly squeezed lime juice (about ½ lime)
- ½ cup packed Thai or regular basil leaves
- ¼ cup roughly chopped fresh cilantro leaves and tender stems
- Prepared cauliflower rice or steamed rice

IN a large, deep skillet or wok, heat the avocado oil over medium-high heat. Add the pork and use the back of a spatula to press the pork down into a single layer. Cook, undisturbed, until one side is crisp and golden brown, about 4 minutes. Add 1 teaspoon of the salt and continue to cook, breaking up the pork with the edge of a spatula, until it is cooked through and no longer pink, about 3 more minutes. Using a slotted spoon, transfer the cooked pork to a clean plate and set aside.

REDUCE the heat to medium and add the toasted sesame oil and shallots to the skillet. Cook, stirring, until shallots are softened, about 2 minutes.

ADD the curry paste, yardlong beans, the remaining ½ teaspoon salt, and the pepper. Cook, tossing often, until the yardlong beans are crisp-tender, about 5 minutes.

ADD the garlic, coconut aminos, fish sauce, and coconut sugar. Stir to combine and bring to a simmer. Continue to cook, tossing, until the yardlong beans are well coated in the sauce, 2 to 3 more minutes.

REDUCE the heat to medium-low and add the pork and any of its juices back into the skillet. Stir in the lime juice, Thai basil, and cilantro. Stir until the herbs are just wilted. Remove from heat and serve immediately with prepared rice.

STORE leftovers in an airtight container in the fridge for up to 3 days. Reheat in a skillet or wok over medium heat to keep the pork tender and yardlong beans crisp, or microwave in 1-minute increments, stirring after each, until warmed through. Serve with rice.

LEFTOVER red curry paste? Try my Chicken Khao Soi–Inspired Soup (page 87), Thai Red Curry Shrimp Noodles (page 110), or Tangy Thai Braised Chicken (page 162).

FROM MY KITCHEN TO YOURS

Yardlong beans, also known as Chinese long beans, are a staple in many Asian dishes and are known for their mild flavor and crisp texture, making them perfect for this recipe. If you can't find yardlong beans, you can substitute French green beans. While they're slightly crisper and waxier, they still work well and complement the dish beautifully.

SLOW COOKER OR PRESSURE COOKER THAI-INSPIRED SHREDDED BEEF BOWLS

MAKES 6 SERVINGS | **TOTAL TIME:** 4 TO 8 HOURS (SLOW COOKER) OR 1 HOUR 15 MINUTES (PRESSURE COOKER)

DIETARY
GLUTEN-FREE
DAIRY-FREE
GRAIN-FREE
PALEO (IF MODIFIED)
MAKE AHEAD

Starting dinner in the slow cooker in the morning is the best trick for a busy day! This recipe features tender, tangy beef that cooks all day and is served over rice with a quick-pickled veggie salad. I always have mini bell peppers on hand for snacking, and slicing them up along with a carrot, onion, and chiles makes for a colorful, crunchy salad that brightens this dish. Prefer the quick convenience of a pressure cooker? You'll find that method here as well!

FOR THE STEAK

4 garlic cloves, minced

1 teaspoon minced fresh ginger

¼ cup coconut sugar

⅓ cup coconut aminos

1 tablespoon fish sauce

2 tablespoons creamy unsweetened peanut butter (sub almond butter for paleo)

1 to 3 Thai chiles, minced (see note, page 122)

2 pounds flap or flank steak, trimmed of excess fat, patted dry, and cut into 4 equal-size pieces

2 teaspoons kosher salt

1 teaspoon freshly ground black pepper

½ cup low-sodium beef broth (pressure cooker only)

Grated zest of ½ lime

2 tablespoons freshly squeezed lime juice (about 1 lime)

SLOW COOKER METHOD

IN a slow cooker, whisk together the garlic, ginger, coconut sugar, coconut aminos, fish sauce, peanut butter, and Thai chiles.

PREPARE THE STEAK: Season the steak evenly with the salt and pepper, then nestle it into the slow cooker. Cook on high for 4 hours or low for 8 hours, until the beef is fall-apart tender.

WHEN the cook time is complete, transfer the steak pieces to a rimmed sheet pan and use two forks to shred the meat. Transfer the meat and its juices back to the slow cooker. Add the lime zest and lime juice and toss to combine. Keep on warm while you prepare the veggie salad.

PRESSURE COOKER METHOD

IN a pressure cooker, whisk together the garlic, ginger, coconut sugar, coconut aminos, fish sauce, peanut butter, Thai chiles, and broth.

SEASON the steak evenly with the salt and pepper, then nestle it into the pressure cooker. Secure the lid on the pressure cooker and ensure the vent is sealed. Press the "manual" or "pressure cook" button (depending on your model) and set the time to 60 minutes.

WHEN the cook time is finished, release the pressure manually by carefully turning the valve and letting it vent completely. When it is done venting, carefully remove the lid. Transfer the steak pieces to a rimmed sheet pan and use two forks to shred the meat. Transfer the meat and its juices back to the pressure cooker. Add the lime zest and lime juice and toss to combine. Keep warm while you prepare the veggie salad.

FOR THE VEGGIE SALAD

12 mini bell peppers, seeded and sliced into thin strips

½ cup halved and thinly sliced red onion (about ½ small onion)

2 cups matchstick-cut carrots

1 to 3 Thai chiles, minced

2 garlic cloves, minced

2 tablespoons rice vinegar

4 teaspoons fish sauce

Pinch of kosher salt

FOR SERVING

Prepared cauliflower rice or steamed rice

Fresh cilantro leaves

Fresh Thai or regular basil leaves

Lime wedges

FOR BOTH METHODS

MAKE THE VEGGIE SALAD: In a large bowl, toss together all the salad ingredients to combine. Set aside for at least 10 minutes to lightly pickle.

TO SERVE: Divide the beef among bowls along with the prepared rice and veggie salad. Top with the cilantro and basil. Serve with lime wedges.

STORE leftovers in an airtight container in the fridge for up to 4 days, keeping the veggie salad separate. Reheat the beef in a skillet over medium heat, or microwave in 1-minute increments, stirring between, until warmed through. Assemble bowls with the veggie salad, rice, desired toppings, and lime wedges.

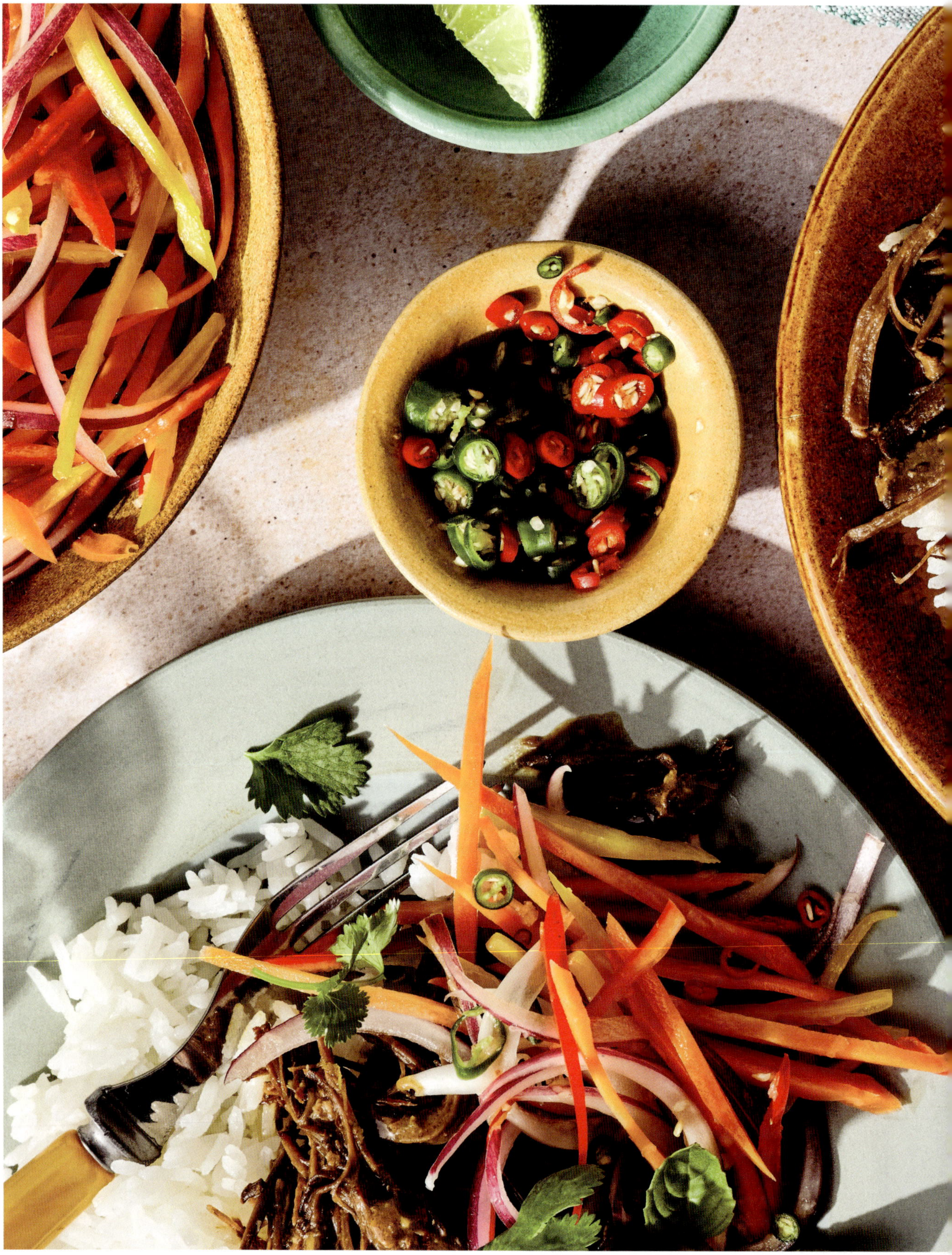

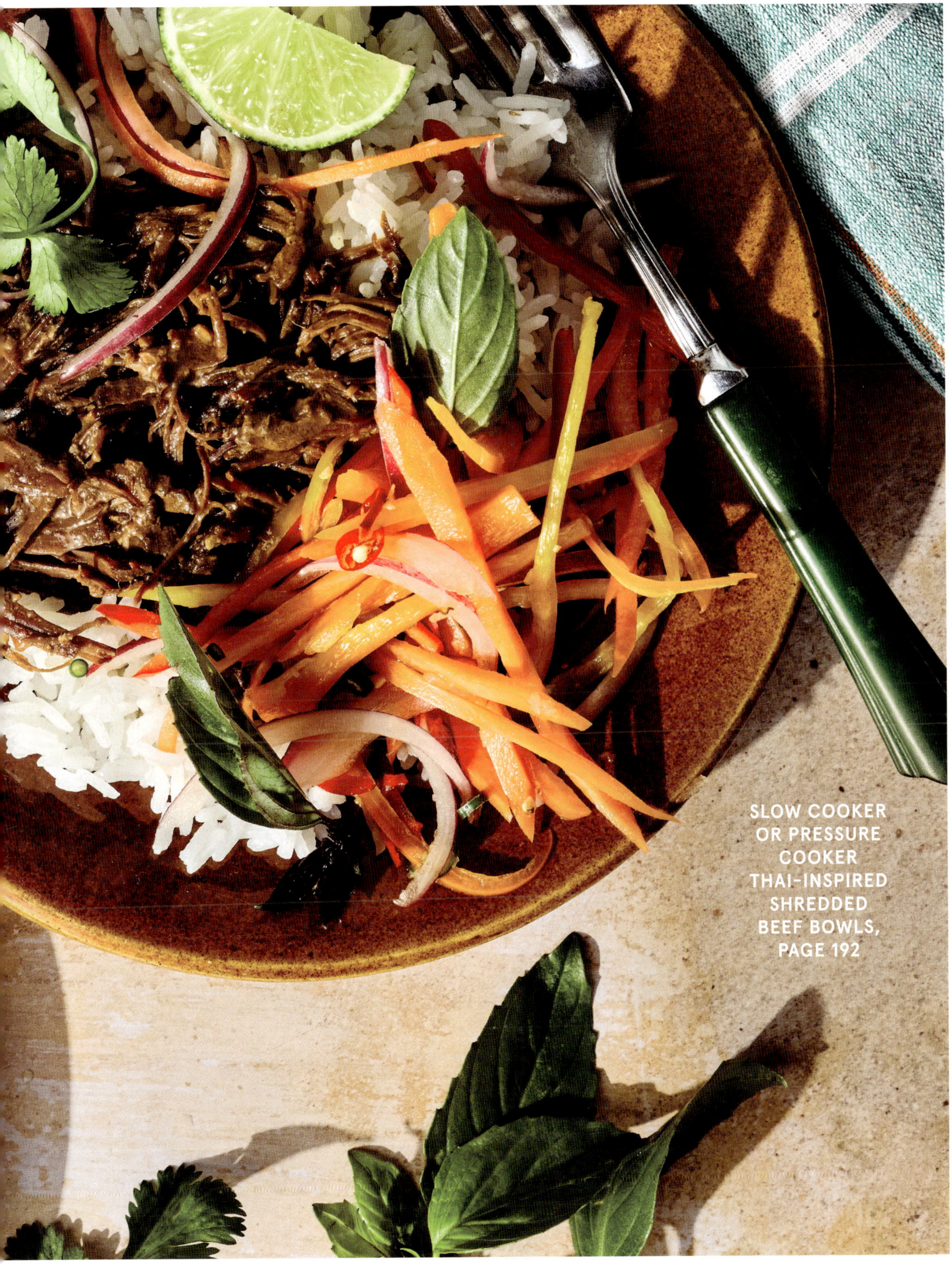

SLOW COOKER OR PRESSURE COOKER THAI-INSPIRED SHREDDED BEEF BOWLS, PAGE 192

SWEET AND SAVORY KOREAN-STYLE BEEF BOWLS

MAKES 4 SERVINGS | **TOTAL TIME:** 35 MINUTES

DIETARY
GLUTEN-FREE
DAIRY-FREE
GRAIN-FREE
MAKE AHEAD

These ground beef bulgogi-inspired bowls are a quick and flavorful take on the Korean classic. Tender beef is coated in a savory-sweet sauce with hints of ginger, garlic, and gochujang, then served over a bed of rice and paired with tangy kimchi. My kiddos don't love kimchi (yet!), so I serve theirs with sliced cucumbers! It's a fantastic meal that brings bold flavors to the table in just thirty-five minutes.

FOR THE SAUCE

1 tablespoon toasted sesame oil

¼ cup coconut aminos

2 teaspoons fish sauce

1 teaspoon grated fresh ginger

2 tablespoons coconut sugar

2 tablespoons gluten-free gochujang (see note, page 92)

1 tablespoon freshly squeezed lime juice (about ½ lime)

3 garlic cloves, minced

FOR THE BEEF

2 tablespoons avocado oil

½ cup finely diced white onion (about ½ small onion)

1½ pounds ground beef (90/10)

1½ teaspoons kosher salt

½ teaspoon freshly ground black pepper

3 green onions thinly sliced on the diagonal, white and green parts kept separate

FOR SERVING

Prepared cauliflower rice or steamed rice

1 tablespoon toasted sesame seeds

2 cups store-bought kimchi

MAKE THE SAUCE: In a small bowl, whisk together all the sauce ingredients. Set aside.

PREPARE THE BEEF: In a large, deep skillet, heat the avocado oil over medium-high heat. Add the white onion and cook, stirring often, until softened, about 2 minutes. Add the ground beef and use the back of a spatula to press the beef down into a single layer. Cook, undisturbed, until one side is crisp and golden brown, about 4 minutes. Continue to cook, breaking up the meat with the edge of a spatula, until it is cooked through and no longer pink, about 3 more minutes. Drain off the excess fat and return the beef to the pan.

ADD the salt, pepper, and white parts of the green onions and pour in the sauce. Cook, stirring, until the sauce has coated the meat and reduced slightly, 3 to 4 more minutes.

TO SERVE: Place some prepared rice in each bowl and spoon the beef and sauce over the top. Garnish with toasted sesame seeds and the green parts of the green onions and nestle in plenty of kimchi on the side.

STORE leftovers in an airtight container in the fridge for up to 3 days, keeping rice and kimchi separate. Reheat the beef in a skillet over medium heat until hot, or microwave in 1-minute increments, stirring between, until warmed through. Assemble bowls with rice, kimchi, and garnishes.

LEFTOVER kimchi or gochujang? Try my Kimchi Ramen (page 92).

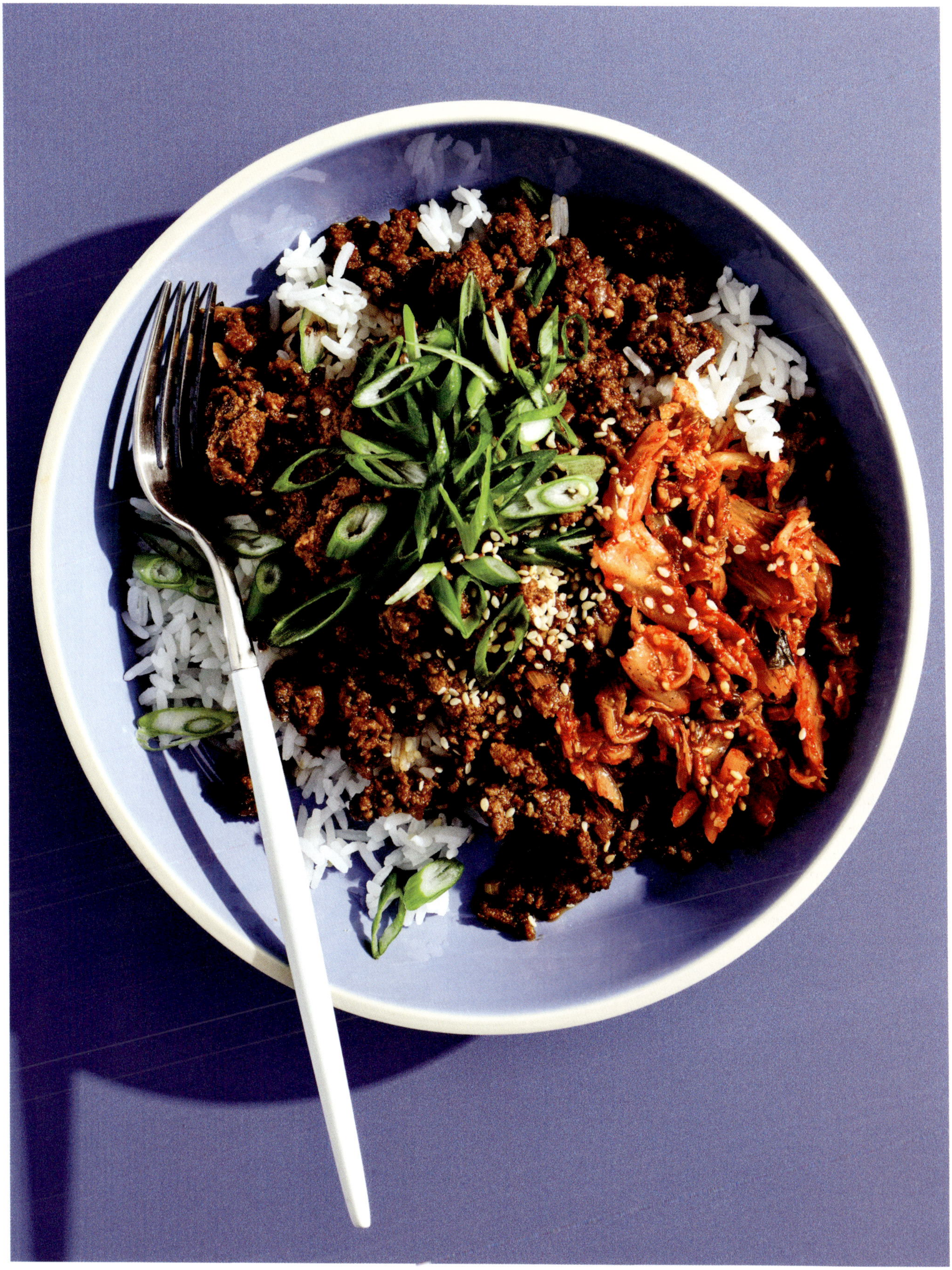

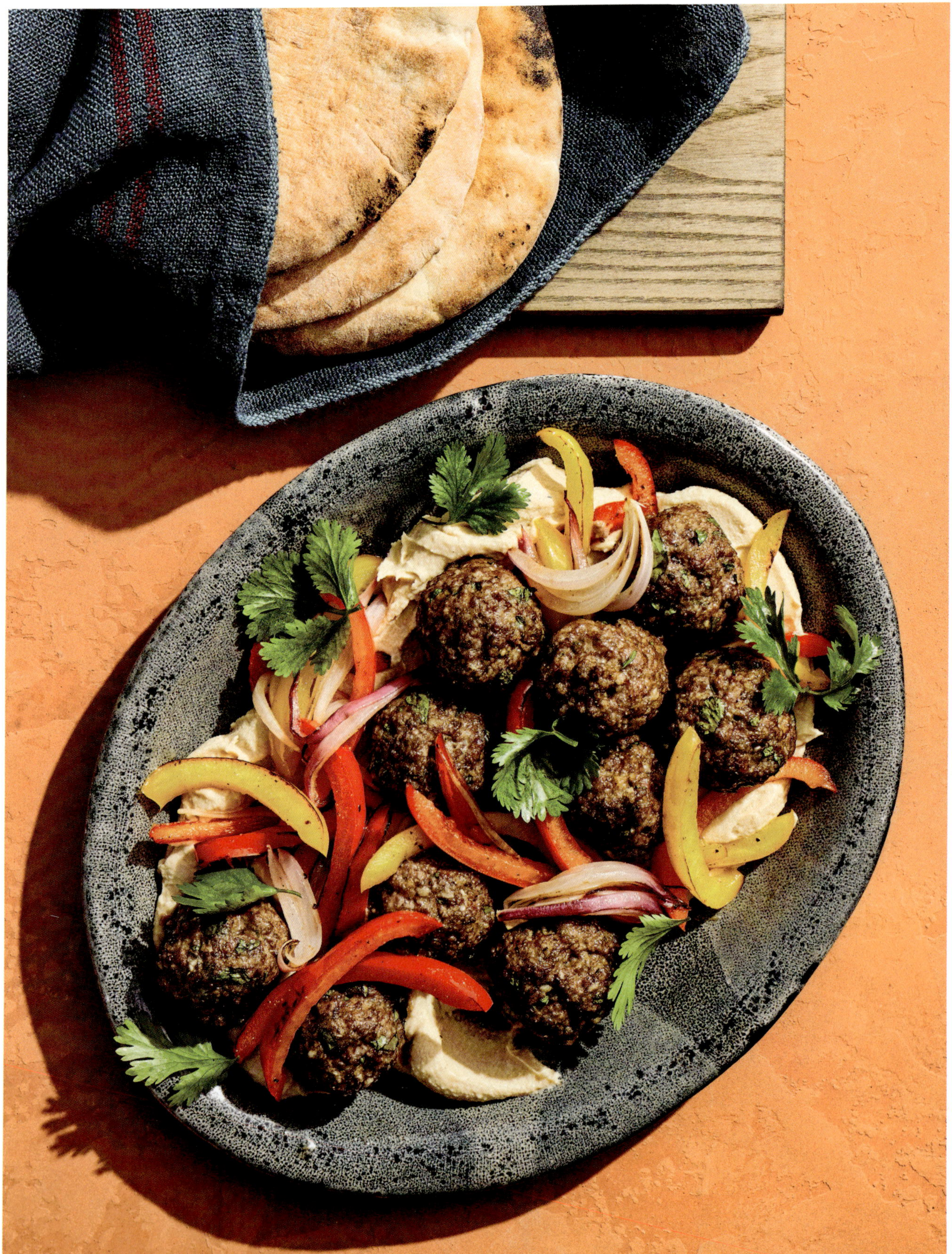

SHEET PAN KOFTA MEATBALLS WITH VEGGIES

MAKES 4 SERVINGS | **TOTAL TIME**: 35 MINUTES

DIETARY
DAIRY-FREE
GLUTEN-FREE (IF MODIFIED)
GRAIN-FREE (IF MODIFIED)
MAKE AHEAD

Kofta, a classic Middle Eastern dish traditionally made with ground lamb or beef, is often shaped into patties or skewers and grilled to perfection. Here, I've turned kofta into easy sheet pan meatballs, roasting them alongside veggies for a no-fuss, flavor-packed dinner. They're fantastic on their own, but I love pairing them with store-bought hummus and warm pita for a quick, satisfying meal.

FOR THE VEGGIES

2 medium red bell peppers, seeded and sliced into ¼-inch strips

1 medium yellow bell pepper, seeded and sliced into ¼-inch strips

½ large red onion, sliced into ¼-inch strips

1 tablespoon extra-virgin olive oil

½ teaspoon kosher salt

¼ teaspoon freshly ground black pepper

½ teaspoon ground cumin

FOR THE MEATBALLS

1 pound ground lamb or ground beef

1 large egg

¼ cup gluten-free panko bread crumbs

3 garlic cloves, minced

2 teaspoons ground cumin

2 teaspoons ground coriander

1 teaspoon allspice

¼ teaspoon cayenne pepper, optional

1 teaspoon kosher salt

½ teaspoon freshly ground black pepper

2 tablespoons finely chopped fresh cilantro leaves

FOR SERVING

⅓ cup store-bought hummus

Fresh cilantro leaves

Warm pita bread (omit for gluten-free and grain-free)

POSITION a rack at the top of the oven and preheat the oven to 425°F.

PLACE the bell peppers and onion on a large sheet pan. Drizzle with the oil and season with the salt, black pepper, and cumin. Toss until well combined. Spread into a single layer.

IN a medium bowl, combine the lamb, egg, panko, garlic, cumin, coriander, allspice, cayenne (if using), salt, black pepper, and cilantro. Using clean hands, mix until well combined, then roll into 1½-inch meatballs. Nestle the meatballs onto the sheet pan with the veggies.

TRANSFER to the top oven rack and bake until the meatballs are golden on the tops and no longer pink in the center, and the veggies are tender, about 15 minutes.

TO SERVE: Place 1 to 2 tablespoons of hummus in a shallow bowl or on a small plate. Plate the meatballs and veggies over the hummus and garnish with cilantro. Serve with warm pita (if using).

STORE leftovers in an airtight container in the fridge for up to 3 days. Reheat on a sheet pan in the oven at 350°F for 10 to 12 minutes, in a skillet over medium heat, or microwave in 1-minute increments, tossing after each, until warmed through. Serve with fresh hummus and pita (if using), and garnish with cilantro.

SKILLET UNSTUFFED CABBAGE ROLLS

MAKES 6 SERVINGS | **TOTAL TIME:** 55 MINUTES

DIETARY
GLUTEN-FREE
DAIRY-FREE (IF MODIFIED)
MAKE AHEAD

If you love the cozy, comforting flavors of traditional cabbage rolls but not the time it takes to roll and bake them, this one-skillet version is for you. It's got all the hearty goodness—savory ground beef, warming spices, tender cabbage, and fluffy rice—cooked together in a flavorful tomato broth until everything is perfectly tender. With fresh herbs stirred in at the end, this easy weeknight dinner is vibrant, satisfying, and just as delicious as the classic, minus the fuss.

- 1 tablespoon avocado oil
- 1 cup small-diced yellow onion (about 1 small onion)
- 1 pound ground beef (90/10)
- 1½ teaspoons kosher salt, plus more to taste
- ½ teaspoon freshly ground black pepper, plus more to taste
- 1 teaspoon allspice
- 2 teaspoons ground cumin
- 2 teaspoons smoked paprika
- 4 cups roughly chopped green cabbage (about ½ medium head)
- 4 garlic cloves, minced
- 3 tablespoons tomato paste
- 3 tablespoons tamari
- 1 cup basmati rice, rinsed until the water runs clear
- One 14.5-ounce can fire-roasted tomatoes
- 2 cups low-sodium beef broth
- 1 tablespoon coconut sugar
- 1 tablespoon freshly squeezed lemon juice (about ½ lemon)
- ¼ cup finely chopped fresh parsley, plus more for serving
- ¼ cup finely chopped fresh dill, plus more for serving
- Whole-milk plain Greek yogurt, optional for topping (omit for dairy-free)
- Lemon wedges, for serving

IN a large, deep skillet or 3.5-quart braiser with fitted lid, heat the oil over medium-high heat. Add the onion and ground beef and cook, breaking up the meat with the edge of a spoon, until the meat is browned and no longer pink and the onions are tender, about 7 minutes. Drain off the excess fat and return the beef and onions to the pan.

REDUCE the heat to medium and add the salt, pepper, allspice, cumin, and paprika. Cook, tossing, to toast the spices until they are fragrant, about 2 minutes.

ADD the cabbage and garlic and continue to cook, tossing, until the cabbage is slightly softened, about 3 minutes. Add the tomato paste and tamari and stir until well combined.

ADD the rice, tomatoes, broth, coconut sugar, lemon juice, parsley, and dill and stir until well combined. Bring to a rapid simmer, then reduce the heat to a gentle simmer, about medium-low heat, cover, and let cook for 20 minutes. Remove the skillet from the heat and keep covered for 10 minutes to let the rice steam until tender.

FLUFF the rice with a fork and garnish with more dill and parsley before serving.

SCOOP into bowls and top with a dollop of yogurt, if desired. Serve with lemon wedges.

STORE leftovers in an airtight container in the fridge for up to 3 days, separate of toppings. Reheat gently in a skillet over medium heat, or microwave in 1-minute increments, stirring after each, until warmed through. Serve with fresh toppings as desired.

LEFTOVER cabbage? Try my Tangy Thai Crunch Salad with Seared Salmon (page 70) or Shortcut Chicken Pozole Verde (page 94).

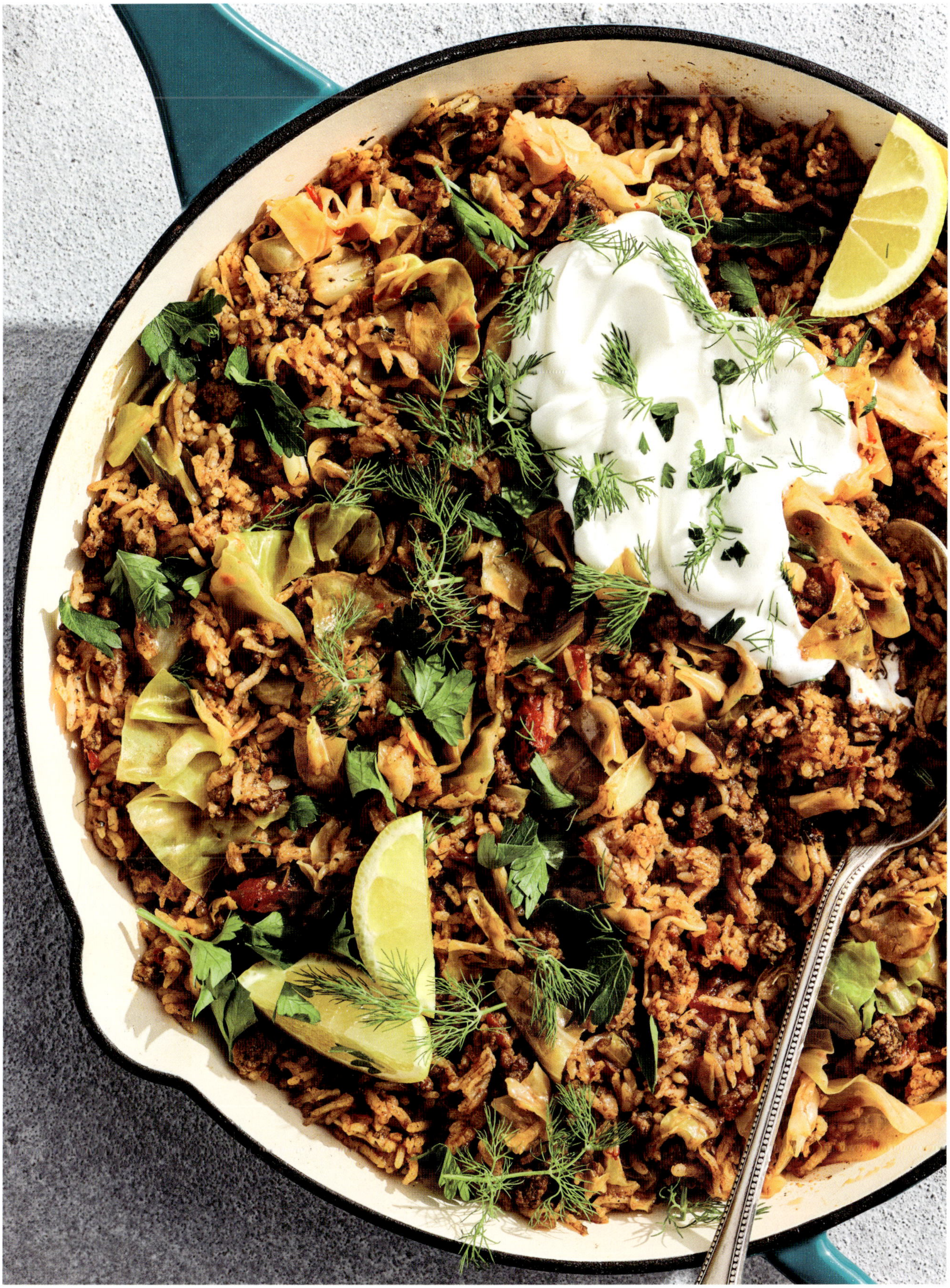

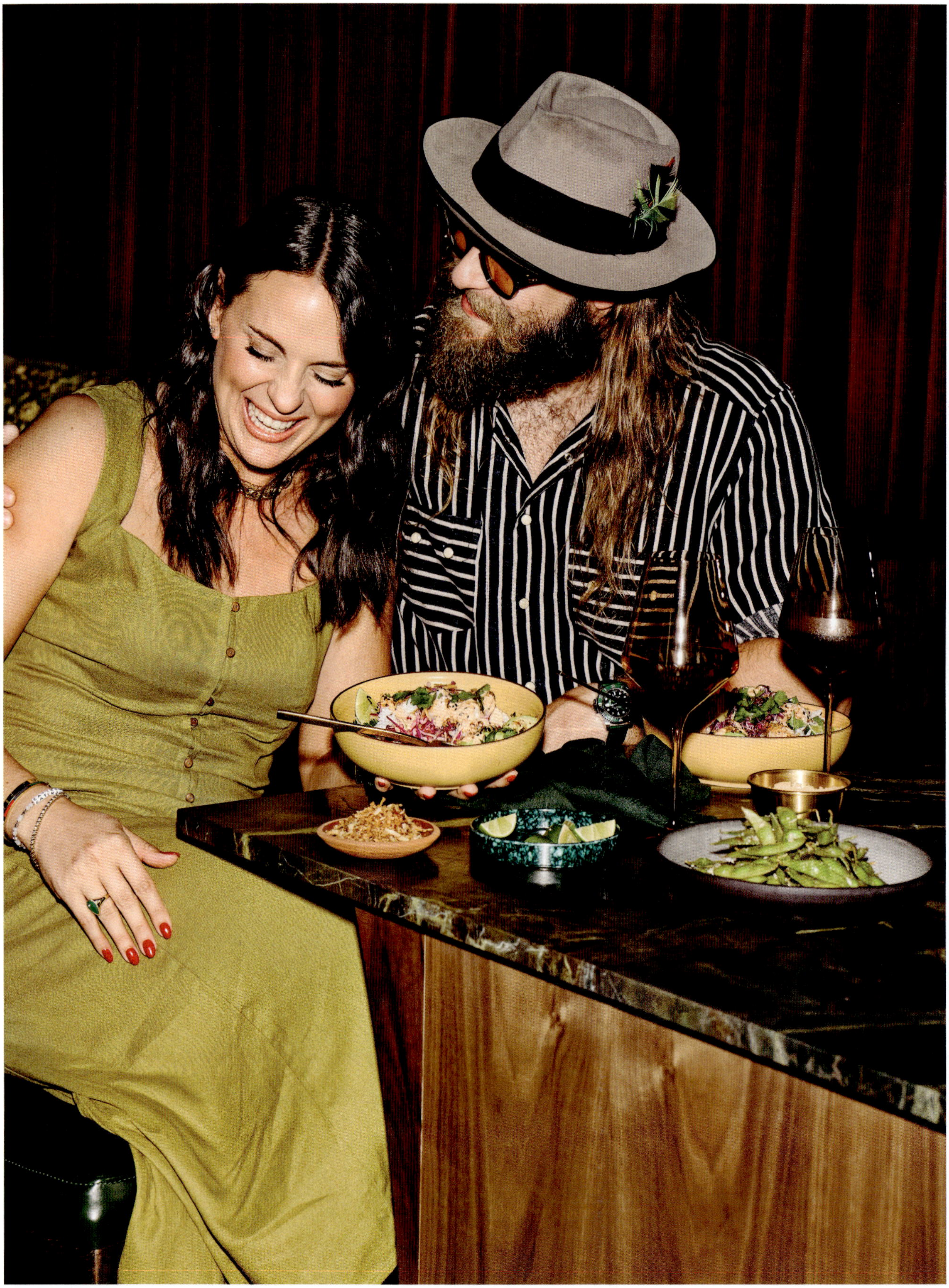

GARLIC SHRIMP STIR-FRY

MAKES 4 SERVINGS | **TOTAL TIME:** 25 MINUTES

DIETARY
GLUTEN-FREE
GRAIN-FREE
DAIRY-FREE
PALEO
MAKE AHEAD

This quick and flavorful stir-fry comes together in twenty-five minutes with juicy shrimp, crisp veggies, and a garlicky, savory-sweet sauce. Serve over rice (or cauliflower rice) and top with chili crisp for a satisfying gluten-free and paleo-friendly meal.

FOR THE SAUCE

¼ cup coconut aminos

1 teaspoon fish sauce

¼ cup low-sodium chicken broth

2 teaspoons toasted sesame oil

1 tablespoon honey

6 garlic cloves, minced

1 teaspoon grated fresh ginger

1 tablespoon tapioca flour

FOR THE STIR-FRY

2 tablespoons avocado oil

3 cups roughly chopped broccoli florets (about 1 medium head)

1 medium red bell pepper, seeded and thinly sliced

1 cup halved and thinly sliced red onion (about 1 small onion)

1 pound peeled, deveined, and tail-off shrimp (31/35 count), patted dry

1 teaspoon kosher salt

½ teaspoon freshly ground black pepper

Prepared cauliflower rice or steamed rice

Chili crisp, optional for serving (see note, page 222)

MAKE THE SAUCE: In a small bowl, whisk together all the sauce ingredients until well combined. Set aside.

MAKE THE STIR-FRY: In a large, deep nonstick skillet, heat the oil over medium heat. Add the broccoli, bell pepper, and onion and cook, stirring, until the veggies are slightly tender, 4 to 5 minutes.

ADD the shrimp, salt, and black pepper to the pan and continue to cook, tossing, until they begin to turn pink. They do not need to be fully cooked through, as they will finish cooking in the sauce.

POUR in the sauce and cook, tossing often, until the shrimp is cooked through and the sauce has thickened, about 4 more minutes. Toss once more to ensure the shrimp are nice and coated.

SERVE over prepared rice with a drizzle of chili crisp, if desired.

STORE shrimp in an airtight container in the fridge for up to 3 days. Reheat in a hot skillet or wok just until warmed through, about 2 minutes, to keep the shrimp tender and veggies crisp. Avoid microwaving, as the shrimp can become rubbery.

LEFTOVER chili crisp? Try my Chili Crisp Citrus Salmon (page 222).

FRESH CATCH

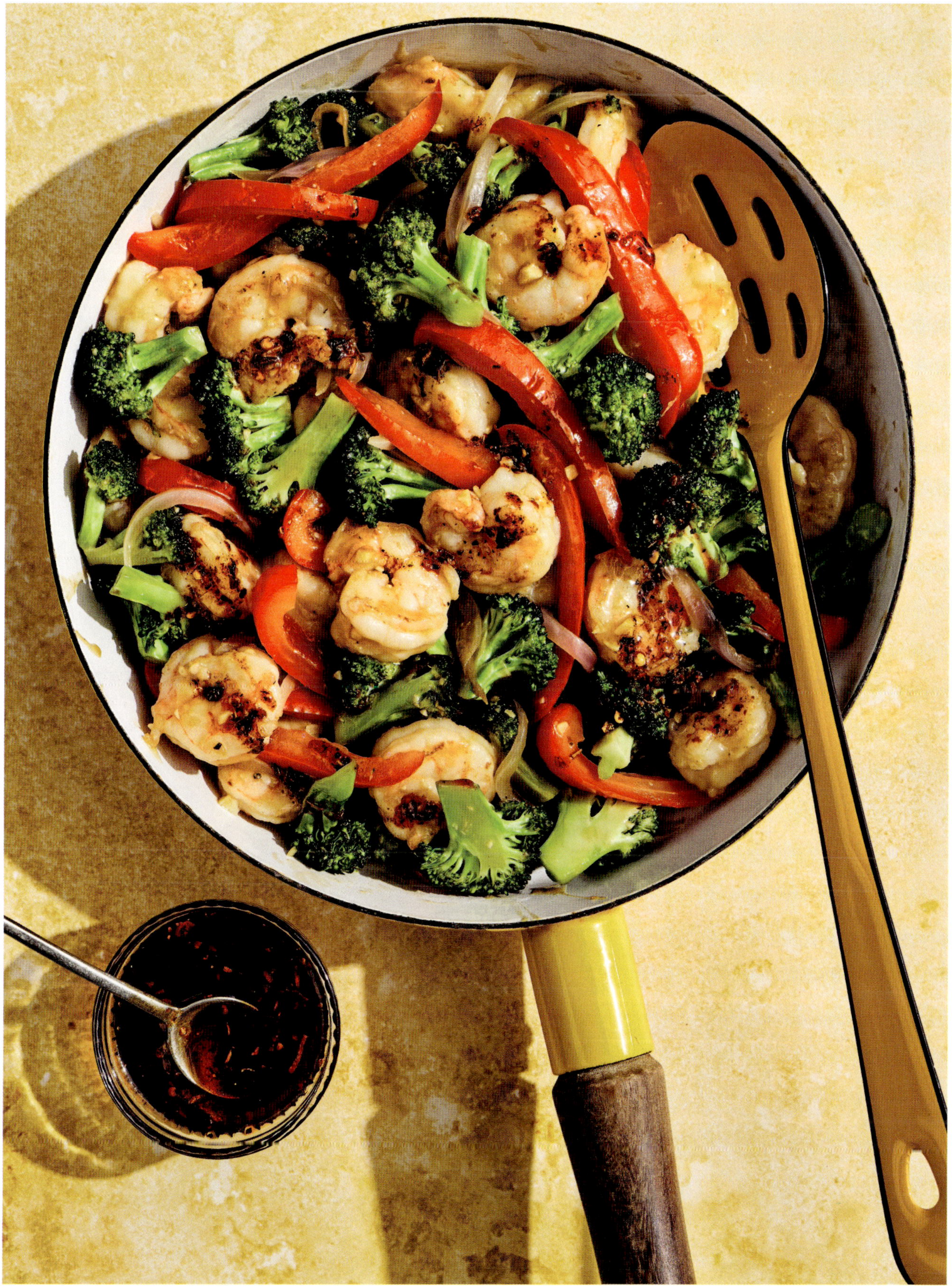

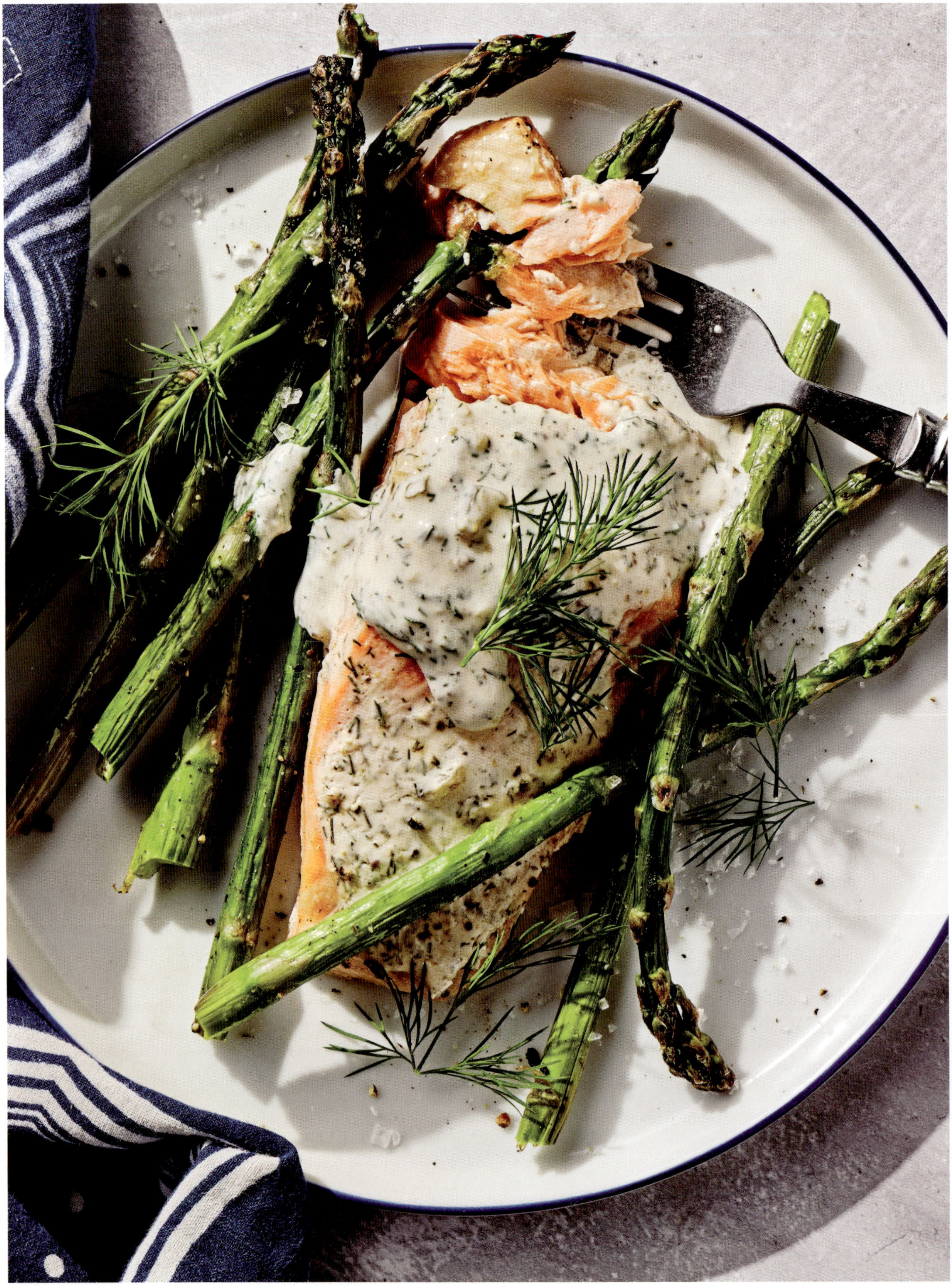

REALLY DILLY SHEET PAN SALMON

MAKES 4 SERVINGS | **TOTAL TIME:** 30 MINUTES

DIETARY
GLUTEN-FREE
GRAIN-FREE
MAKE AHEAD

This salmon dish is a weeknight favorite, featuring a yogurt sauce loaded with both dill relish and fresh dill for a tangy, tartar-like twist. Roasted alongside asparagus, it's a light one-pan meal with minimal cleanup. Perfect for busy weeknights!

FOR THE DILLY SAUCE

- ½ cup whole-milk plain Greek yogurt
- 1 tablespoon dill relish
- 1 teaspoon whole-grain Dijon mustard
- 2 tablespoons finely chopped fresh dill
- 1 teaspoon Louisiana-style hot sauce
- 2 tablespoons freshly squeezed lemon juice (about 1 lemon)
- 1 garlic clove, minced
- ¼ teaspoon kosher salt
- ¼ teaspoon freshly ground black pepper

FOR THE ASPARAGUS AND SALMON

- 1 bunch asparagus, woody ends trimmed
- 2 tablespoons extra-virgin olive oil
- 1½ teaspoons kosher salt, divided
- ¾ teaspoon freshly ground black pepper
- 4 skin-on center-cut salmon fillets (6 ounces each), patted dry and pin bones removed
- Finely chopped fresh dill, for garnish
- Lemon wedges, for serving

PREHEAT the oven to 400°F. Line a sheet pan with parchment paper and set aside.

MAKE THE DILLY SAUCE: In a medium bowl, stir together all the sauce ingredients until well combined. In a small bowl, set aside 2½ tablespoons of the sauce for the salmon, reserving the rest for serving.

PREPARE THE ASPARAGUS AND SALMON: Place the asparagus on the prepared sheet pan and drizzle with the oil. Season with ½ teaspoon of the salt and ½ teaspoon of the pepper. Toss until the asparagus is well coated. Push the asparagus to the sides of the sheet pan, making enough room in the center for the salmon fillets.

PLACE the salmon fillets in the center of the sheet pan. Sprinkle the tops evenly with the remaining 1 teaspoon of the salt and ¼ teaspoon of the pepper. Evenly distribute the reserved 2½ tablespoons of the dilly sauce on top of each fillet and spread to evenly coat the tops of the salmon.

TRANSFER to the oven and bake until the asparagus is tender and the salmon is cooked through and flakes easily with a fork, 12 to 14 minutes.

DIVIDE the salmon fillets and asparagus among four plates. Top with fresh dill and serve with the remaining dilly sauce and lemon wedges on the side.

STORE leftovers in an airtight container in the fridge for up to 3 days, keeping the sauce separate. Reheat on a sheet pan in the oven at 325°F for 10 to 12 minutes, in the air fryer at 350°F for 4 to 6 minutes, or microwave in 1-minute increments until warmed through. Top with fresh dill and serve with dilly sauce and lemon wedges.

LEFTOVER dill relish? Try my Classic Tuna Salad (page 62).

HALIBUT IN WHITE WINE TOMATO-BASIL SAUCE

MAKES 4 SERVINGS | **TOTAL TIME**: 25 MINUTES

DIETARY
GLUTEN-FREE
GRAIN-FREE
DAIRY-FREE
PALEO (IF MODIFIED)

Tender halibut fillets are gently poached in a fragrant sauce crafted from white wine, juicy tomatoes, and fresh basil—all in a single skillet. With minimal prep and cooking time, this dish is a breeze to make, yet it's brimming with light, refreshing flavors that are sure to delight your palate.

- 2 tablespoons extra-virgin olive oil
- ½ cup halved and thinly sliced shallot (about 1 large shallot)
- 2 garlic cloves, minced
- 1 pint cherry tomatoes, halved
- ½ teaspoon crushed red pepper flakes
- 1½ teaspoons kosher salt, divided
- 1 teaspoon freshly ground black pepper, divided
- ½ cup dry white wine (sub fish stock for paleo)
- 4 skinless halibut, cod, or other flaky white fish fillets (6 ounces each), patted dry
- Grated zest of ½ lemon
- 1 tablespoon freshly squeezed lemon juice (about ½ lemon)
- ⅓ cup thinly sliced fresh basil leaves

IN a large, deep skillet or 3.5-quart braiser with a fitted lid, heat the oil over medium heat. Add the shallot, garlic, tomatoes, pepper flakes, 1 teaspoon of the salt, and ½ teaspoon of the black pepper. Sauté, stirring, until the tomatoes begin to burst open, about 4 minutes.

POUR in the wine and bring to a rapid simmer. Cook until the liquid in the pan reduces by half, 1 to 2 minutes.

REDUCE the heat to a gentle simmer, about medium-low heat. Nestle the halibut fillets into the sauce. Sprinkle the tops of the fish evenly with the remaining ½ teaspoon salt, ½ teaspoon black pepper, and the lemon zest. Pour the lemon juice around the fish. Cover and cook until the fish is cooked through and flakes easily, about 8 minutes.

REMOVE from the heat and top with the basil. Divide the fillets among four plates and spoon the tomato sauce over and around the fillets.

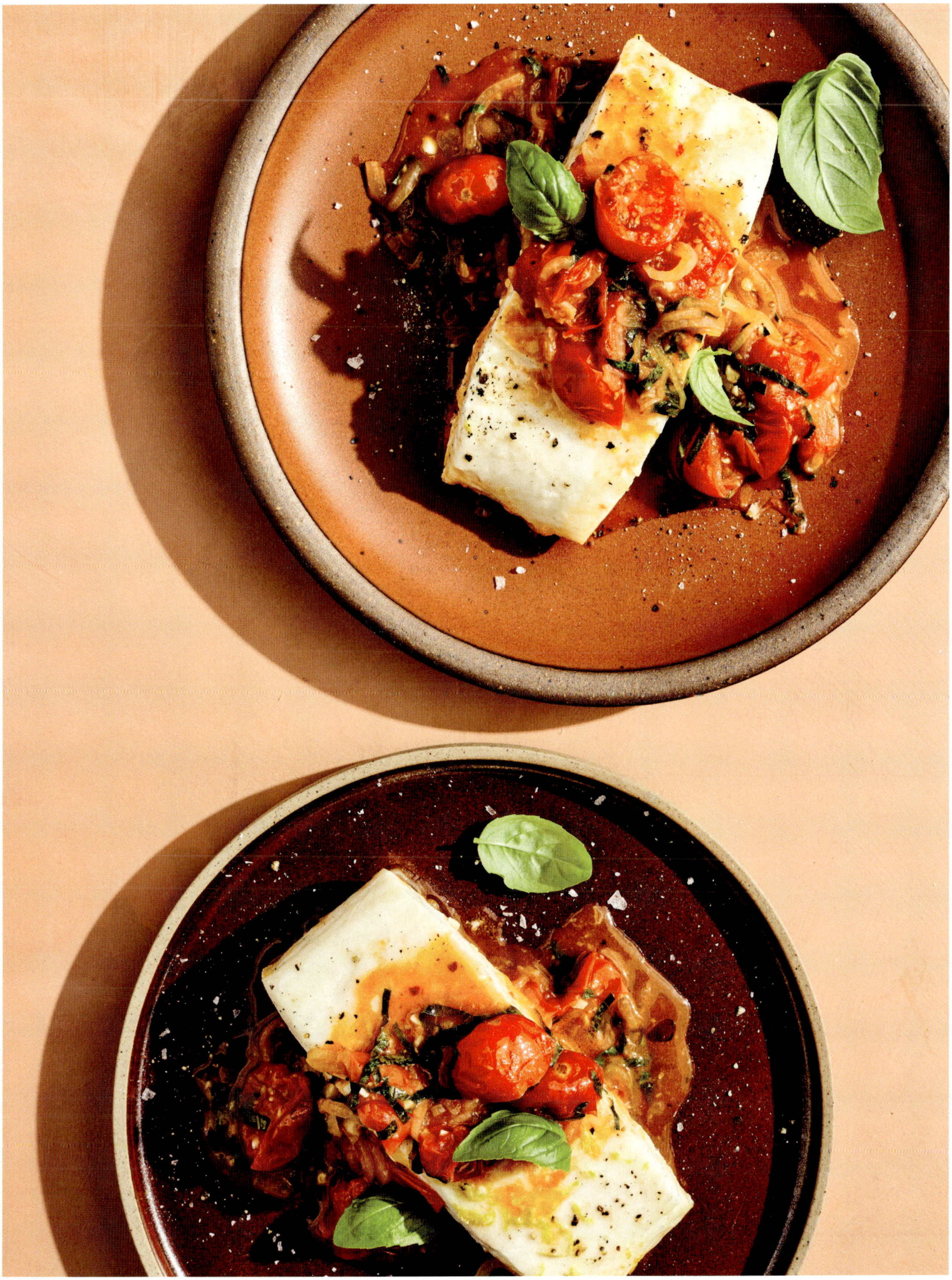

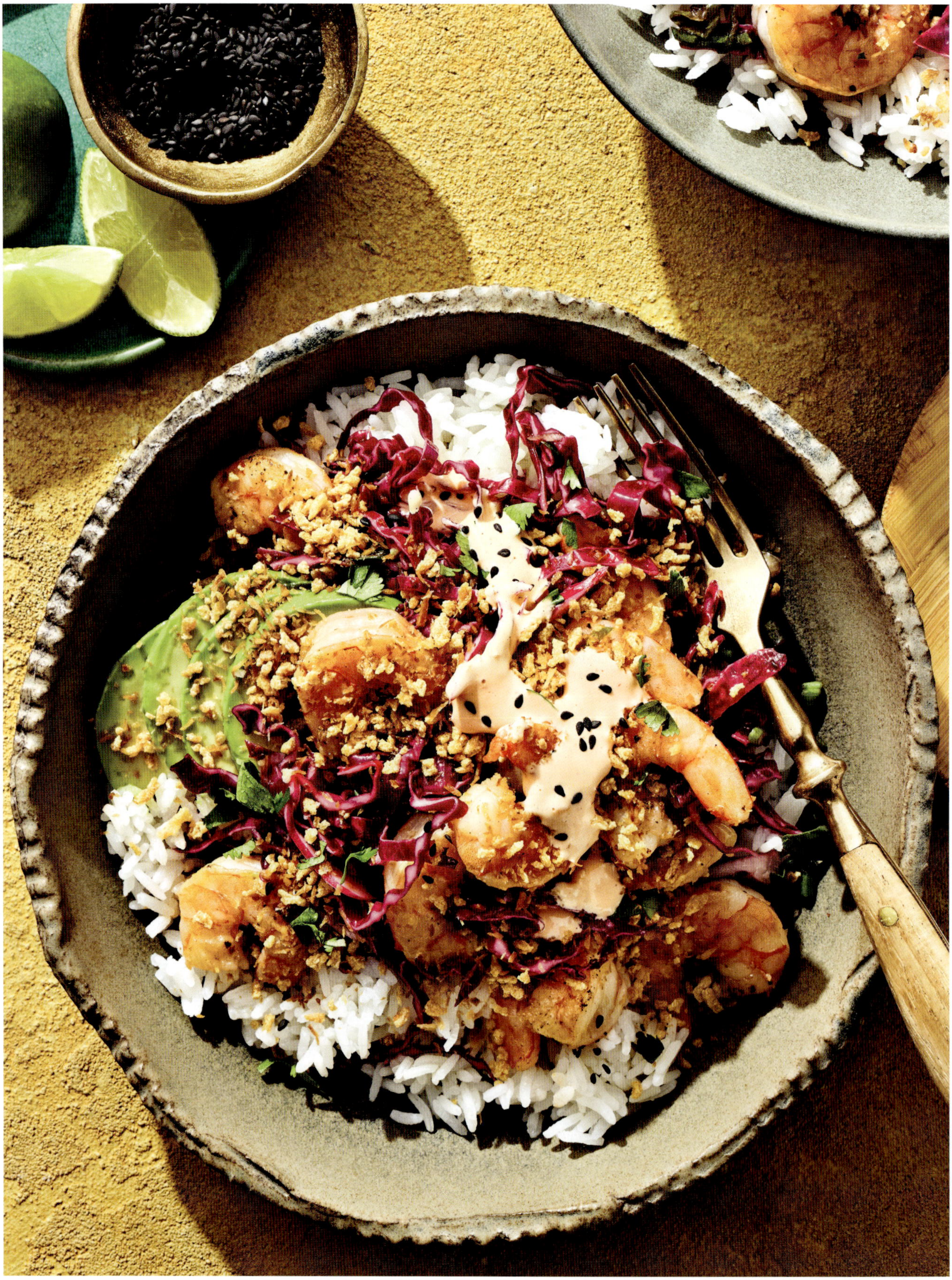

CRUNCHY COCONUT SHRIMP BOWLS WITH SPICY AIOLI

MAKES 4 SERVINGS | **TOTAL TIME:** 30 MINUTES

DIETARY
GLUTEN-FREE
DAIRY-FREE

This recipe brings the festive flavors of coconut-crusted shrimp into a deconstructed weeknight dinner that's sure to become a favorite. With a base of rice and vibrant sesame slaw, perfectly seared shrimp is topped with a crunchy panko-coconut blend and drizzled with a creamy, spicy aioli. Every bite delivers a satisfying mix of textures!

FOR THE SPICY AIOLI

2 tablespoons avocado oil mayo

1 to 2 tablespoons sriracha (depending on your heat preference)

1 tablespoon freshly squeezed lime juice (about ½ lime)

¼ teaspoon kosher salt

FOR THE SESAME SLAW

4 cups finely shredded red cabbage (about ½ medium head)

3 green onions, thinly sliced on the diagonal

2 teaspoons toasted sesame oil

1 tablespoon rice vinegar

½ teaspoon kosher salt

FOR THE COCONUT CRISPY SHRIMP

2 tablespoons avocado oil

1 pound peeled, deveined, and tail-off shrimp (36/40 count), patted dry

1½ teaspoons kosher salt, divided

½ teaspoon freshly ground black pepper

½ cup gluten-free panko bread crumbs

⅓ cup shredded unsweetened coconut

FOR SERVING

2 cups prepared steamed rice

1 avocado, thinly sliced

Chopped fresh cilantro leaves

Black sesame seeds, optional for garnish

Lime wedges

MAKE THE AIOLI: In a small bowl, whisk together all the aioli ingredients until well combined. Set aside.

MAKE THE SESAME SLAW: In a medium bowl, toss together the cabbage, green onions, toasted sesame oil, vinegar, and salt until well combined. Set aside.

COOK THE SHRIMP: Line a plate with paper towels. In a large skillet, heat the avocado oil over medium-high heat. Add the shrimp and sprinkle with 1 teaspoon of the salt and the pepper. Cook until golden brown on each side and cooked through, 2 to 3 minutes per side. Using a slotted spoon, transfer the shrimp to the prepared plate and set aside.

REDUCE the heat to medium. Add the panko, coconut, and the remaining ½ teaspoon salt and toast, tossing, until the panko and coconut are golden brown, 2 to 3 minutes. Watch carefully so as not to burn. Set aside.

TO SERVE: Divide the rice among four bowls. Top with the sesame slaw and shrimp. Sprinkle the coconut bread crumbs over the top and place the sliced avocado to the side. Generously drizzle the spicy aioli over the top, followed by some cilantro. Finish with sesame seeds, if desired. Serve with lime wedges.

LEFTOVER shredded coconut? Try my Almond Joyful Bites (page 246).

BROTHY SAFFRON AND LEMON FISH OVER RICE

MAKES 4 SERVINGS | **TOTAL TIME:** 35 MINUTES

DIETARY
GLUTEN-FREE
DAIRY-FREE (IF MODIFIED)

If you're anything like me and love brothy dishes served over rice, this bright, fragrant fish dish will become a favorite. It's infused with white wine and saffron, creating a rich yet light base to gently poach flaky fish to perfection. Serve with brown rice and you have a simple but elegant meal that feels comforting yet refined, making it ideal for either a healthy weeknight dinner or a special occasion.

½ cup dry white wine

1 teaspoon saffron threads

4 skinless halibut, cod, salmon, or other flaky fish fillets (6 ounces each), patted dry

1½ teaspoons kosher salt, divided

½ teaspoon freshly ground black pepper

2 tablespoons cassava flour

2 tablespoons extra-virgin olive oil

2 tablespoons unsalted butter (sub vegan butter for dairy-free)

½ cup halved and thinly sliced shallot (about 1 large shallot)

3 garlic cloves, minced

½ teaspoon crushed red pepper flakes

1 tablespoon tomato paste

½ teaspoon smoked paprika

½ teaspoon ground turmeric

1 cup low-sodium chicken broth

Grated zest of ½ lemon

2 tablespoons freshly squeezed lemon juice (about 1 lemon)

2 tablespoons capers, drained

¼ cup finely chopped fresh parsley leaves

2 cups prepared brown rice

¼ cup finely chopped fresh dill, for serving

IN a small bowl, stir together the white wine and saffron. Set aside and allow the saffron to bloom for at least 5 minutes.

SEASON the fish fillets evenly with 1 teaspoon of the salt and the black pepper. Place the flour in a large, shallow bowl and dredge the fish on all sides to evenly coat in the flour, shaking off any excess.

IN a large, deep skillet or 3.5-quart braiser with fitted lid, heat the oil over medium-high heat. Add the fish and sear until golden brown on both sides, about 2 minutes per side. The fish does not need to be cooked through, as it will finish cooking in the broth. Remove from the pan and set aside on a clean plate.

REDUCE the heat to medium and melt the butter. Add the shallot, garlic, and pepper flakes and cook, stirring, until the shallot is tender, 2 to 3 minutes.

ADD the tomato paste, the remaining ½ teaspoon salt, the paprika, and turmeric and stir to combine. Pour in the wine and saffron mixture and stir to combine. Cook, stirring, until the wine reduces by half, 2 to 3 more minutes.

ADD the broth, lemon zest, lemon juice, capers, and parsley. Stir to combine and bring to a rapid simmer.

REDUCE to a gentle simmer, about medium-low heat, and nestle the fish fillets into the broth. Cover and cook until the fish is cooked through and flakes easily with a fork, 4 to 5 minutes.

TO SERVE: Divide the rice among four shallow bowls. Top with the fish and spoon the broth over and around the fish. Finish with fresh dill.

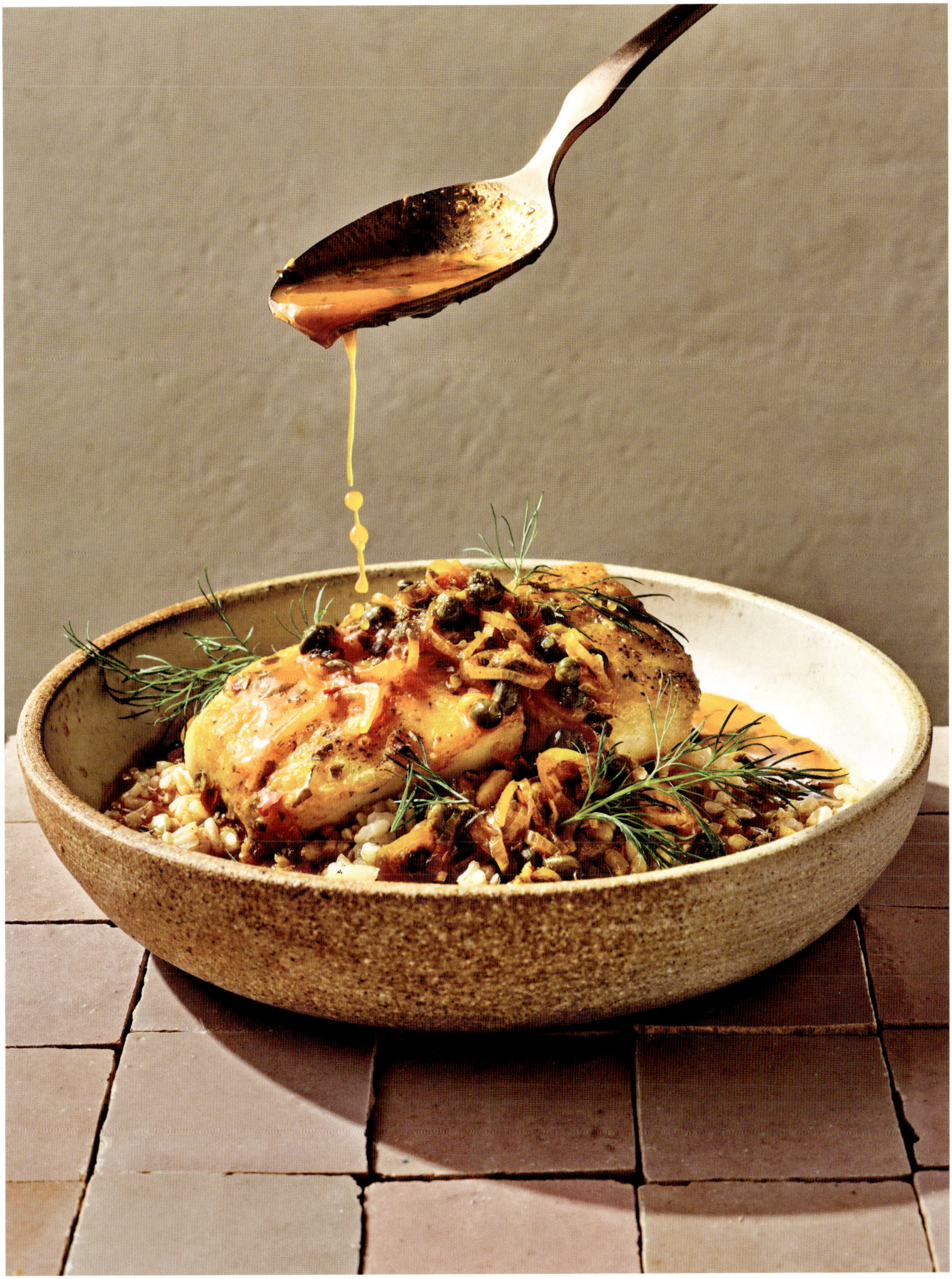

HARISSA SALMON BITES WITH SESAME CUCUMBER SALAD

MAKES 4 SERVINGS | **TOTAL TIME:** 25 MINUTES

DIETARY
GLUTEN-FREE
GRAIN-FREE

A key component of many weeknight meals is a well-stocked pantry with ingredients that provide a depth of flavor with little work. Here, I rely on flavorful harissa, Mediterranean spices you likely have in your cabinet, and nutty tahini to make this less-than-thirty-minute meal feel elevated. With fresh salmon and a cool cucumber salad, this is the perfect light meal that will impress the whole family.

FOR THE SESAME CUCUMBER SALAD

¼ cup whole-milk plain Greek yogurt

1 tablespoon tahini

2 teaspoons toasted sesame oil

2 tablespoons freshly squeezed lemon juice (about 1 lemon)

1 garlic clove, minced

½ teaspoon kosher salt

½ teaspoon freshly ground black pepper

2 medium English cucumbers

1 cup halved and thinly sliced red onion (about 1 small onion)

½ cup roughly chopped fresh cilantro leaves, plus more for garnish

½ cup roughly chopped fresh dill

2 tablespoons toasted sesame seeds, plus more for garnish

FOR THE SALMON

1½ pounds skinless center-cut salmon, patted dry and pin bones removed, cut into 1-inch cubes

1 tablespoon arrowroot flour

2 teaspoons smoked paprika

2 teaspoons garlic powder

½ teaspoon dried oregano

1½ teaspoons kosher salt

½ teaspoon freshly ground black pepper

1 tablespoon avocado oil

3 tablespoons mild harissa paste

2 tablespoons freshly squeezed lemon juice (about 1 lemon)

1 tablespoon honey

Prepared cauliflower rice, steamed rice, or gluten-free orzo

POSITION racks in the center and at the top of the oven. Preheat the oven to 425°F. Line a sheet pan with parchment paper and set aside.

PREPARE THE SALAD: In a large bowl, combine the yogurt, tahini, toasted sesame oil, lemon juice, garlic, salt, and pepper. Whisk to combine. The dressing will look very thick, but it will thin out once the veggies are added.

CUT the cucumbers in half lengthwise. Using a small spoon, scoop out the seeds. Thinly slice the cucumber halves crosswise into half-moons (you should have around 4 cups) and add them to the bowl with the dressing. Add the onion and toss to combine, continuing to stir until the cucumbers begin to release some of their liquid and the dressing thins a bit. Add the cilantro, dill, and sesame seeds and toss once more. Place in the fridge until the salmon is ready.

PREPARE THE SALMON: In a medium bowl, combine the salmon, arrowroot, paprika, garlic powder, oregano, salt, pepper, and avocado oil. Toss until all pieces are evenly coated. Transfer the salmon to the prepared sheet pan and spread into a single layer, ensuring there is ample space between each piece. Transfer to the oven on the middle rack and bake for 10 minutes.

LEFTOVER tahini? Try my Chicken Shawarma Salad (page 52). Leftover harissa? Try my Spiced Chicken and Chickpea Skillet (page 150) or Smashed Lamb Burger Tacos with Harissa-Yogurt Sauce (page 183).

MEANWHILE, in a small bowl, whisk together the harissa, lemon juice, and honey. Set aside.

AFTER 10 minutes, remove the sheet pan from the oven and pour the harissa mixture over the salmon. Toss to combine, ensuring the salmon is evenly coated. Turn the broiler on high. Transfer back to the oven on the top rack. Broil until the salmon bites are slightly charred, about 3 more minutes, watching closely so as to not burn it. Remove from the oven and allow to cool slightly.

TO SERVE: Divide the prepared rice or orzo among four shallow bowls. Top with the sesame cucumber salad and divide the salmon on top. Garnish with more cilantro and a sprinkle of sesame seeds.

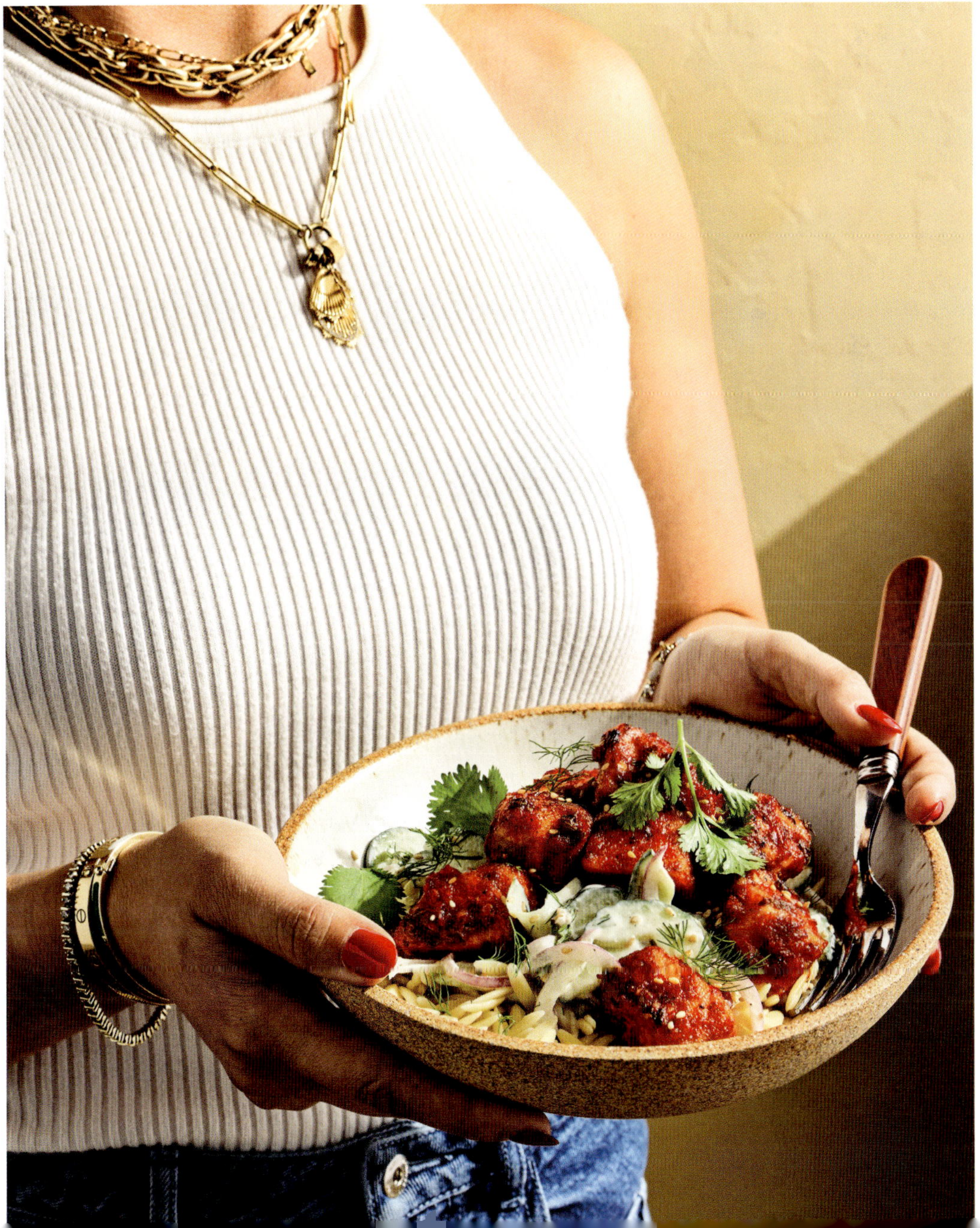

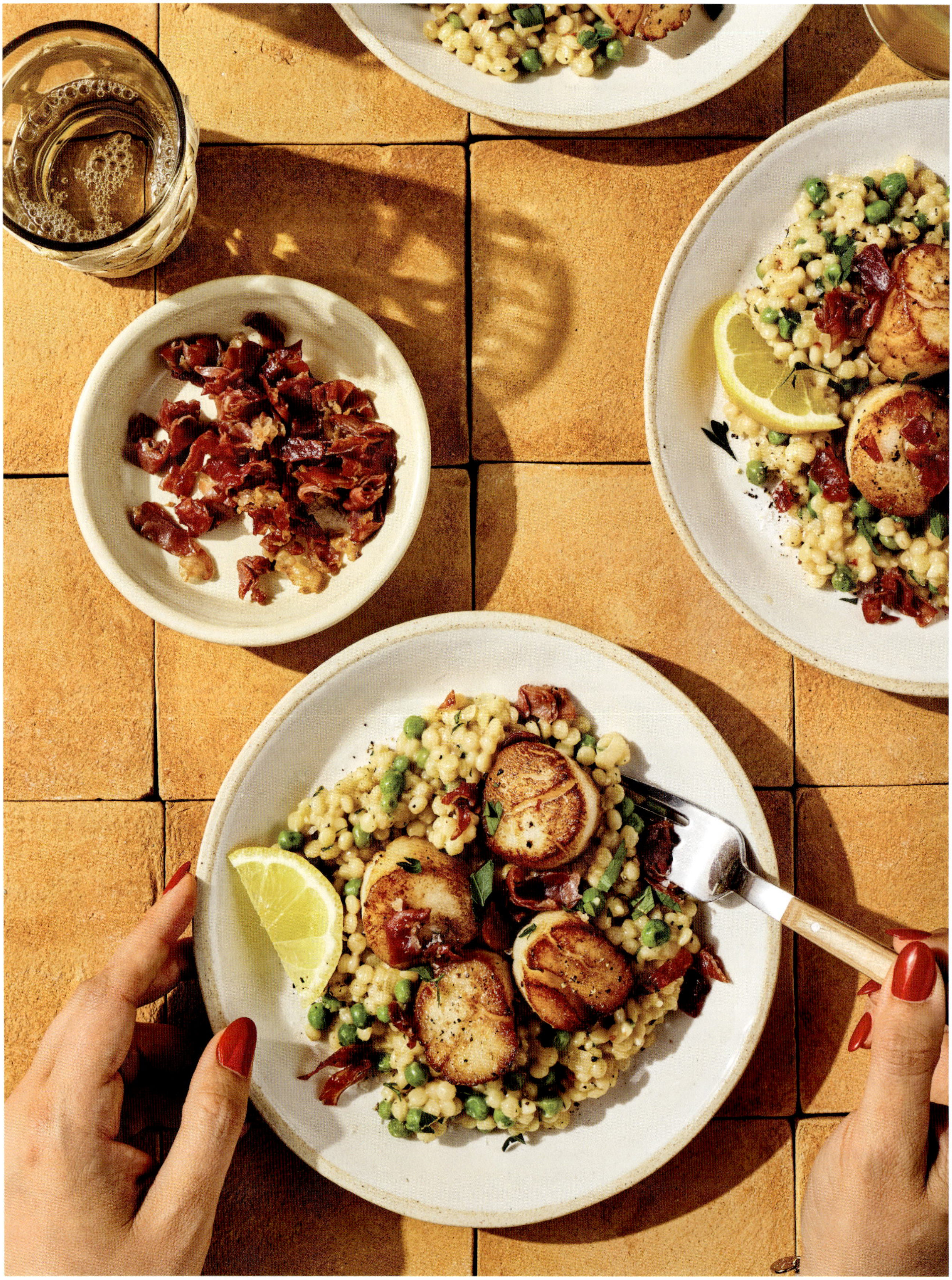

SEARED SCALLOPS WITH CREAMY PEA COUSCOUS AND CRISPY PROSCIUTTO

MAKES 4 SERVINGS | **TOTAL TIME:** 30 MINUTES

I don't buy scallops often, but when I do, I'm feeling fancy. So I like to lean into that—elevating the presentation to make it feel like a restaurant-worthy experience. But the best part? As elegant as they seem, scallops are surprisingly simple to cook. Here, I serve them over creamy pea couscous that mimics the richness of risotto, then top it all off with crispy prosciutto for a perfect bite. It's the kind of dish you'd expect at a nice restaurant, but you can have it on the table in just thirty minutes.

FOR THE COUSCOUS

½ cup diced prosciutto (about 3 ounces, see note)

2 tablespoons extra-virgin olive oil

½ cup finely diced yellow onion (about ½ small onion)

2 garlic cloves, minced

½ teaspoon crushed red pepper flakes

1½ cups Israeli or pearl couscous

3 cups low-sodium vegetable broth

1 teaspoon kosher salt

½ teaspoon freshly ground black pepper

1 cup frozen peas

2 tablespoons unsalted butter

½ cup grated parmesan cheese

2 tablespoons freshly squeezed lemon juice (about 1 lemon)

2 tablespoons finely chopped fresh parsley leaves, plus more for garnish

FOR THE SCALLOPS

1 pound jumbo sea scallops, patted dry

1 teaspoon kosher salt

½ teaspoon freshly ground black pepper

2 tablespoons extra-virgin olive oil

Lemon wedges, for serving

MAKE THE COUSCOUS: Line a plate with paper towels. In a medium saucepan, cook the prosciutto over medium heat, stirring occasionally, until just crisp, 3 to 4 minutes. Using a slotted spoon, transfer to the prepared plate and set aside.

PLACE the oil, onion, garlic, and pepper flakes in the saucepan and cook, stirring, until the onion softens, about 4 minutes.

ADD the couscous, broth, salt, and black pepper and bring to a rapid simmer. Reduce the heat to a gentle simmer, about medium-low heat, and cook, uncovered, stirring often, until most of the liquid has been absorbed and the couscous is tender, 8 to 10 minutes.

REMOVE from the heat and stir in the peas, butter, parmesan, lemon juice, and parsley until well combined and creamy. Cover to keep warm while you cook the scallops.

COOK THE SCALLOPS: Line a plate with paper towels and set aside. Season the scallops evenly with the salt and black pepper.

IN a large skillet, heat the oil over medium-high heat until it shimmers. Add the scallops to the skillet and cook, undisturbed, until a golden-brown crust forms on one side and the scallops are opaque one-third of the way up, about 2 minutes. Gently flip the scallops and continue to cook until the rest of the scallop is opaque and the center is gently cooked, about 2 minutes. Transfer the cooked scallops to the prepared plate.

TO SERVE: Divide the creamy pea couscous among four shallow bowls. Top with 3 to 4 seared scallops and some of the crispy prosciutto. Finish with a sprinkle of parsley and serve with lemon wedges.

FROM MY KITCHEN TO YOURS

To dice the prosciutto, stack a few slices, then roll them up tightly like a cigar. Use a sharp knife to slice crosswise into thin ribbons, then run your knife through the ribbons to create small bite-size pieces.

SHEET PAN CHIPOTLE-HONEY BUTTER SALMON

MAKES 4 SERVINGS | **TOTAL TIME:** 45 MINUTES

DIETARY
GLUTEN-FREE
GRAIN-FREE
DAIRY-FREE (IF MODIFIED)
MAKE AHEAD

Smoky-sweet chipotle-honey butter melts over tender salmon fillets, paired with caramelized sweet potatoes and Brussels sprouts, in this simple sheet pan meal. It's vibrant, wholesome, and perfect for easy weeknight dinners—or impressing guests without the fuss!

1 pound Brussels sprouts, trimmed, halved lengthwise

1 large sweet potato, unpeeled and cut into ½-inch dice (about 2 cups)

2 tablespoons avocado oil

2 teaspoons kosher salt, divided

½ teaspoon freshly ground black pepper

1 teaspoon smoked paprika

3 tablespoons unsalted butter, softened (sub vegan butter for dairy-free)

2 garlic cloves, minced

2 canned chipotle peppers in adobo sauce, minced (about 2 tablespoons)

3 tablespoons honey

Grated zest of ½ lime

2 tablespoons freshly squeezed lime juice (about 1 lime)

1 tablespoon finely chopped fresh cilantro leaves, plus more for garnish

4 skinless center-cut salmon fillets (6 ounces each), patted dry and pin bones removed

Lime wedges, for serving

LEFTOVER chipotles in adobo? Try my Saucy Chipotle Chicken Tacos (page 142) or Chipotle Chimichurri Steak Bite Bowls (page 166).

PREHEAT the oven to 400°F. Line a sheet pan with parchment paper.

ADD the Brussels sprouts and sweet potato to the prepared sheet pan. Drizzle with the oil and season with 1 teaspoon of the salt, the black pepper, and paprika. Toss to coat and spread into an even layer. Bake for 20 minutes.

MEANWHILE, MAKE THE CHIPOTLE-HONEY BUTTER: In a small bowl, combine the softened butter, garlic, chipotle peppers, honey, lime zest, lime juice, and cilantro. Stir until well combined.

AFTER 20 minutes, remove the veggies from the oven. Add 2 tablespoons of the chipotle-honey butter to the sheet pan and toss so that the veggies are well coated. Push the veggies to the edges of the sheet pan, making room in the center for the salmon.

PLACE the salmon fillets in the center of the sheet pan. Evenly distribute the remaining chipotle-honey butter on top of each fillet and spread to evenly coat the tops of the salmon. Sprinkle the tops of the salmon evenly with the remaining 1 teaspoon salt.

TRANSFER to the oven and bake until the salmon is cooked through and flakes easily with a fork, about 12 minutes.

TO SERVE: Divide the fish among four plates along with the Brussels sprouts and sweet potatoes. Garnish with fresh cilantro and serve with lime wedges.

STORE leftovers in an airtight container in the fridge for up to 3 days. Reheat on a sheet pan in the oven at 325°F for 10 to 12 minutes, in the air fryer at 350°F for 4 to 6 minutes, or microwave in 1-minute increments, tossing the veggies after each, until warmed through.

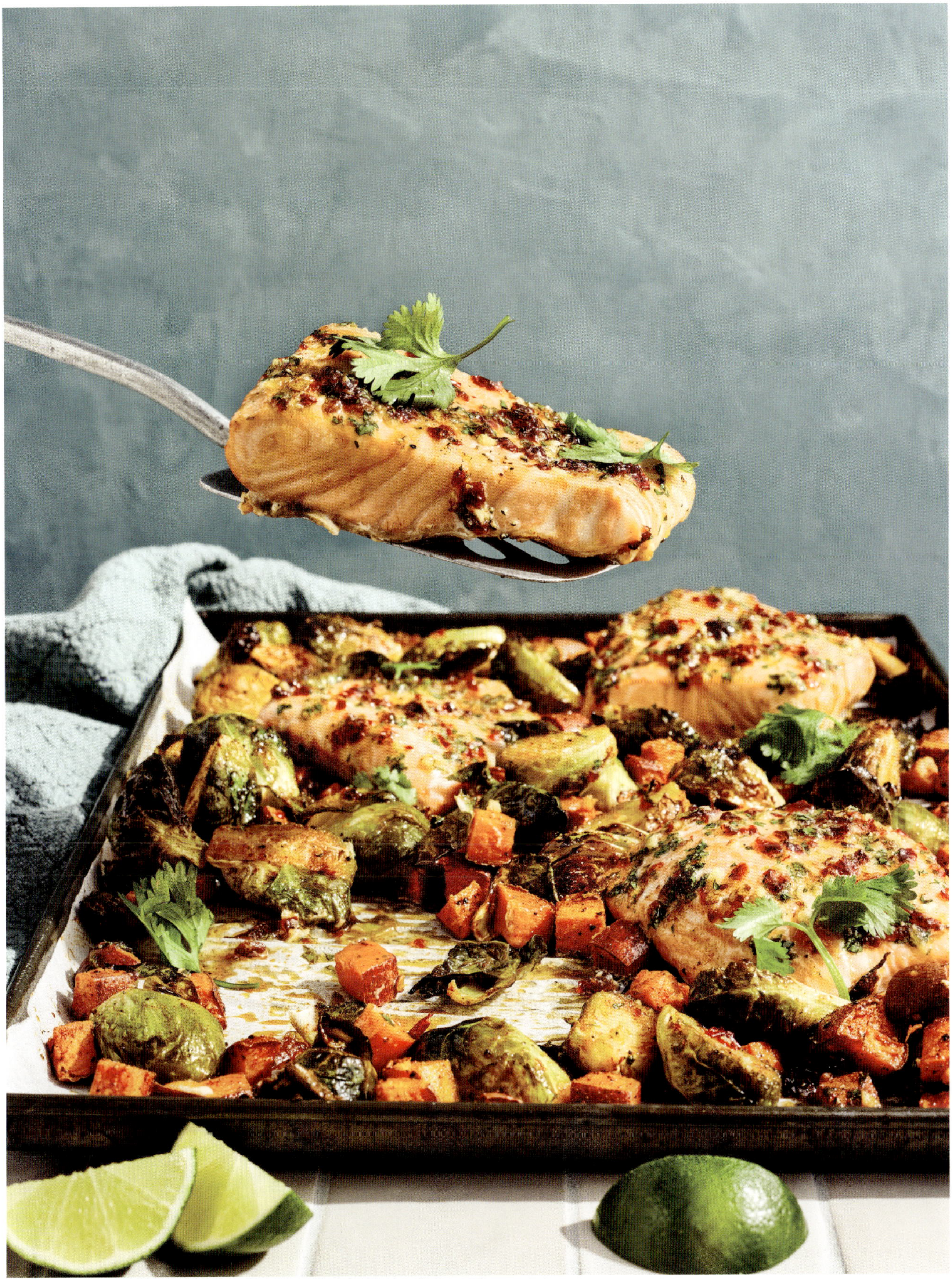

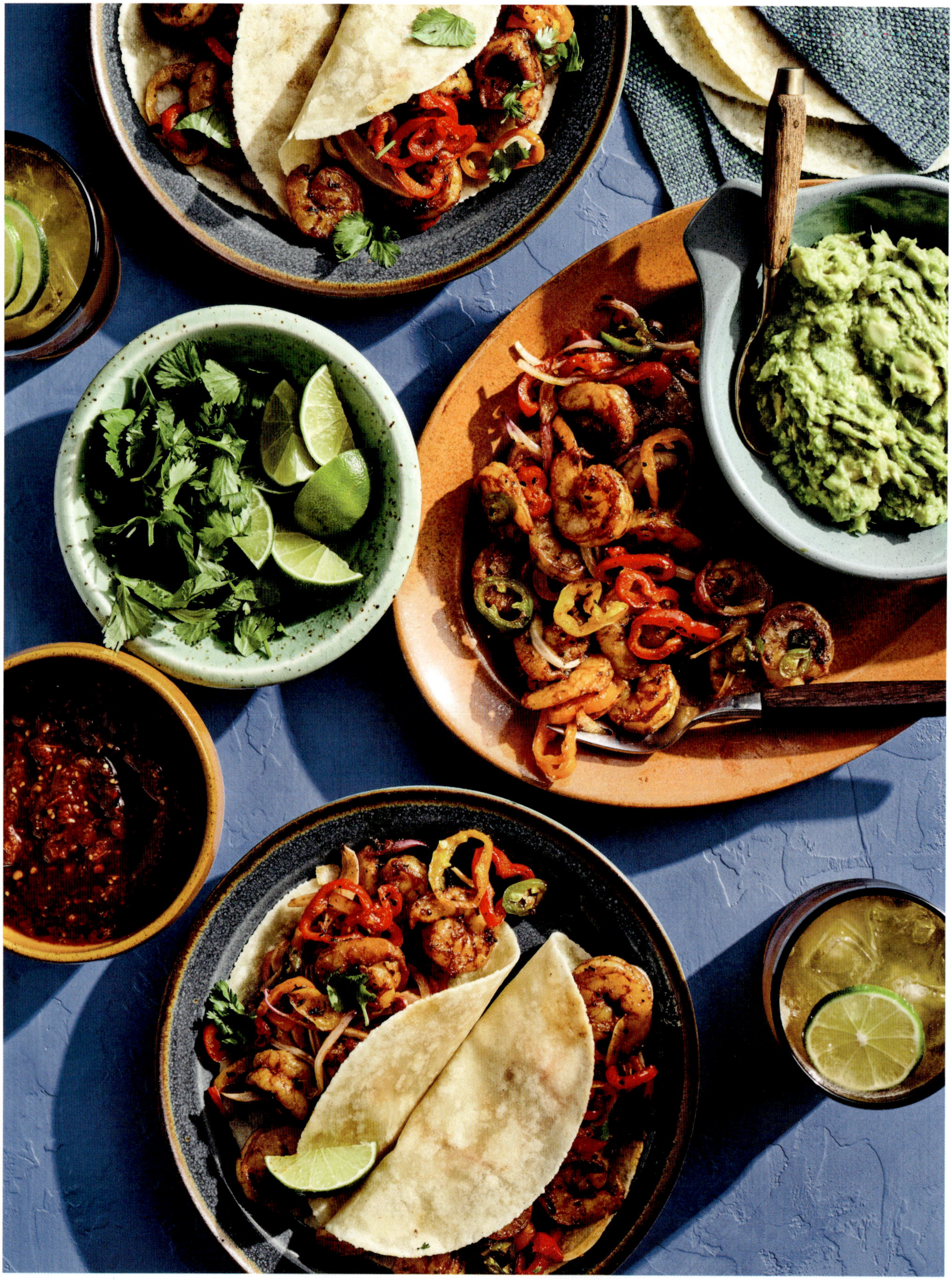

SHEET PAN SHRIMP FAJITA TACOS

MAKES 4 SERVINGS | **TOTAL TIME:** 40 MINUTES

DIETARY
GLUTEN-FREE
GRAIN-FREE
DAIRY-FREE
PALEO
MAKE AHEAD

This light and flavorful sheet pan dinner is perfect for a fuss-free fajita night at home. Juicy shrimp, vibrant bell peppers, and onion are tossed with bold spices and roasted until sizzling. Simply scoop them into warm tortillas for classic fajitas or switch things up by serving over rice.

FOR THE FAJITAS

1 pound mini bell peppers, seeded and sliced into thin rounds

1 cup halved and thinly sliced red onion (about 1 small onion)

1 serrano pepper, thinly sliced into rounds, optional

4 tablespoons avocado oil, divided

2 teaspoons kosher salt, divided

1 teaspoon freshly ground black pepper, divided

1½ pounds peeled, deveined, and tail-off shrimp (36/40 count), patted dry

2 teaspoons chili powder

1 teaspoon garlic powder

1 teaspoon smoked paprika

½ teaspoon ground cumin

1 tablespoon finely chopped fresh oregano leaves

Grated zest of ½ lime

FOR THE TACOS

10 grain-free tortillas or lettuce cups

2 avocados, mashed

¼ cup freshly chopped cilantro leaves

Salsa, for serving

Lime wedges, for serving

PREHEAT the oven to 425°F. Line a sheet pan with parchment paper.

MAKE THE FAJITAS: Place the bell peppers, onion, and serrano pepper (if using) on the prepared sheet pan. Drizzle with 2 tablespoons of the oil, ½ teaspoon of the salt, and ½ teaspoon of the black pepper and toss until well combined. Spread into an even layer, transfer to the oven, and roast until just softened, about 10 minutes.

MEANWHILE, place the shrimp in a large bowl. Add the remaining 2 tablespoons oil, 1½ teaspoons salt, ½ teaspoon black pepper, the chili powder, garlic powder, paprika, cumin, oregano, and lime zest and toss until well combined and the shrimp is evenly coated. Set aside.

REMOVE the veggies from the oven and add the shrimp to the pan. Toss until combined and spread into an even layer. Return to the oven and roast until the shrimp is cooked through, about 10 minutes.

ASSEMBLE THE TACOS: If using tortillas, one at a time place the tortillas in a dry (no oil) skillet over medium heat and cook for about 30 seconds on each side. Alternatively, you can use tongs to char the tortillas directly over a gas flame for a few seconds.

FOR each taco, spread the mashed avocado on the bottom of a tortilla (or inside a lettuce cup) and fill with the shrimp fajitas and veggies. Finish with a sprinkle of cilantro and a drizzle of salsa. Serve with lime wedges.

STORE leftovers in an airtight container in the fridge for up to 2 days, keeping tortillas and toppings separate. Reheat quickly in a skillet over medium heat or in the air fryer at 350°F for 3 to 4 minutes to keep the shrimp tender. Avoid microwaving, as the shrimp can become rubbery. Assemble tacos as desired.

CHILI CRISP CITRUS SALMON

MAKES 4 SERVINGS | **TOTAL TIME:** 30 MINUTES

DIETARY
GLUTEN-FREE
GRAIN-FREE
DAIRY-FREE
PALEO

This quick skillet dinner combines zesty citrus, spicy chili, savory coconut aminos, and a touch of toasted sesame oil over salmon for a dish that is packed with flavor. Perfect for busy weeknights, this healthy option is bursting with deliciousness, perfect for when you're craving something easy yet satisfying. And let's not forget the magic of chili crisp, the secret weapon for turning a weeknight meal into a flavorful adventure.

- 2 tablespoons avocado oil
- 2 teaspoons toasted sesame oil
- ½ cup halved and thinly sliced shallot (about 1 large shallot)
- 4 green onions, cut into 2-inch pieces
- 1 teaspoon kosher salt, divided
- ½ teaspoon freshly ground black pepper, divided
- 2 medium navel oranges, peeled and cut into ¼-inch rounds (see note)
- ¼ cup coconut aminos
- 1 tablespoon honey
- 1 tablespoon rice vinegar
- 2 tablespoons chili crisp, plus more for serving (see note)
- 4 skinless center-cut salmon fillets (6 ounces each), patted dry and pin bones removed
- Fresh mint leaves, for garnish
- Prepared cauliflower rice or steamed rice

LEFTOVER chili crisp? Try my Garlic Shrimp Stir-Fry (page 204).

POSITION a rack in the center of the oven and preheat the oven to 400°F.

IN a large, deep, oven-safe skillet or 3.5-quart braiser, heat the avocado oil and toasted sesame oil over medium-high heat. Add the shallot, green onions, ½ teaspoon of the salt, and ¼ teaspoon of the pepper. Cook, stirring, until veggies are just tender, about 2 minutes.

ADD the orange rounds, coconut aminos, honey, vinegar, and chili crisp. Stir to combine and bring to a simmer. Nestle the salmon fillets into the skillet and spoon some of the sauce over the salmon. Sprinkle the tops of the fillets with the remaining ½ teaspoon salt and ¼ teaspoon pepper.

TRANSFER to the oven and bake until the salmon is cooked through and flakes easily with a fork, 8 to 10 minutes.

REMOVE from the oven and garnish with fresh mint. Serve over prepared rice with a drizzle of additional chili crisp.

FROM MY KITCHEN TO YOURS

FOR THE ORANGES: To peel the orange, I recommend using a paring knife so that you can better remove the white pith. To do this, slice off the top and bottom of the orange. Using the middle of the blade, make gentle curving slices down the side of the orange to remove the rind and pith, then cut into rounds.

FOR THE CHILI CRISP: This is a spicy, crunchy condiment made with crispy bits of fried garlic, shallots, and chili flakes suspended in oil, adding both heat and texture. Unlike chili oil, which is smooth and mainly used for infusing flavor, chili crisp brings a satisfying crunch that makes it a perfect topping for everything from noodles to eggs. You can find it in most grocery stores in the international aisle, at Asian markets, or online.

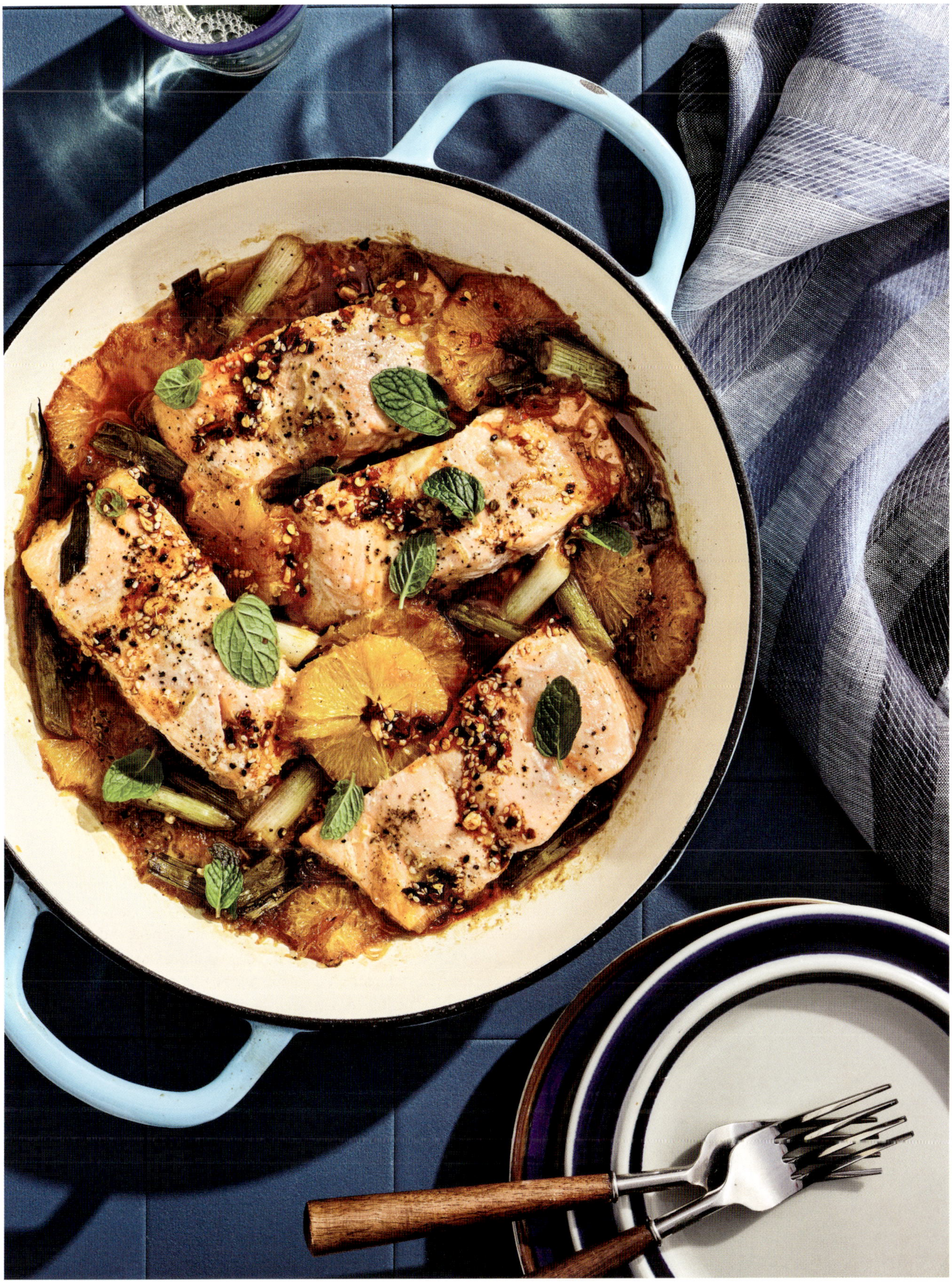

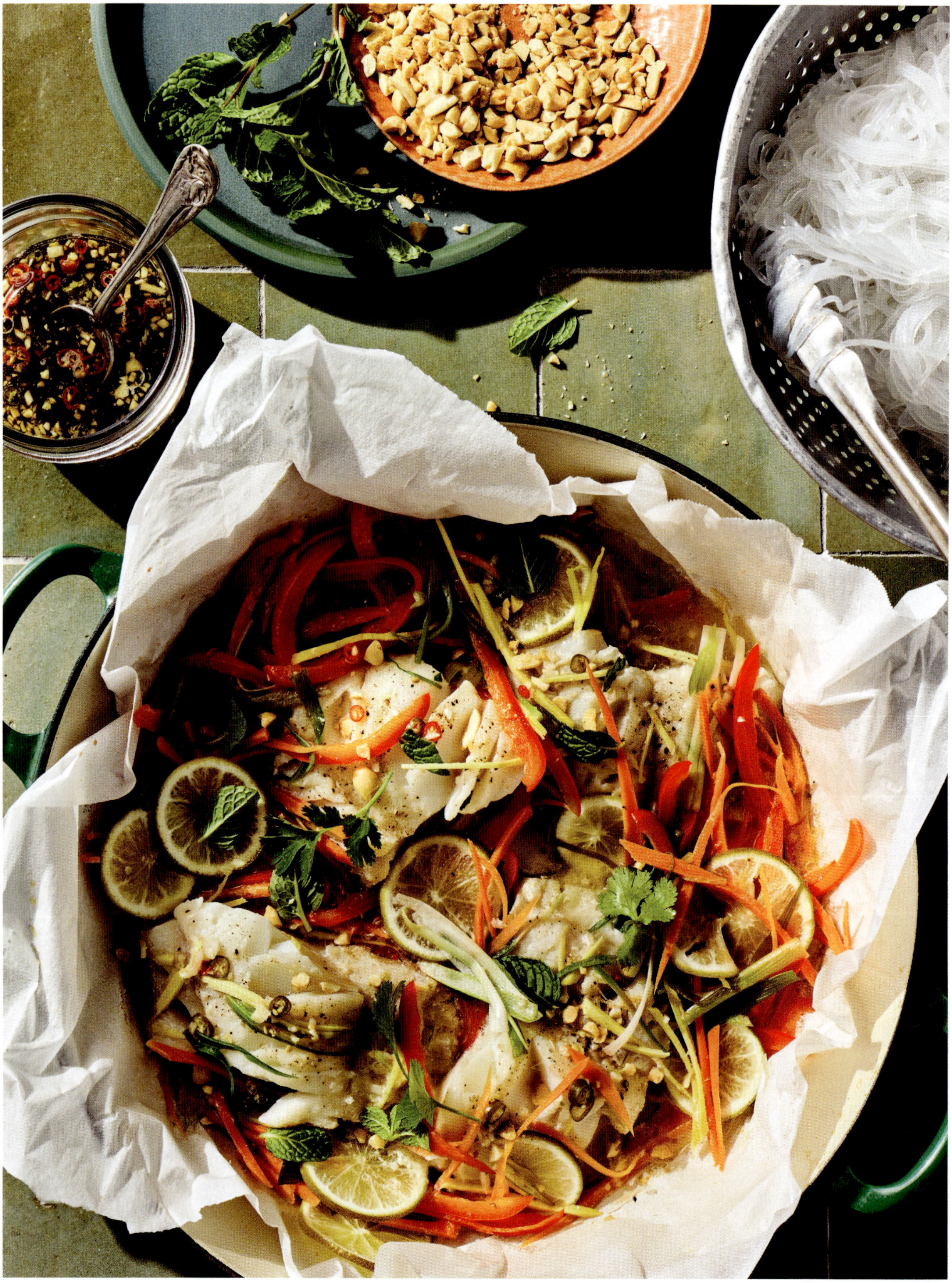

VIETNAMESE-INSPIRED STEAMED FISH WITH RICE NOODLES AND HERBS

DIETARY
GLUTEN-FREE
DAIRY-FREE

MAKES 4 SERVINGS | **TOTAL TIME:** 40 MINUTES

In the past, I've cooked fish in individual parchment paper packets, which, while foolproof, can feel a bit tedious to prepare. Then one day I was introduced to this game-changing method: Simply line a skillet with parchment paper, add the fish and aromatics, cover, and let it all steam together in one pan. It's so much easier and the results are just as delicious! This version, bursting with tangy, fresh, and slightly spicy Vietnamese flavors, is a real standout.

FOR THE NUOC CHAM SAUCE

3 tablespoons avocado oil

1 tablespoon coconut sugar

2 tablespoons fish sauce

¼ cup freshly squeezed lime juice (about 2 limes)

2 tablespoons coconut aminos

1 garlic clove, minced

1 to 2 Thai chiles, thinly sliced (1 for mild, 2 for medium)

FOR THE FISH AND BOWLS

4 skinless halibut, cod, or other flaky fish fillets (6 ounces each), patted dry

½ teaspoon kosher salt

½ teaspoon freshly ground black pepper

1 small lime, thinly sliced

1-inch piece fresh ginger, peeled and cut into very thin matchsticks

3 green onions, cut into 2-inch pieces and sliced into thin matchsticks

1 large red bell pepper, seeded and thinly sliced

1 cup matchstick-cut carrots

8 ounces vermicelli rice noodles

¼ cup fresh cilantro leaves

¼ cup fresh mint leaves

¼ cup roughly chopped dry-roasted peanuts

FILL a medium saucepan with water and bring to a boil.

MAKE THE NUOC CHAM SAUCE: In a small bowl, combine all the sauce ingredients and whisk until the sugar is dissolved. Set aside.

PREPARE THE FISH: Place a 12-inch sheet of parchment paper in the center of a 10-inch heavy-bottom skillet or 3.5-quart braiser with fitted lid.

PLACE the fillets on the parchment in the skillet and sprinkle the tops evenly with the salt and pepper. Nestle the lime around the fillets, then evenly distribute the ginger, green onions, bell pepper, and carrots on and around the fish. Spoon 5 tablespoons of the nuoc cham sauce over the fish and veggies, being careful to not touch the fish with the spoon, and reserve the rest of the sauce for serving.

COVER the pan with the lid (do not remove the lid during the cooking process). Cook over medium-high heat for 5 minutes. Reduce the heat to medium and continue to cook, covered, for another 8 to 10 minutes, until the fish is cooked through and flakes easily with a fork. Remove the pan from the heat and let it rest, covered, for 5 minutes.

WHILE the fish is resting, add the rice noodles to the pot of boiling water and cook according to the package directions. Drain and rinse with water.

TO SERVE: Divide the noodles among four bowls. Top each bowl with the steamed fish and veggies, the cilantro, mint, and some roughly chopped peanuts. Finish by spooning more of the nuoc cham sauce over the bowls.

CURRIED SALMON AND CHICKPEA BAKE

MAKES 4 SERVINGS | **TOTAL TIME:** 45 MINUTES

DIETARY
GLUTEN-FREE
GRAIN-FREE
DAIRY-FREE
MAKE AHEAD

This flavorful one-pan meal is as easy as it is impressive. Creamy coconut milk, aromatic spices, and roasted tomatoes create a luscious base for tender chickpeas and perfectly cooked salmon fillets. It's a vibrant dish that's weeknight-friendly yet elegant enough for entertaining. Serve with warm naan or fluffy rice to soak up the spiced golden sauce!

Two 15-ounce cans chickpeas, drained and rinsed

1 cup halved and thinly sliced shallot (about 2 large shallots)

1½ cups halved grape tomatoes

2 garlic cloves, minced

Grated zest of ½ lemon

1 teaspoon grated fresh ginger

1 teaspoon ground cumin

1 teaspoon ground turmeric

1 tablespoon curry powder

¼ teaspoon cayenne pepper, optional

2 teaspoons kosher salt, divided

½ teaspoon freshly ground black pepper

1 cup unsweetened full-fat coconut milk

4 skinless center-cut salmon fillets (6 ounces each), patted dry and pin bones removed

¼ cup freshly chopped cilantro, for garnish

Lemon wedges, for serving

POSITION a rack at the top of the oven and preheat the oven to 400°F.

IN a 9 × 13-inch baking dish or 1-quart oval roasting pan, combine the chickpeas, shallots, tomatoes, garlic, lemon zest, ginger, cumin, turmeric, curry powder, cayenne (if using), 1 teaspoon of the salt, the black pepper, and the coconut milk. Gently toss until well combined.

TRANSFER to the oven and bake for 20 minutes, until the chickpeas get hot and bubbly and the tomatoes are tender.

SEASON both sides of the salmon fillets evenly with the remaining 1 teaspoon salt, pressing it into the fillets. Set aside.

CAREFULLY remove the baking dish from the oven and toss the chickpeas. Nestle the fish fillets into the chickpeas, spooning some of the mixture over the tops of the salmon. Transfer back to the oven and bake until the salmon is cooked through and flakes easily with a fork, 12 to 15 more minutes.

REMOVE from the oven. Place the fillets in four shallow bowls and spoon the curried chickpeas over and around the fillets. Sprinkle with cilantro and serve with lemon wedges.

STORE leftovers in an airtight container in the fridge for up to 3 days. Reheat in the oven at 325°F for 10 to 12 minutes, or microwave in 1-minute increments, stirring the chickpeas after each, until warmed through.

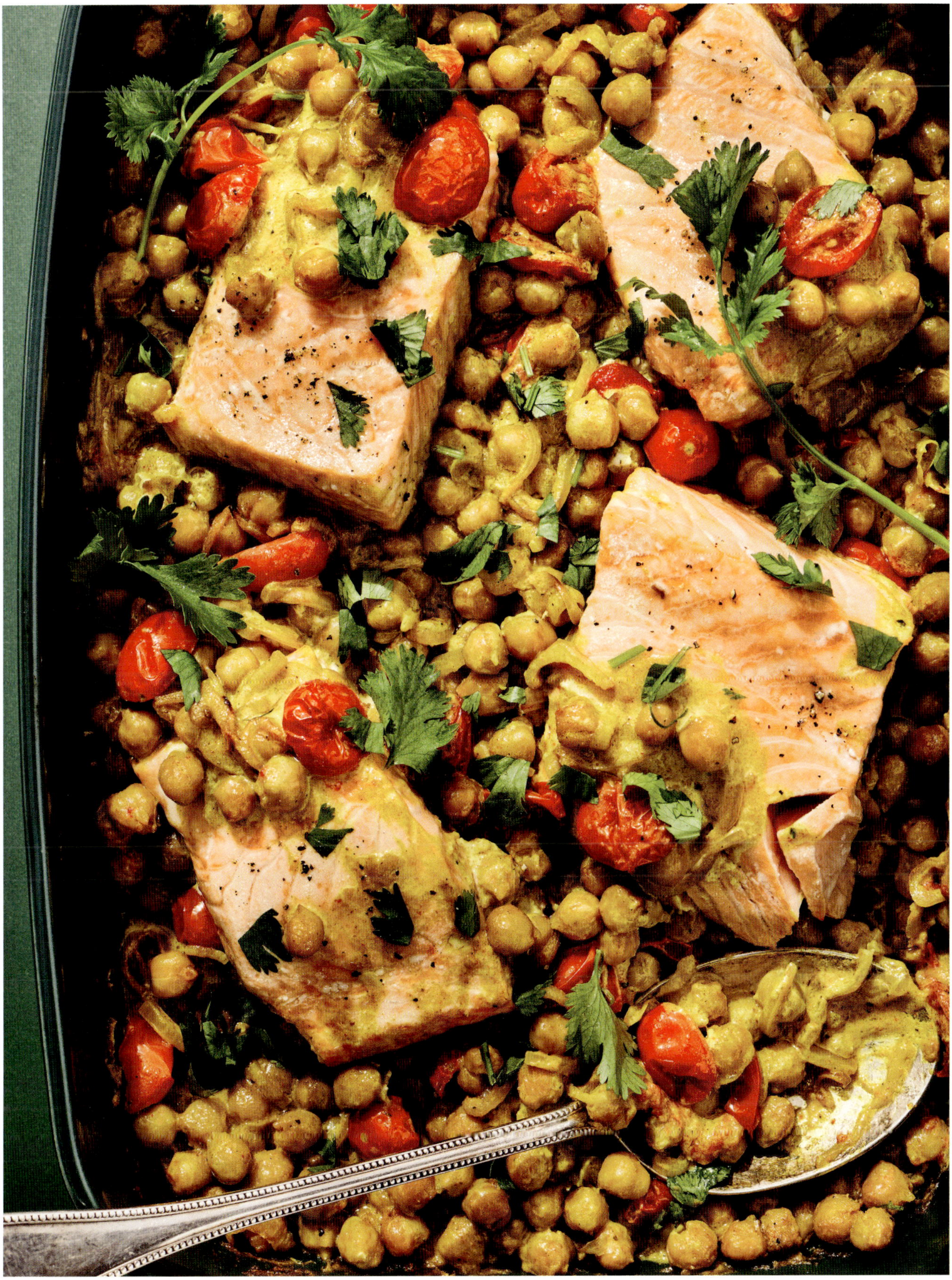

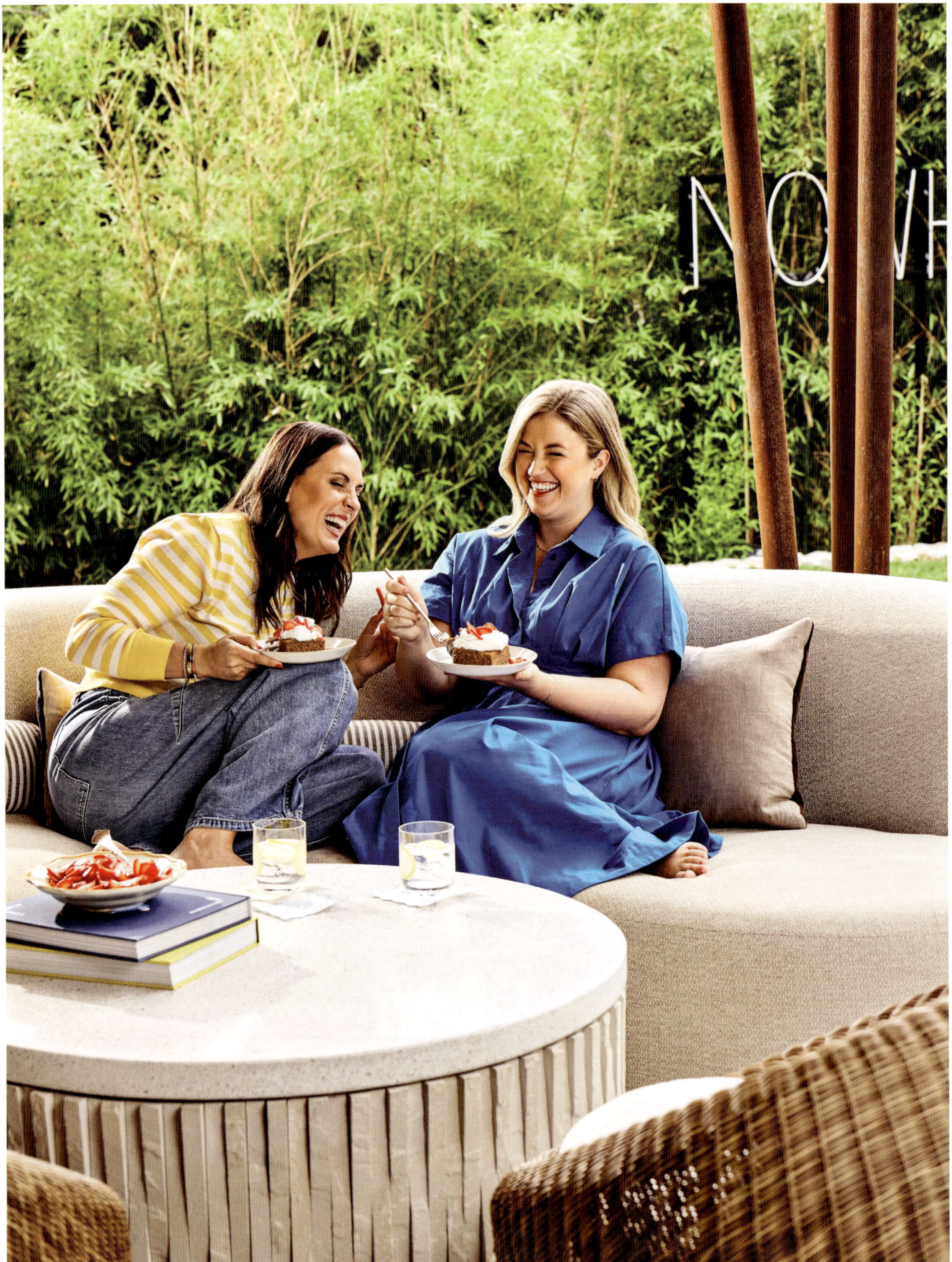

EASY SWEETS

SKILLET PEACH CRUMBLE

MAKES 8 SERVINGS | **TOTAL TIME:** 40 MINUTES

DIETARY

GLUTEN-FREE

VEGETARIAN

DAIRY-FREE (IF MODIFIED)

As a Southern girl, I know there's nothing quite like a bubbling peach crumble for dessert. Using frozen sliced peaches brings this dish together in no time (plus allows you to make this year-round) and the quick crumble topping is a breeze to make. Top it with a scoop of ice cream and you've got an easy yet impressive sweet treat that never fails to delight.

FOR THE PEACHES

2 tablespoons unsalted butter (sub vegan butter for dairy-free)

32 ounces frozen sliced peaches or 8 to 10 fresh peaches (see note)

1 teaspoon ground cinnamon

¼ teaspoon kosher salt

¼ cup coconut sugar

¼ cup pure maple syrup

1 teaspoon pure vanilla extract

Grated zest of ½ lemon

2 tablespoons tapioca flour or arrowroot flour

FOR THE CRUMBLE TOPPING

1½ cups gluten-free old-fashioned oats

½ cup gluten-free all-purpose flour

¼ cup coconut sugar

1 tablespoon pure maple syrup

6 tablespoons cold unsalted butter, cut into ¼-inch dice (sub vegan butter for dairy-free)

Vanilla ice cream, optional for serving (sub dairy-free ice cream for dairy-free)

PREHEAT the oven to 400°F.

START THE PEACHES: In a 10- or 12-inch cast-iron skillet, melt the butter over medium-high heat. Add the peaches, cinnamon, and salt and cook, stirring, until the peaches thaw and begin to release their juices, about 5 minutes.

ADD the coconut sugar, maple syrup, vanilla extract, and lemon zest. Increase the heat to a simmer and cook, tossing the peaches, until well coated, 1 to 2 minutes. Remove from the heat and sprinkle in the tapioca flour. Stir until well combined and smooth. Spread the peaches into a single layer in the pan and set aside to cool slightly.

MEANWHILE, MAKE THE CRUMBLE TOPPING: In a medium bowl, combine the oats, all-purpose flour, coconut sugar, maple syrup, and butter. Using clean hands or a pastry cutter, mash until the butter is fully incorporated and the mixture is coarse and crumbly. Sprinkle the topping evenly over the peaches.

BAKE THE CRUMBLE: Transfer the skillet to the oven and bake until the crumble is golden brown and the peaches are bubbling, about 20 minutes.

REMOVE from the oven and let cool slightly before serving, 5 to 10 minutes. Serve as is or finish with a scoop of ice cream, if desired.

FROM MY KITCHEN TO YOURS

Frozen peaches allow this recipe to be enjoyed all year long, but if you find some fantastic fresh peaches, those will work great. Just watch them closely and adjust the time they spend in the pan at the beginning so they are not too soft ahead of baking. You will likely only need to sauté for 2 to 3 minutes instead of 5 minutes.

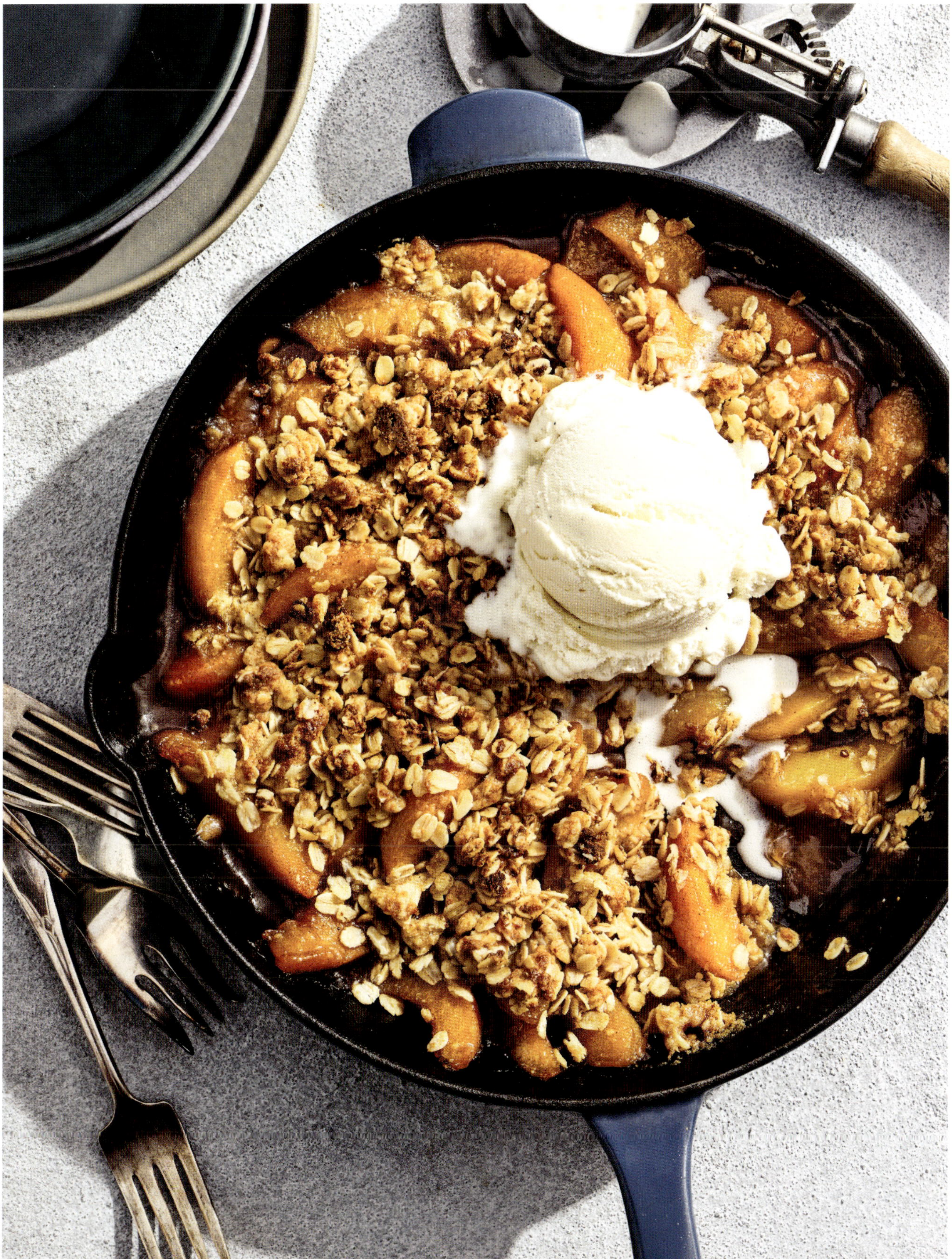

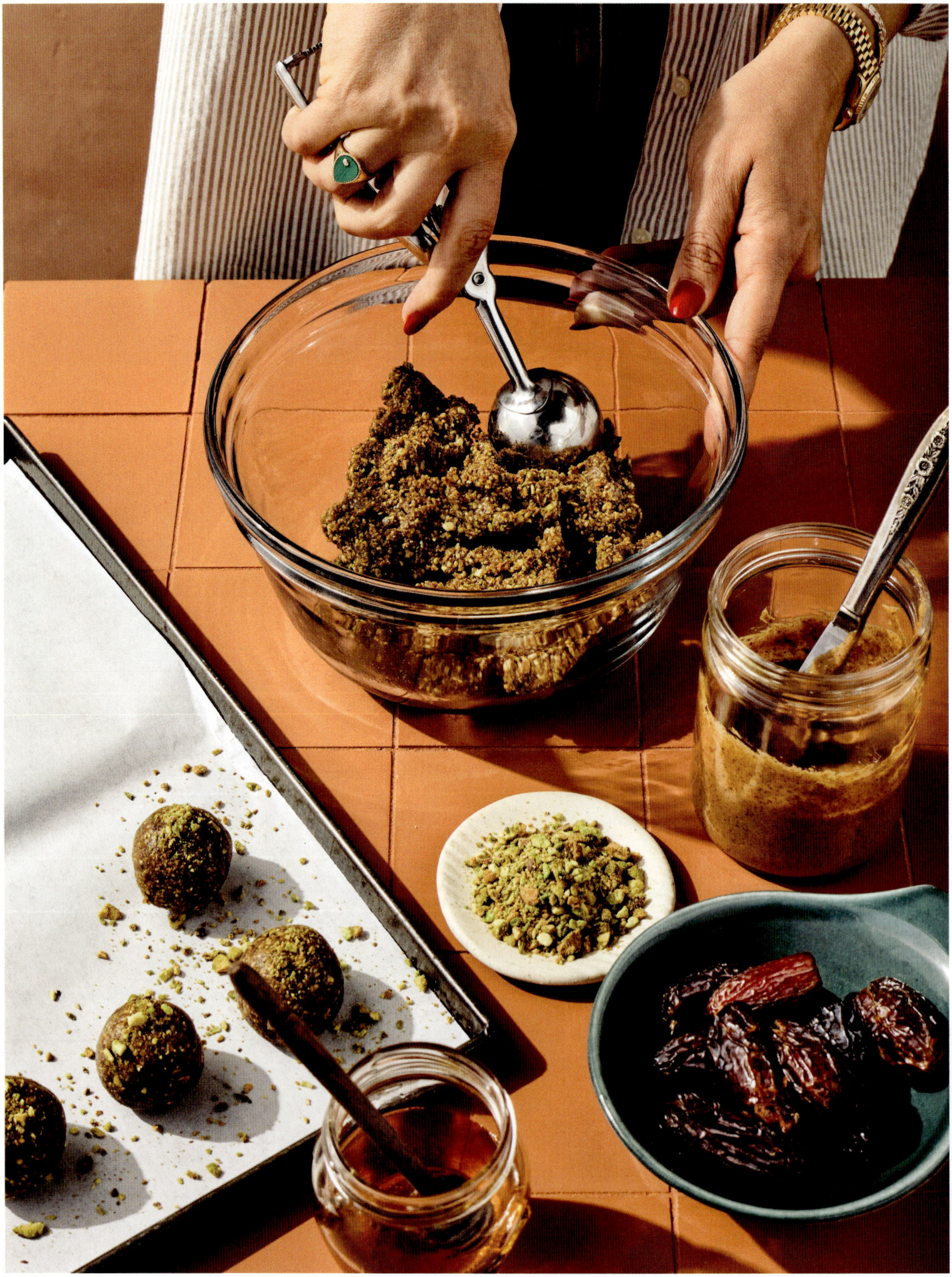

BAKLAVA-INSPIRED ENERGY BITES

MAKES 20 BITES | **PREP TIME:** 20 MINUTES | **CHILL TIME:** 30 MINUTES

DIETARY
GLUTEN-FREE
DAIRY-FREE
PALEO
VEGETARIAN
MAKE AHEAD

Packed with pistachios, walnuts, warm spices, dates, and honey, these energy bites are inspired by the flavors of baklava and are the perfect, nutritious sweet snack. Not only are they full of protein, fiber, and healthy fats, but they also have a subtle sweetness from dates and honey that makes them dessert-ready.

- 4 Medjool dates, pitted
- ½ cup plus 2 tablespoons roasted unsalted pistachios
- ½ cup walnut halves and pieces
- 1 cup gluten-free old-fashioned oats
- ½ cup almond flour
- ⅓ cup flaxseed meal
- 1½ teaspoons ground cinnamon
- ½ teaspoon kosher salt
- ¼ teaspoon allspice
- ¼ cup creamy unsweetened almond butter
- ½ teaspoon orange zest
- 3 tablespoons honey
- 1 teaspoon pure vanilla extract

LINE a sheet pan with parchment paper and set aside.

PLACE the dates in a small bowl and cover with hot water. Set aside.

IN a food processor or blender, pulse the pistachios until they form a sandy texture. Remove 2 tablespoons of the mixture and set aside for garnish.

ADD the walnuts, oats, flour, flaxseed meal, cinnamon, salt, and allspice to the food processor. Blend on low speed for 30 seconds, until the mixture is sandy. Scrape down the sides of the bowl and blend for another 10 seconds, until the mixture is well combined and the nuts are well chopped.

DRAIN the water off the dates and add the dates to the food processor along with the almond butter, orange zest, honey, and vanilla extract. Blend on low speed, working in 10-second increments and scraping the sides of the bowl between each interval, until a dough forms. The mixture will be thick and sticky.

TRANSFER the dough to a medium bowl. Using clean hands, knead the mixture for about 30 seconds to ensure all the ingredients are well incorporated.

USING a small cookie scoop, scoop out the dough into approximately 20 tablespoon-size portions. Roll each portion into a ball and set it on the prepared sheet pan. If needed, wet your hands a bit to keep the dough from sticking to them. Sprinkle the reserved pistachio bits over the energy bites.

TRANSFER to the fridge and chill for at least 30 minutes to firm up.

STORE in the fridge in an airtight container for up to 1 week or in the freezer for up to 3 months. Place a small piece of parchment paper between each layer to prevent sticking.

MINI CHOCOLATE RASPBERRY TARTS

MAKES 24 TARTS | **PREP TIME:** 40 MINUTES | **CHILL TIME:** 30 MINUTES

DIETARY
GLUTEN-FREE
GRAIN-FREE
DAIRY-FREE
PALEO
VEGETARIAN
MAKE AHEAD

These tarts are the perfect decadent treat and great to store in the freezer to grab on days you need something sweet. Not only are they super cute, but they're also packed with dark chocolate, healthy fats from the almond and coconut, and a bit of raspberry jam for a surprising fruity touch in the center.

FOR THE COOKIE BASE

Nonstick cooking spray
¼ cup coconut sugar
¼ cup coconut oil, melted
1 large egg, at room temperature
¼ cup pure maple syrup
1¼ cups almond flour
¾ cup tapioca flour
⅓ cup cocoa powder
½ teaspoon baking soda
½ teaspoon kosher salt
1 teaspoon instant espresso powder

FOR THE FILLING

¼ cup no-sugar-added raspberry jam
½ cup dairy-free dark chocolate chips
¼ cup unsweetened full-fat coconut milk
2 tablespoons pure maple syrup
½ teaspoon instant espresso powder
½ teaspoon pure vanilla extract
24 fresh raspberries
Flaky sea salt

POSITION a rack in the center of the oven and preheat the oven to 350°F. Thoroughly grease a mini muffin pan with the nonstick cooking spray. Set aside.

MAKE THE COOKIE BASE: In a large bowl, combine the coconut sugar, coconut oil, egg, and maple syrup. Whisk until smooth.

IN a medium bowl, combine the almond flour, tapioca flour, cocoa powder, baking soda, salt, and espresso powder. Whisk to combine and break up any clumps. Add the flour mixture to the coconut sugar mixture. Using a rubber spatula, stir to combine until a dough begins to form.

USING clean hands, work the dough until it is well combined and forms into a ball. The dough will be a bit sticky. If needed, wet your hands a bit to keep the dough from sticking to them.

ROLL the dough into 24 equal-size balls, about 1 tablespoon each. Place each in a muffin cup. Using your fingers, press each ball down in the center, bringing the dough up the sides of the muffin cups about three-quarters of the way, to make a small crust.

TRANSFER to the oven and bake for 9 minutes. Remove from the oven. The cookie base will have puffed up a bit; use the back of a small cookie scoop or tablespoon measure to press a well into each one. Transfer back to the oven and bake for 2 more minutes.

REMOVE from the oven and again press down on the bases as needed, ensuring there is a well in each crust for the filling. Allow to cool entirely.

MAKE THE FILLING: When the cookie bases have cooled, start the filling. Place ½ teaspoon of raspberry jam in the center of each crust.

IN a microwave-safe bowl, combine the chocolate chips, coconut milk, and maple syrup. Microwave in 30-second increments, stirring after each, until the chocolate is smooth. Add the espresso powder and vanilla and stir to combine.

USING a spoon, drizzle about 1 tablespoon of the chocolate mixture into each crust, filling it up to the top of the well. Top with a fresh raspberry, gently pressing it into the chocolate to adhere. Sprinkle with flaky salt.

TRANSFER to the fridge and chill for 30 minutes, until set. Using a butter knife, gently remove each tart from the tin. Transfer to an airtight container and store in the fridge for up to 1 week or in the freezer for up to 1 month.

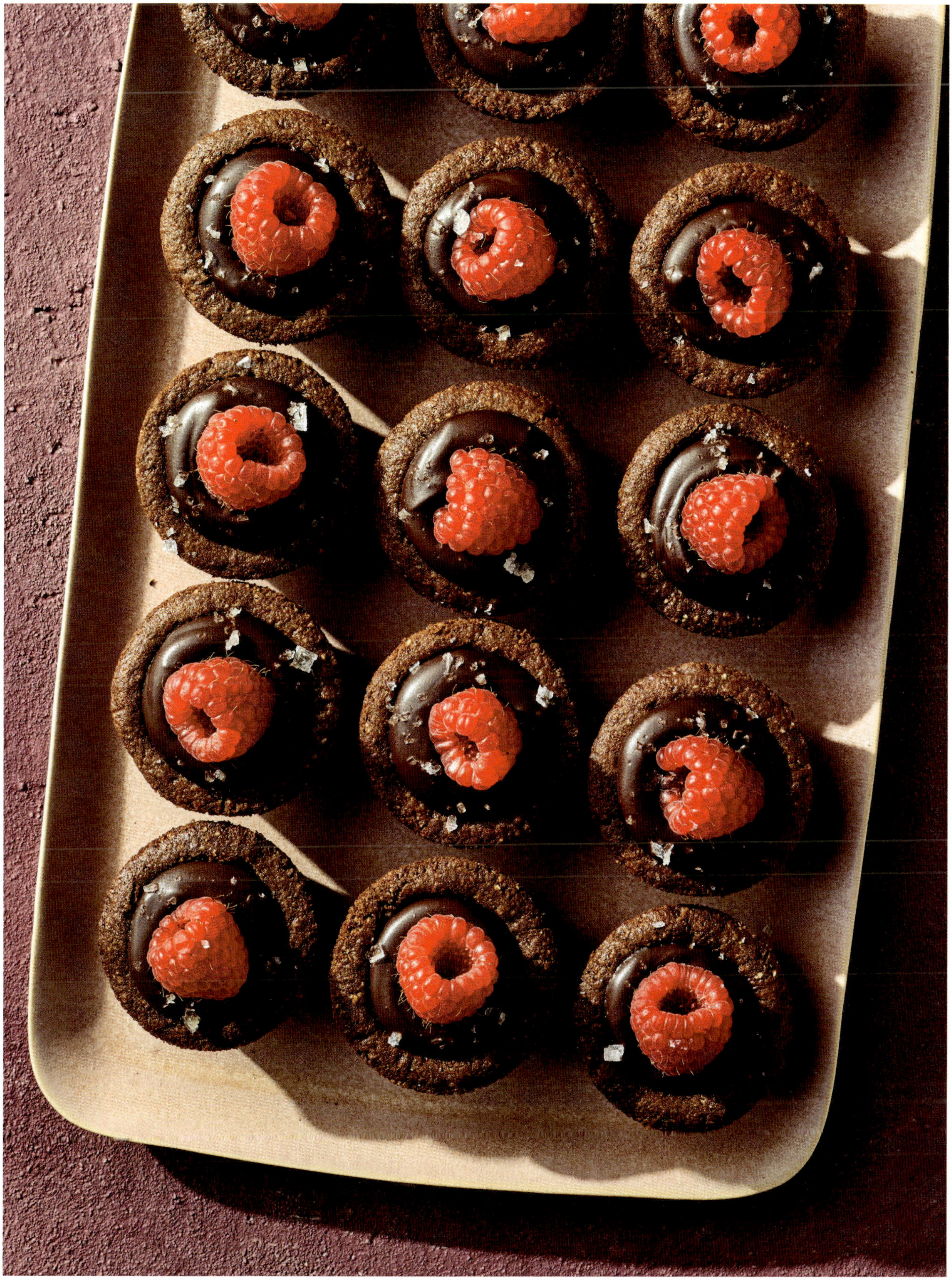

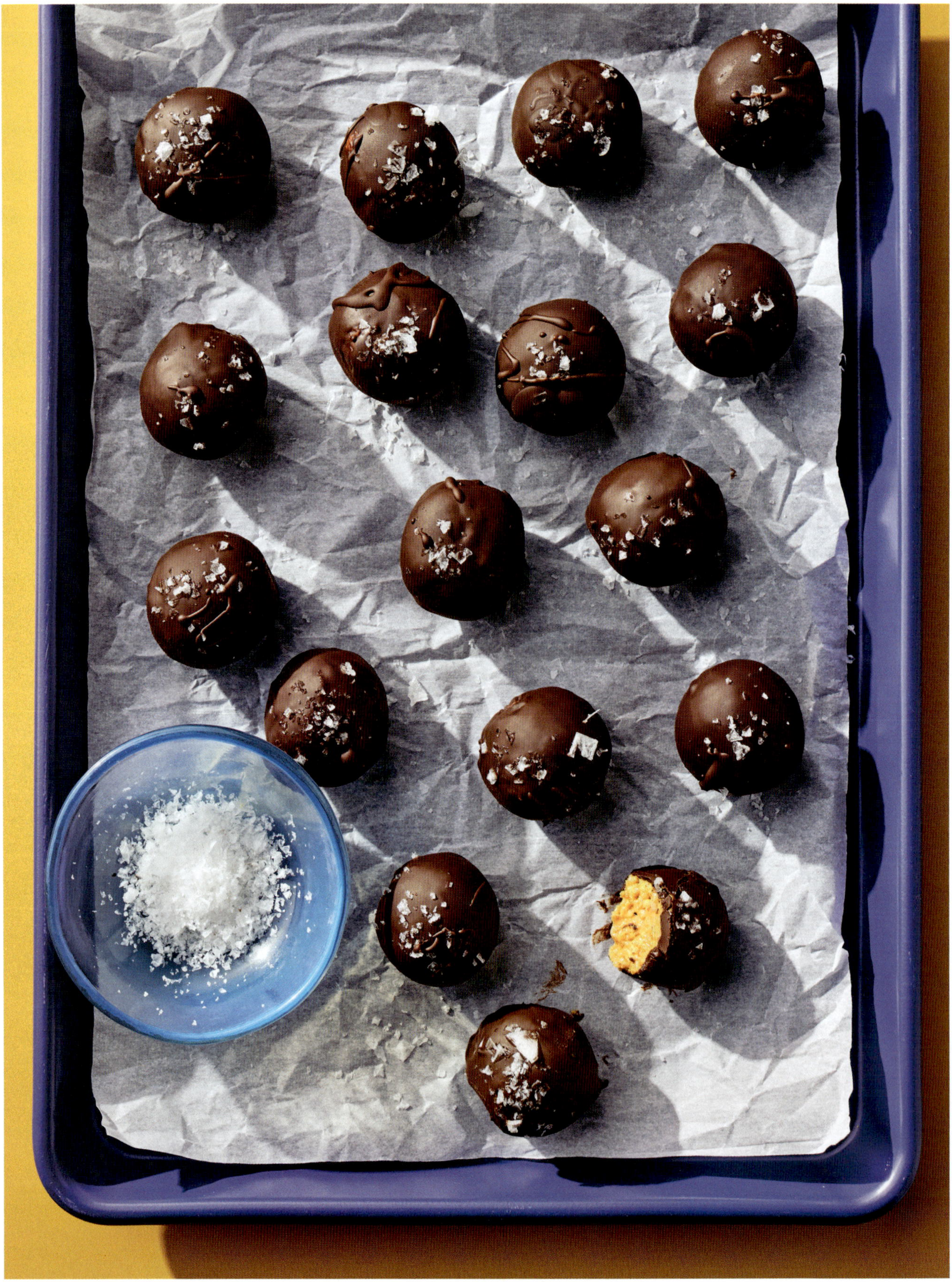

EASY NO-BAKE CRUNCHY PEANUT BUTTER BITES

MAKES 18 BITES | **PREP TIME:** 20 MINUTES | **CHILL TIME:** 30 MINUTES

DIETARY
GLUTEN-FREE
DAIRY-FREE
VEGETARIAN
MAKE AHEAD

These tasty no-bake bites are a hit in our house! With just a few ingredients and no oven required, they're simple enough for my kids to make on their own, but we all enjoy them. We love keeping a batch in the freezer for a quick sweet treat whenever the candy bar craving strikes.

- 1 cup creamy peanut butter
- 2 tablespoons honey
- 2 cups cornflakes cereal
- 2 tablespoons hemp hearts
- ½ cup dairy-free dark chocolate chips
- 1 teaspoon liquid coconut oil (see note, page 24)
- 1 tablespoon flaky sea salt

LINE a sheet pan with parchment paper and set aside.

IN a medium bowl, combine the peanut butter and honey. Stir until well combined.

PLACE the cereal in a zip-top bag and, using your hands or rolling pin, crush the cereal until it is coarsely crumbled. Add the cereal and the hemp hearts to the bowl with the peanut butter–honey mixture. Stir until well combined.

USING clean damp hands, roll the mixture into about eighteen 1-inch round balls and place them on the prepared sheet pan. Transfer to the freezer to chill slightly while you melt the chocolate.

IN a microwave-safe bowl, combine the chocolate chips and coconut oil. Microwave in 30-second increments, stirring after each, until the chocolate is completely melted and smooth, taking care not to burn it. Set aside to cool slightly.

REMOVE the bites from the freezer. Using a fork and a spoon, coat each of the bites in the melted chocolate, using the spoon to help coat the top of the bite and the fork to pull it out of the chocolate and allow excess chocolate to drip off. Transfer the dipped bite back to the sheet pan and top with a sprinkle of flaky salt. Repeat with the remaining bites until all are coated.

PLACE in the freezer and let chill until the chocolate is set, at least 30 minutes. Store in an airtight container in the fridge for up to 1 week or in the freezer for up to 3 months.

CADY'S STRAWBERRY SHORTCAKE

MAKES 9 SQUARES | **TOTAL TIME:** 1 HOUR

DIETARY
GLUTEN-FREE
GRAIN-FREE
DAIRY-FREE
VEGETARIAN

Cady is my right hand at the Defined Dish—and she happens to be a total whiz at baking. She's shared cake recipes in my last two books, so naturally we needed another Cady classic here! This one is light, simple, and topped with juicy strawberries—basically my dream dessert when the weather warms up. It's the perfect not-too-sweet treat, and with store-bought whipped topping, it comes together in no time. You could even skip the berries and whipped topping and frost this instead for an easy twist on a celebration cake!

FOR THE SHORTCAKE

- Nonstick cooking spray
- 2½ cups almond flour
- 1¼ cups tapioca flour
- ½ tablespoon ground cinnamon
- 1 teaspoon kosher salt
- 3 large eggs, at room temperature
- ¾ cup liquid coconut oil (see note, page 24)
- ½ cup pure maple syrup
- 2½ teaspoons baking soda
- 1½ teaspoons pure vanilla extract
- Grated zest of 1 lemon
- ⅓ cup freshly squeezed lemon juice, strained (about 2 lemons)

FOR THE STRAWBERRY TOPPING

- 3 cups thinly sliced strawberries (about 1 pound)
- 1 teaspoon freshly squeezed lemon juice, strained
- 1½ teaspoons pure maple syrup
- Dairy-free whipped topping, for serving

POSITION a rack in the center of the oven and preheat the oven to 350°F. Line a 9 × 9-inch baking pan with parchment paper, letting it hang over two opposite sides of the pan (you'll use it to lift out the cake later). Lightly mist it with nonstick cooking spray and set aside.

MAKE THE SHORTCAKE: In a medium bowl, sift together the almond flour, tapioca flour, cinnamon, and salt. Set aside.

IN a large bowl with a hand mixer or in a stand mixer fitted with the whisk attachment, beat the eggs on medium-high speed until pale yellow and fluffy, 3 to 4 minutes. Lower the speed to medium and beat in the coconut oil, maple syrup, baking soda, vanilla extract, lemon zest, and lemon juice until combined.

ADJUST the mixer speed to medium-low and, working in 1-cup increments, slowly add the dry ingredients, scraping down the sides of the bowl as needed. Mix until everything is well combined, 1 to 2 minutes.

POUR the batter into the prepared baking pan and gently tap the pan on the counter to remove any air bubbles. Bake until the top of the cake is lightly browned and a cake tester inserted into the middle comes out clean, about 35 minutes. If the top starts to get overly browned, place a sheet of foil over the top, but note that this will be a darker cake.

ALLOW the cake to cool in the pan for 10 minutes, then use the parchment sling to carefully transfer the cake to a wire rack to cool completely.

MEANWHILE, MAKE THE STRAWBERRY TOPPING: In a large bowl, stir together the strawberries, lemon juice, and maple syrup. Place the bowl in the fridge until you're ready to assemble the cake.

TO SERVE: When the cake is cooled, transfer it to a serving platter and cut it into squares using a serrated knife. Plate each slice and top with a dollop of the whipped topping, then the strawberries. Serve immediately for best results.

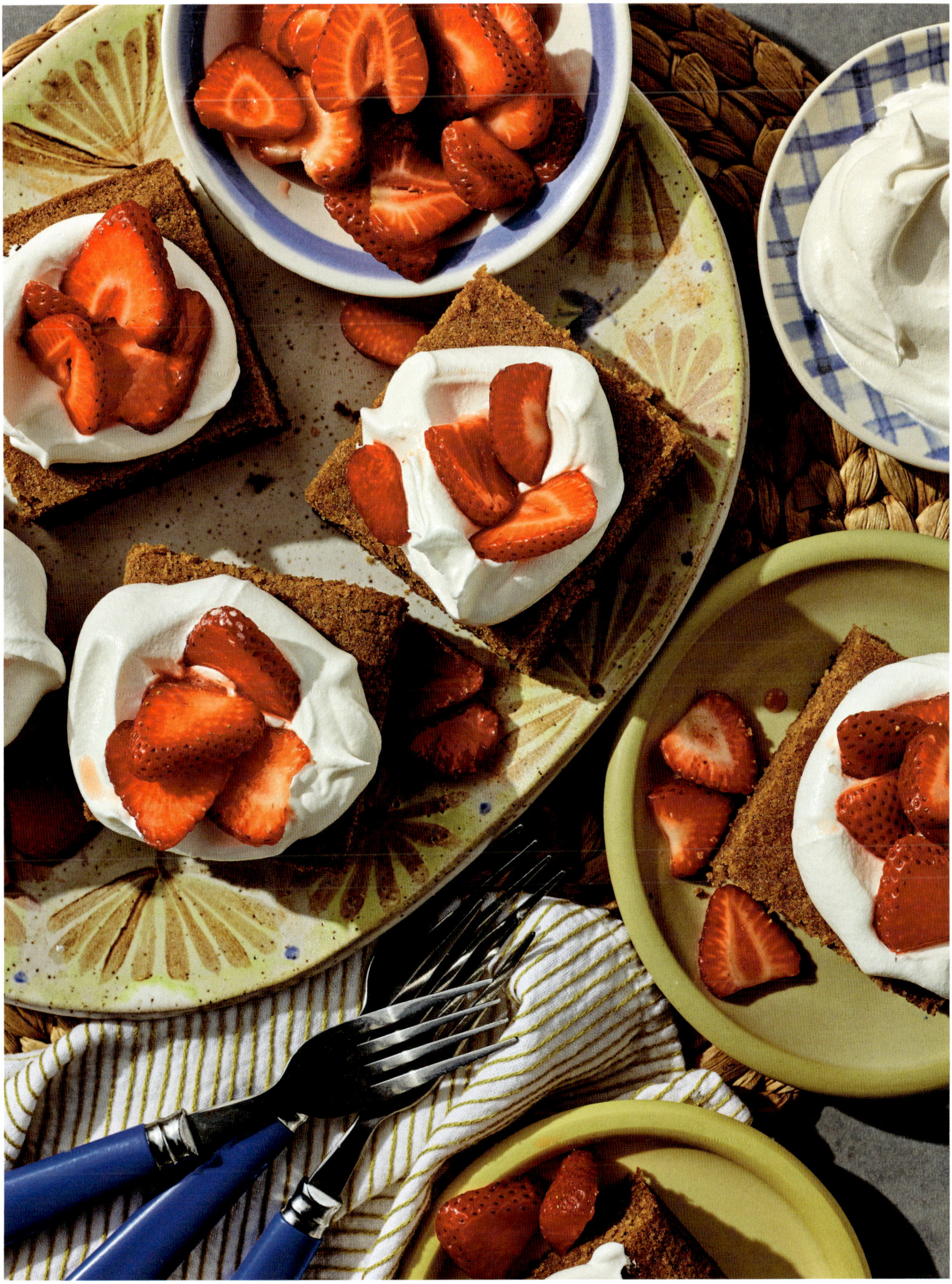

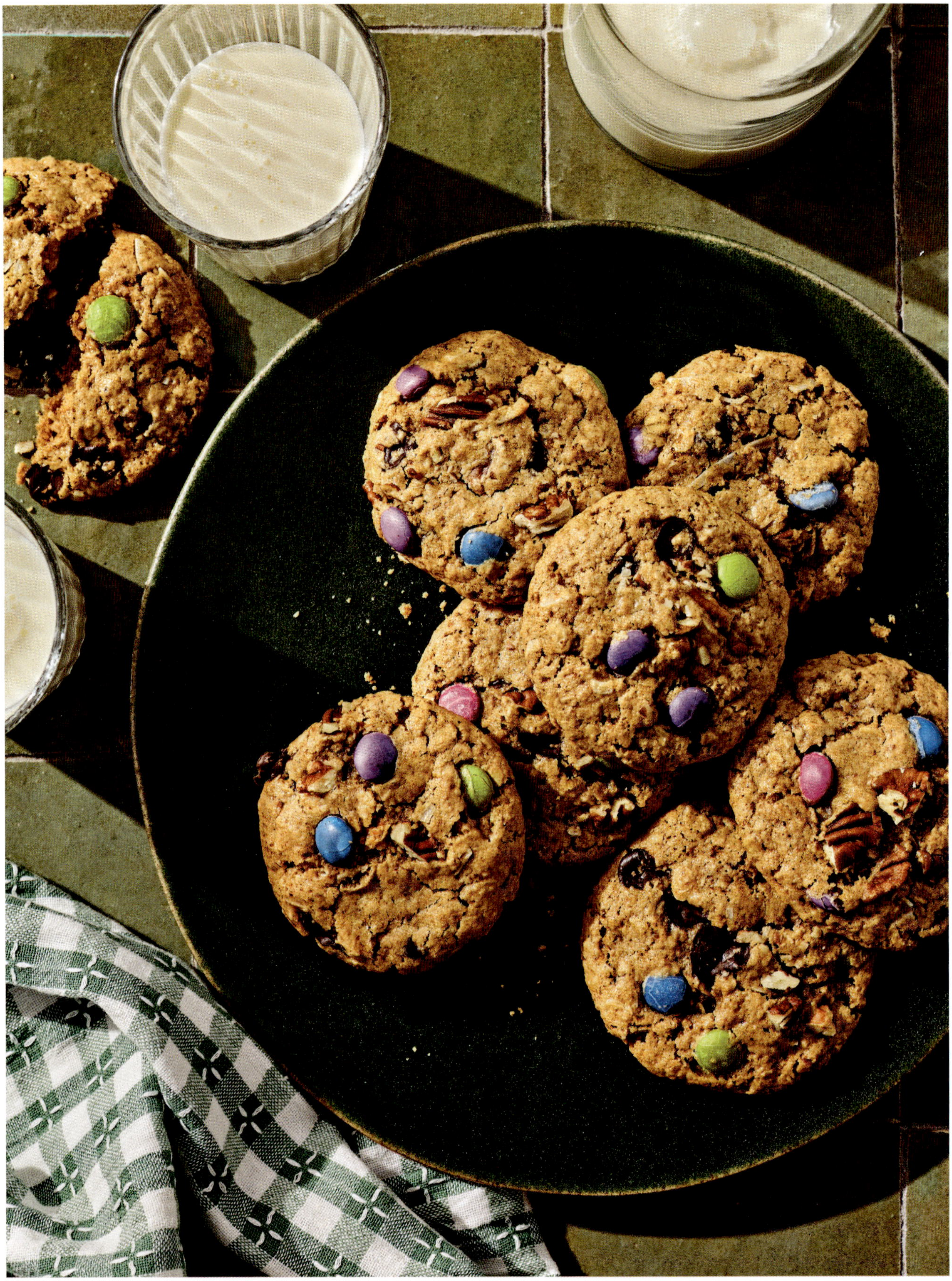

COWBOY COOKIES

MAKES: 25 COOKIES | **TOTAL TIME:** 1 HOUR (INCLUDES CHILLING)

DIETARY
GLUTEN-FREE
DAIRY-FREE
VEGETARIAN

MAKE AHEAD

Cowboy cookies are a nostalgic classic, perfect for turning pantry staples into a salty, nutty, and sweet treat. This gluten-free version keeps the essentials like oats, chocolate chips, and pecans. I love having the dough in my freezer for when my sweet tooth strikes or unexpected company arrives. It's an easy, crowd-pleasing delight!

- 2 cups gluten-free old-fashioned oats
- 1½ cups almond flour
- 1 cup arrowroot flour
- 1 teaspoon baking powder
- ½ teaspoon baking soda
- ½ teaspoon ground cinnamon
- ¼ teaspoon kosher salt
- 2 large eggs, at room temperature
- ½ cup liquid coconut oil (see note, page 24)
- ½ cup creamy unsweetened almond butter
- 2 teaspoons pure vanilla extract
- 1 cup coconut sugar
- ¼ cup pure maple syrup
- ½ cup chopped toasted pecans
- ½ cup unsweetened shredded coconut
- ½ cup dairy-free dark chocolate chips
- ½ cup dairy-free candy-coated chocolate gems, divided

IN a food processor or blender, combine the oats, almond flour, arrowroot flour, baking powder, baking soda, cinnamon, and salt. Pulse for 20 seconds, just until the oats begin to break down slightly. You still want some texture. Set aside.

IN a large bowl, combine the eggs, coconut oil, almond butter, vanilla extract, coconut sugar, and maple syrup. Whisk vigorously until the mixture is smooth and resembles a caramel sauce.

SLOWLY add the oat mixture into the bowl with the wet ingredients and stir until well combined and a dough has formed. The dough will be thick and sticky. Fold in the pecans, shredded coconut, chocolate chips, and ¼ cup of the candy-coated chocolate gems.

LINE a sheet pan with parchment paper. Using a large cookie scoop, portion the dough into about twenty-five 2-inch balls and place them on the prepared sheet pan (you don't need to separate them much at this step). Press a few of the remaining candy-coated chocolate gems into each cookie. Transfer to the freezer and allow the dough to set for 30 minutes.

ONCE set, position two racks in the center of the oven and preheat the oven to 350°F. Line another sheet pan with parchment paper. Divide the dough balls between the two prepared sheet pans, spacing them about 2 inches apart.

TRANSFER the sheet pans to the center racks of the oven and bake until the cookies are golden brown and soft in the middle, 10 to 12 minutes. Remove from the oven, gently tap the sheet pans on the counter to slightly deflate the cookies and allow them to cool completely on the sheet pans.

STORE in an airtight container at room temperature for up to 3 days.

FROM MY KITCHEN TO YOURS

FREEZER TIP: Once the cookie dough balls are frozen, you can store them in a freezer-safe zip-top bag in the freezer. I like to bake them off in smaller batches if I don't think we will go through the entire batch in a week. If you bake them straight from the freezer, you will need to add 1 to 2 minutes to the baking time.

PECAN SANDIES

MAKES 18 COOKIES | **TOTAL TIME:** 35 MINUTES

DIETARY
GLUTEN-FREE
GRAIN-FREE
VEGETARIAN
DAIRY-FREE (IF MODIFIED)
MAKE AHEAD

Named pecan sandies for their crumbly texture, these classic, old-fashioned shortbread cookies are slightly sweet, decadent, and buttery—perfect for the holidays or alongside a cup of coffee for a mid-morning treat. This gluten-free version has just a few ingredients and comes together quickly!

1 stick unsalted butter, at room temperature (sub vegan butter for dairy-free)
⅓ cup coconut sugar
1 teaspoon pure vanilla extract
½ cup plus 2 tablespoons tapioca flour
1¼ cups almond flour
½ teaspoon kosher salt
¼ teaspoon ground cinnamon
½ cup finely chopped pecans
18 pecan halves

IN a large bowl with a hand mixer or in a stand mixer fitted with the paddle attachment, cream together the butter, coconut sugar, and vanilla extract on medium speed until fluffy, 2 to 3 minutes, scraping down the sides of the bowl as needed. Beating until fluffy is an important step for the final texture of the cookies.

ADD the tapioca flour, almond flour, salt, and cinnamon. Mix on low until just combined and the dough starts to form. Add the chopped pecans and continue mixing on low until the pecans are well distributed throughout the dough.

POSITION two racks in the center of the oven. Preheat the oven to 350°F. Line two sheet pans with parchment paper.

USING a 1½-tablespoon cookie scoop, scoop out the dough and roll it into 18 balls. Place the dough balls onto one of the prepared sheet pans (you don't need to separate them much at this step). Transfer the sheet pan to the fridge to chill while the oven preheats.

DIVIDE the dough balls between the two prepared sheet pans, spacing them about 2 inches apart. Using two fingers, gently press down the dough balls to flatten to about ½ inch thick. Top each cookie with a pecan half, gently pressing it into the dough.

TRANSFER the sheet pans to the center racks of the oven and bake until golden brown and firm, 12 to 14 minutes. Transfer to a wire rack and let cool for 8 to 10 minutes before serving.

STORE in an airtight container at room temperature for up to 5 days.

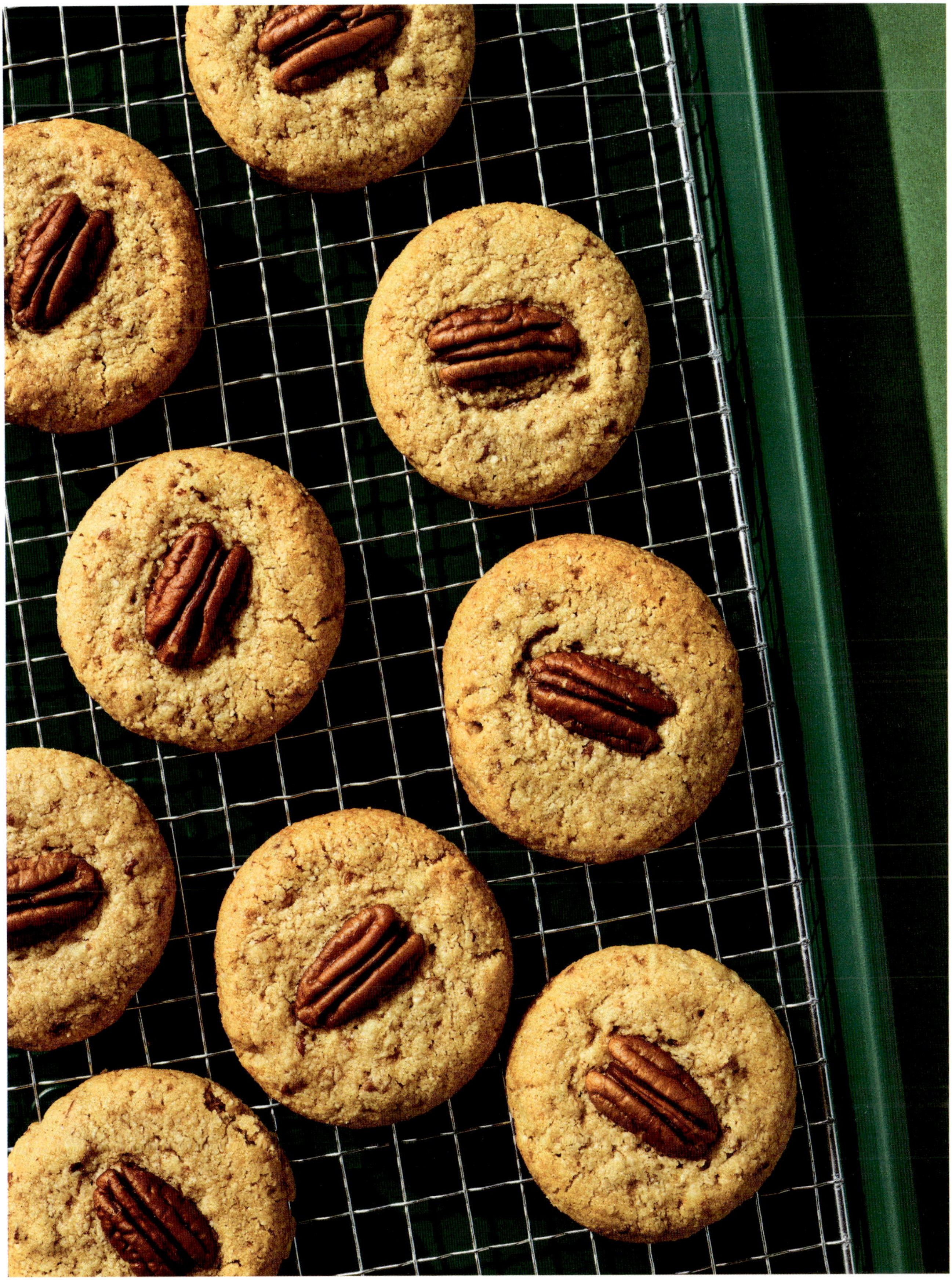

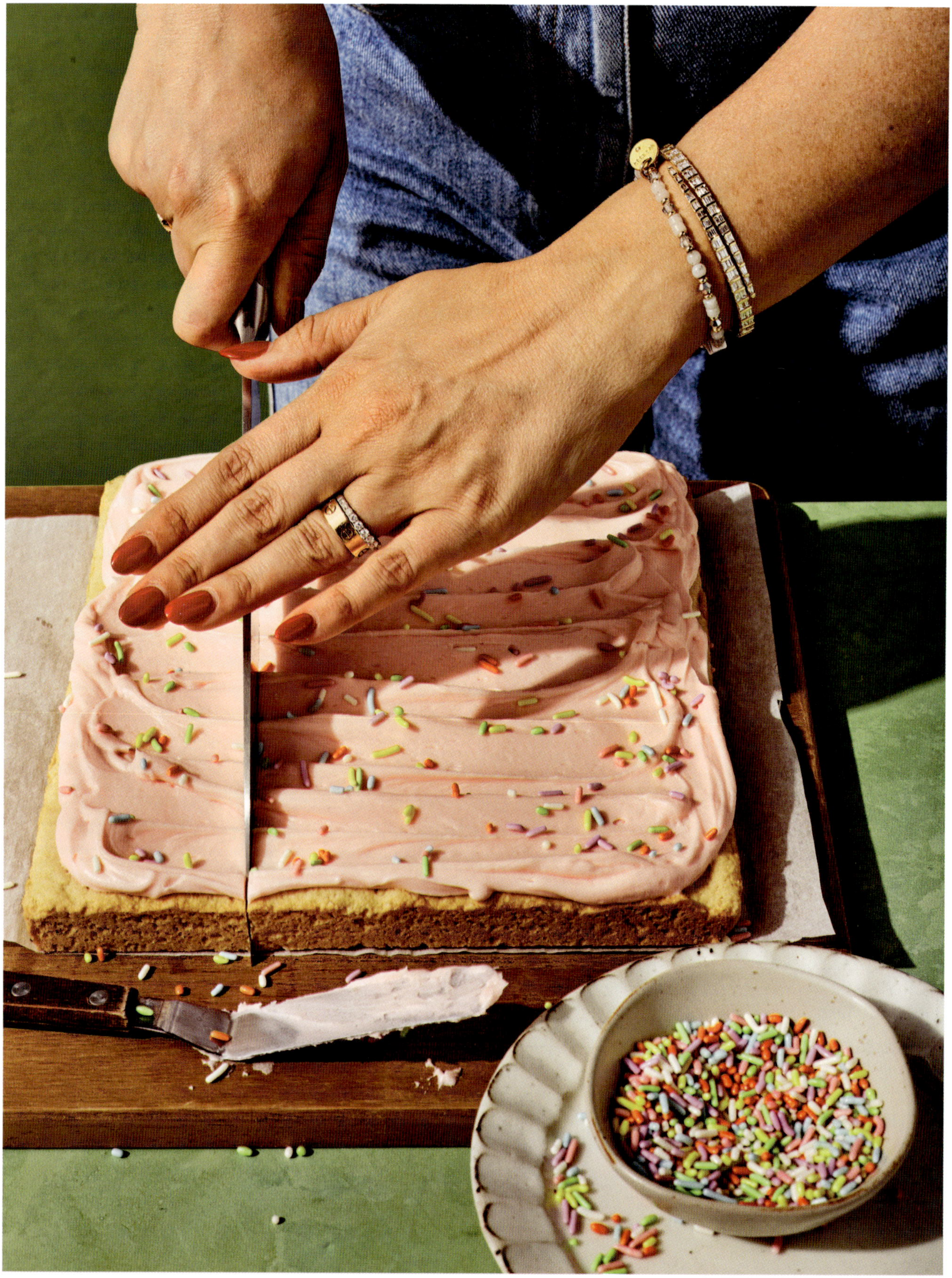

FROSTED COOKIE BARS

MAKES 12 SQUARES | **TOTAL TIME:** 1 HOUR 15 MINUTES

DIETARY

GLUTEN-FREE

GRAIN-FREE

VEGETARIAN

DAIRY-FREE (IF MODIFIED)

Have you ever tried Lofthouse cookies? The classic grocery store frosted cookie was a staple in my childhood—one of my absolute favorites! I decided to make a foolproof bar version of these delicious cookies. The only dreadful part? Waiting for the cookie base to completely cool! But trust me, it'll be worth the wait.

FOR THE COOKIE BASE

Nonstick cooking spray

3 cups almond flour

1 cup tapioca flour

½ teaspoon kosher salt

½ teaspoon baking powder

¼ teaspoon baking soda

6 tablespoons unsalted butter, melted (sub vegan butter for dairy-free)

½ cup pure maple syrup

1½ teaspoons pure vanilla extract

½ teaspoon pure almond extract

1 large egg, at room temperature

FOR THE FROSTING

4 ounces cream cheese, softened (sub dairy-free cream cheese for dairy-free)

2 tablespoons unsalted butter, softened (sub vegan butter for dairy-free)

1 teaspoon pure vanilla extract

2 cups powdered sugar

Pink gel food coloring (see note)

2 tablespoons rainbow sprinkles

PREHEAT the oven to 350°F. Line a 9 × 9-inch baking pan with parchment paper, letting it hang over two opposite sides of the pan (you'll use it to lift out the bars later). Lightly mist it with nonstick cooking spray and set aside.

MAKE THE COOKIE BASE: In a large bowl, combine the almond flour, tapioca flour, salt, baking powder, and baking soda. Stir to combine and break up any clumps.

ADD the melted butter, maple syrup, vanilla extract, almond extract, and egg. Using a rubber spatula, stir until well combined and a sticky dough forms.

TRANSFER the dough into the prepared baking pan and press it into an even layer using a rubber spatula or clean damp hands. Bake until golden brown and a cake tester comes out clean when inserted in the middle of the pan, about 20 minutes. Remove from the oven and let cool slightly in the pan, about 5 minutes, then use the parchment sling to transfer to a wire rack. Let cool completely before frosting, at least 30 minutes.

MAKE THE FROSTING: In a stand mixer with the paddle attachment, combine the cream cheese, butter, and vanilla extract. Beat on medium until light and fluffy, 2 to 3 minutes. Slowly add the powdered sugar and beat on high until combined, 2 to 3 more minutes.

ADD a drop of the gel food coloring to the frosting and mix until well combined. Add more coloring as desired.

TRANSFER the icing to the fridge until the cookie base is completely cooled.

ASSEMBLE THE BARS: Once cooled, use a small offset spatula or the back of a butter knife to frost the cooled cookie base with the frosting. Top with the rainbow sprinkles. Allow the bars to set at room temperature for 15 more minutes, so the frosting can firm up, before cutting into squares and serving.

STORE in an airtight container at room temperature for up to 2 days.

FROM MY KITCHEN TO YOURS

A little amount of food gel goes a long way! Add a small amount to start until you achieve the color you prefer. I also love switching up the color I use depending on the occasion!

ALMOND JOYFUL BITES

MAKES 12 BITES | **PREP TIME:** 15 MINUTES | **CHILL TIME:** 1 HOUR 30 MINUTES

DIETARY
GLUTEN-FREE
GRAIN-FREE
DAIRY-FREE
PALEO
VEGETARIAN
MAKE AHEAD

Candy bar lovers, here is a fun one for you! Dairy-free, gluten-free, grain-free, and refined-sugar-free almond bites made with fewer than ten ingredients—and no baking required! I love these bites for a perfectly portioned sweet treat and healthier alternative to the real thing. They keep well in the freezer and can be stored for weeks, ensuring you always have a little dessert on hand!

FOR THE BASE

1½ cups unsweetened shredded coconut

½ cup almond flour

¼ cup coconut oil, melted

¼ cup honey

1 teaspoon pure vanilla extract

2 tablespoons almond milk or other nondairy milk alternative

¼ teaspoon kosher salt

12 raw almonds

FOR THE COATING

1 cup dairy-free dark chocolate chips

1 tablespoon liquid coconut oil

LEFTOVER shredded coconut? Try my Crunchy Coconut Shrimp Bowls with Spicy Aioli (page 211).

LINE a sheet pan with parchment paper and set aside.

MAKE THE BASE: In a medium bowl, combine the shredded coconut and almond flour. Stir to combine. Add the coconut oil, honey, vanilla extract, almond milk, and salt. Using a rubber spatula, stir to combine until the base is evenly mixed. The mixture will be a bit sticky.

USING a 1½-tablespoon cookie scoop, scoop out the dough into 12 portions. Roll them into balls. If needed, wet your hands a bit to keep the dough from sticking to them. Using your fingers, gently press down on each ball, carefully forming into an oval shape that is about ½ inch thick. Top each piece with one almond, pressing it lightly into the center. Transfer to the freezer and chill for at least 30 minutes, preferably 1 hour, until they have hardened.

MAKE THE COATING: In a microwave-safe bowl, combine the chocolate chips and coconut oil. Microwave in 30-second increments, stirring after each, until the chocolate is completely melted and smooth, taking care not to burn it. Set aside to cool slightly.

REMOVE the sheet pan from the freezer. Using a fork and a spoon, coat each of the bites in the melted chocolate, using the spoon to help coat the top of the bite and the fork to pull it out of the chocolate and allow excess chocolate to drip off. Transfer the dipped bite back to the sheet pan and repeat with the remaining bites until all are coated.

PLACE in the freezer and let chill until the chocolate is set, at least 30 minutes.

STORE in an airtight container in the fridge for up to 1 week or in the freezer for up to 3 months.

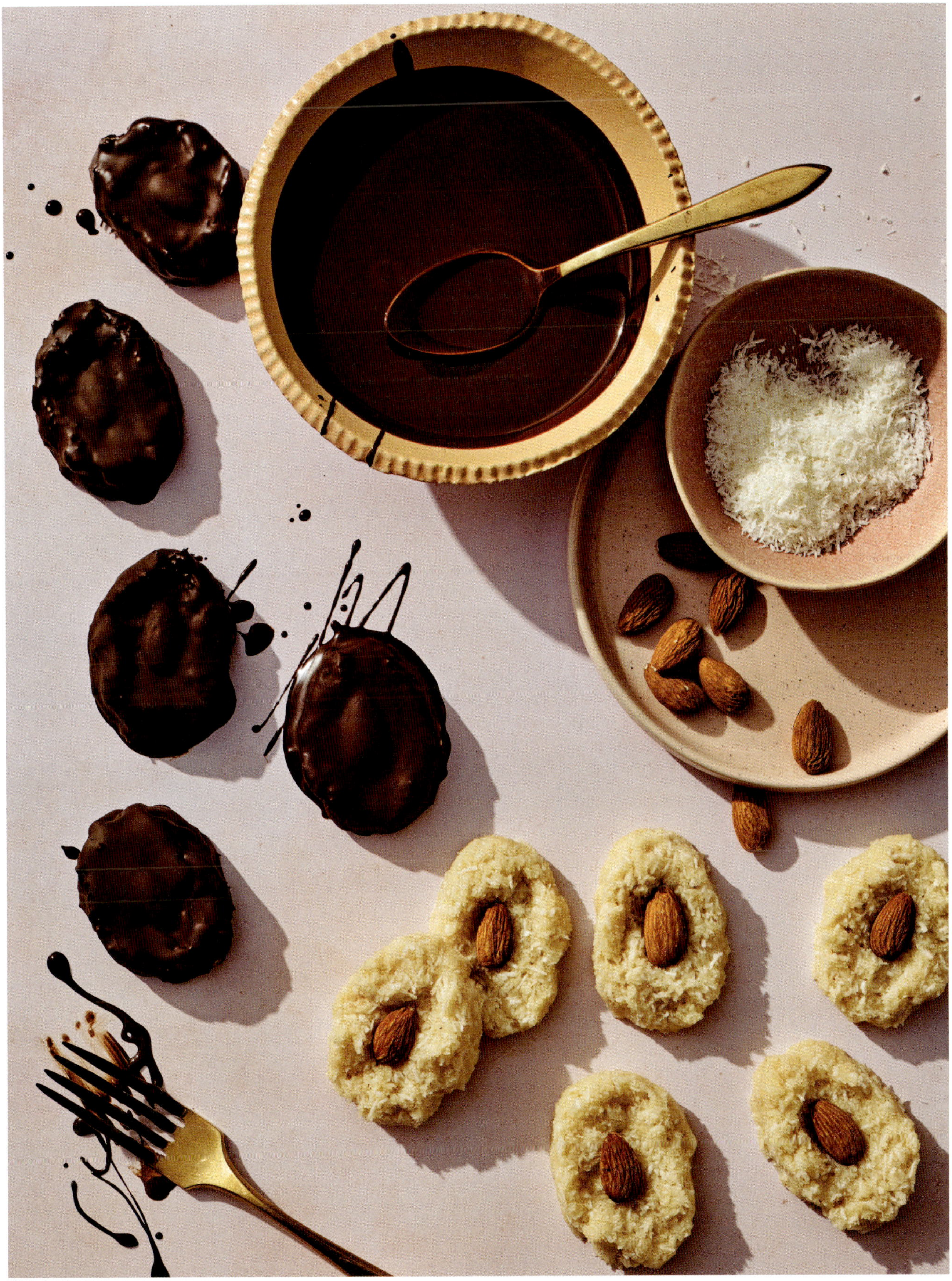

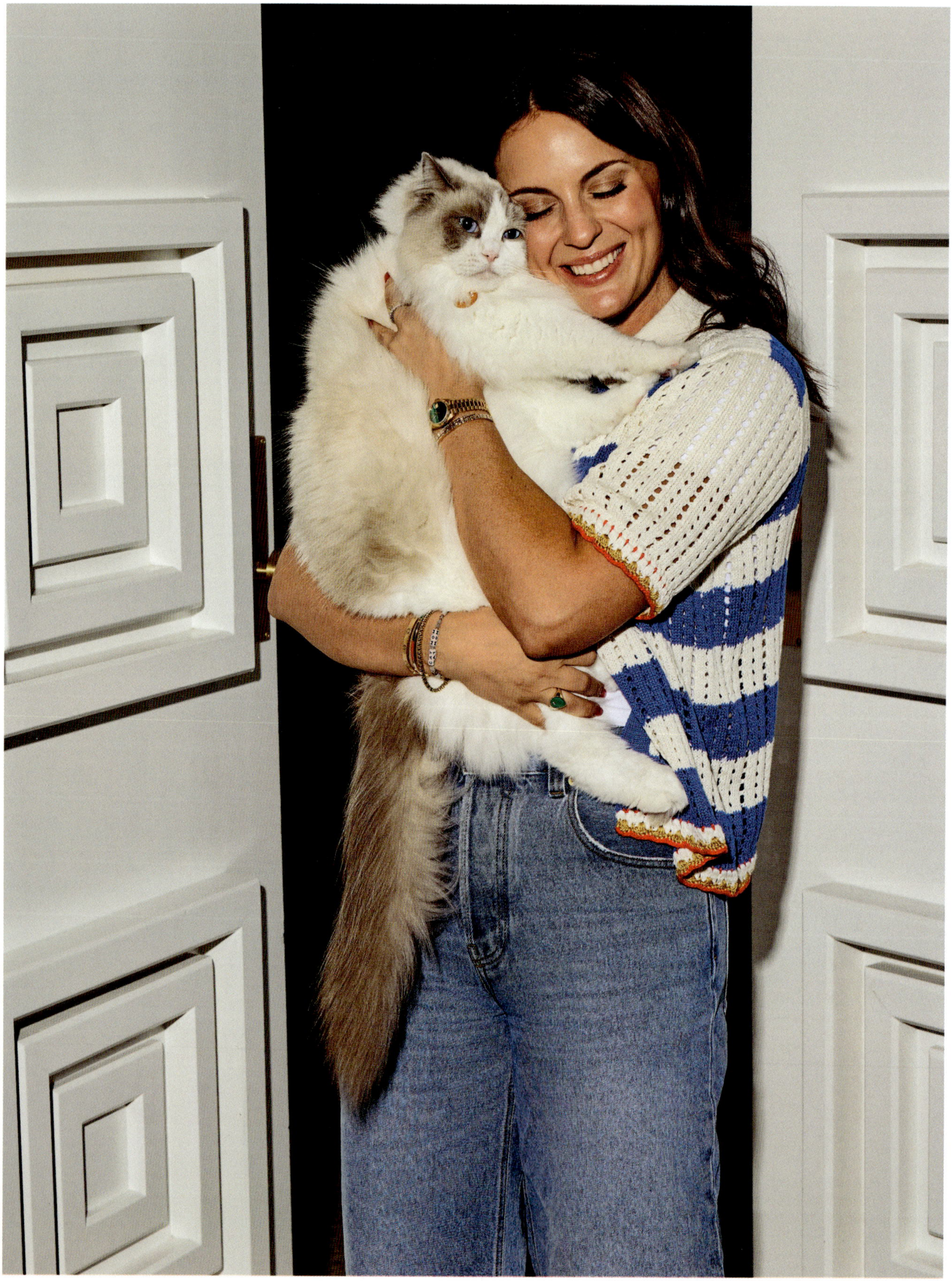

TO THE DEFINED DISH COMMUNITY—Wow! Look how far we have come together. From the early days to book four! I hope you know the gratitude that beats through my heart and soul for your continued love and support. Thank you times a million.

CLAYTON, SUTTON, AND WINNIE—The three of you are my whole world. I could be at any dinner table and be happy as long as you're there with me. While creating and sharing these recipes brings me so much joy, it's gathering around the table with you three that fills my heart the most.

CADY—My right hand, my rock. We both know none of this would get done with as much grace without you. Thank you for making this book better, my business stronger, and me a better person. I'll forever be grateful to the angels above who dropped you into my life.

MCKENZIE—I'll never stop thanking the social media gods for connecting us. Your expert recipe testing and thoughtful feedback made this book better than I ever imagined. I'm so grateful for you.

EVA—What a dream it's been to bring this book to life with you. Your creativity and vision go beyond anything I could have dreamed of. It was an honor to work alongside you.

ADAM—Thank you for just getting it. Your craftsmanship and dedication to these recipes have resulted in beautiful dishes that still feel like me.

GENESIS—Your creative eye is pure magic. Thank you for lending your talent to this project.

DENISE—We've been through so much together and I know the road ahead will still have you in the passenger seat, always rooting for me.

NICOLE—The best lit agent in the business. I'm so lucky to have you by my side on this journey.

CASSIE AND THE WILLIAM MORROW TEAM—Working with you is a dream. Thank you for letting me be myself and for supporting my books, which continue to feel true to who I am.

TO MY PARENTS AND SIBLINGS—Thank you for instilling in me a love for gathering around the dinner table. Those moments we've shared (and continue to share) spark my passion for creating and publishing recipes.

AND TO MY DEAREST FRIENDS AND TRUSTY RECIPE TESTERS—Thank you for the unwavering support, the laughter, and the endless taste testing. Especially my "Alex's Test Kitchen" crew whose love, feedback, and "dumb questions" (which are never actually dumb!) make my work better and my life fuller. I'm a better person because of each of you.

THANK YOU

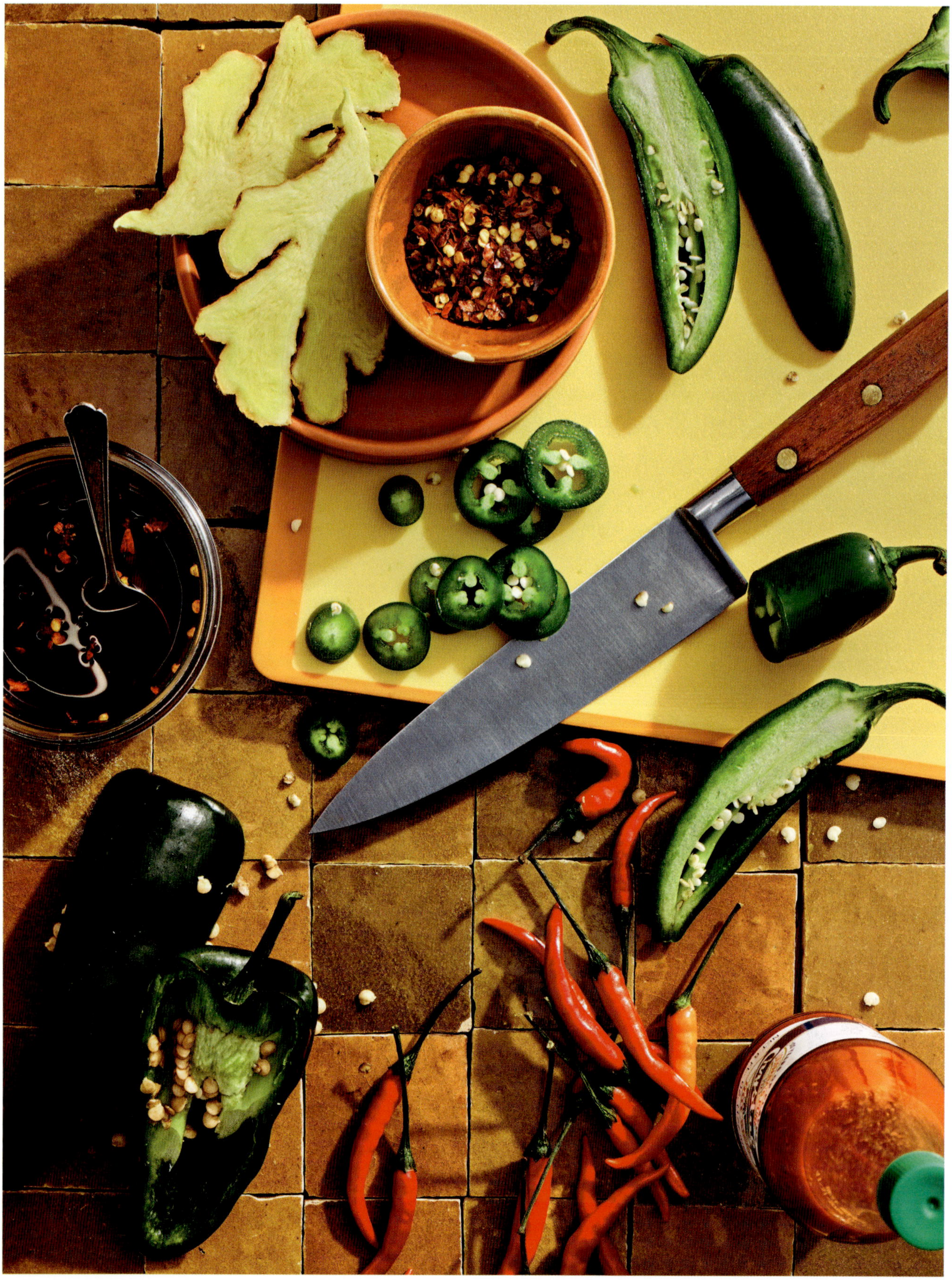

UNIVERSAL CONVERSION CHART

OVEN TEMPERATURE EQUIVALENTS

250°F = 120°C

275°F = 135°C

300°F = 150°C

325°F = 160°C

350°F = 180°C

375°F = 190°C

400°F = 200°C

425°F = 220°C

450°F = 230°C

475°F = 240°C

500°F = 260°C

MEASUREMENT EQUIVALENTS

Measurements should always be level unless directed otherwise.

⅛ teaspoon = 0.5 mL

¼ teaspoon = 1 mL

½ teaspoon = 2 mL

1 teaspoon = 5 mL

1 tablespoon = 3 teaspoons = ½ fluid ounce = 15 mL

2 tablespoons = ⅛ cup = 1 fluid ounce = 30 mL

4 tablespoons = ¼ cup = 2 fluid ounces = 60 mL

5⅓ tablespoons = ⅓ cup = 3 fluid ounces = 80 mL

8 tablespoons = ½ cup = 4 fluid ounces = 120 mL

10⅔ tablespoons = ⅔ cup = 5 fluid ounces = 160 mL

12 tablespoons = ¾ cup = 6 fluid ounces = 180 mL

16 tablespoons = 1 cup = 8 fluid ounces = 240 mL

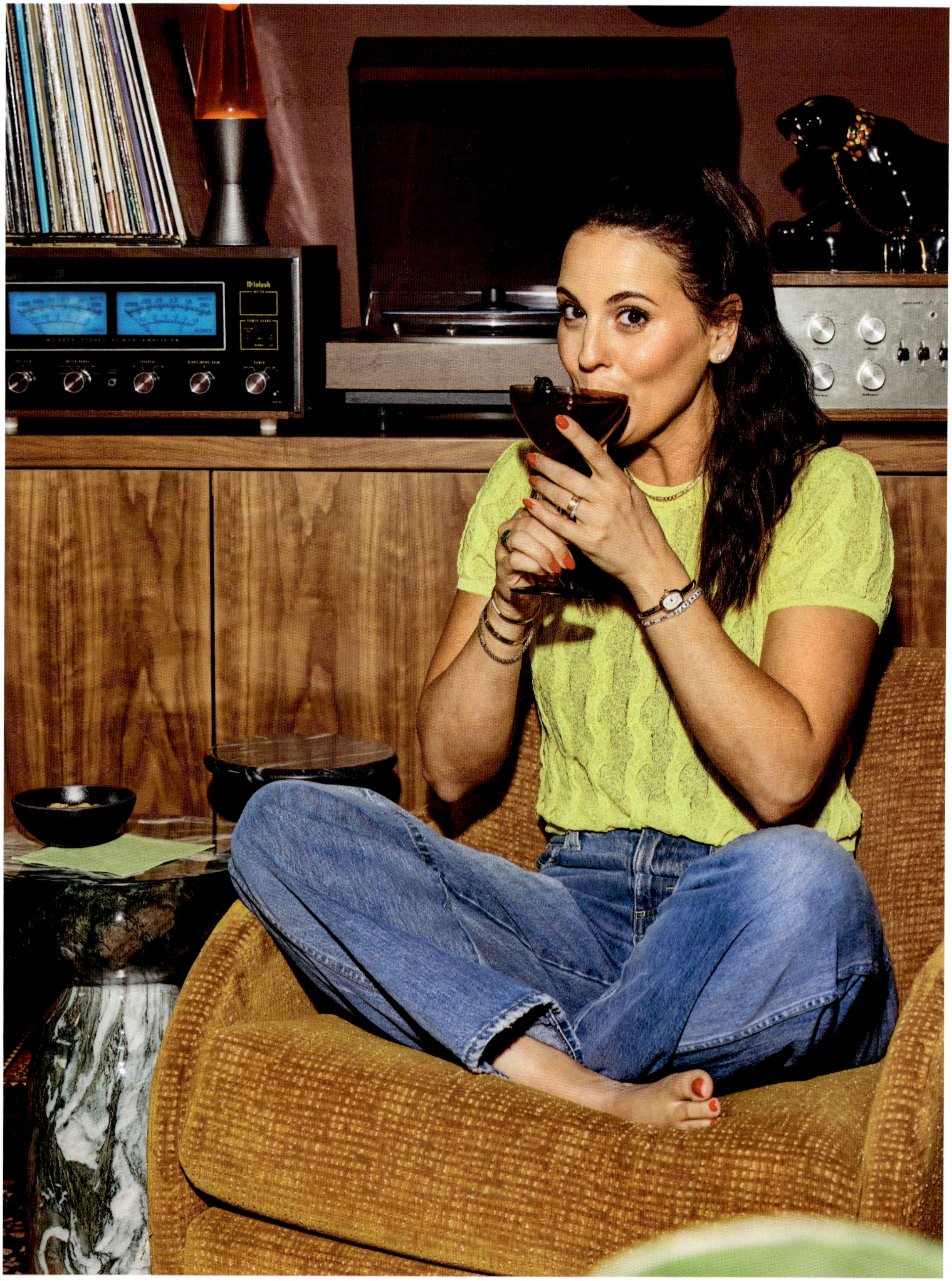

INDEX

Note: Page references in *italics* indicate photographs.

C

O

P

R

S

T

V

W

Y

Z

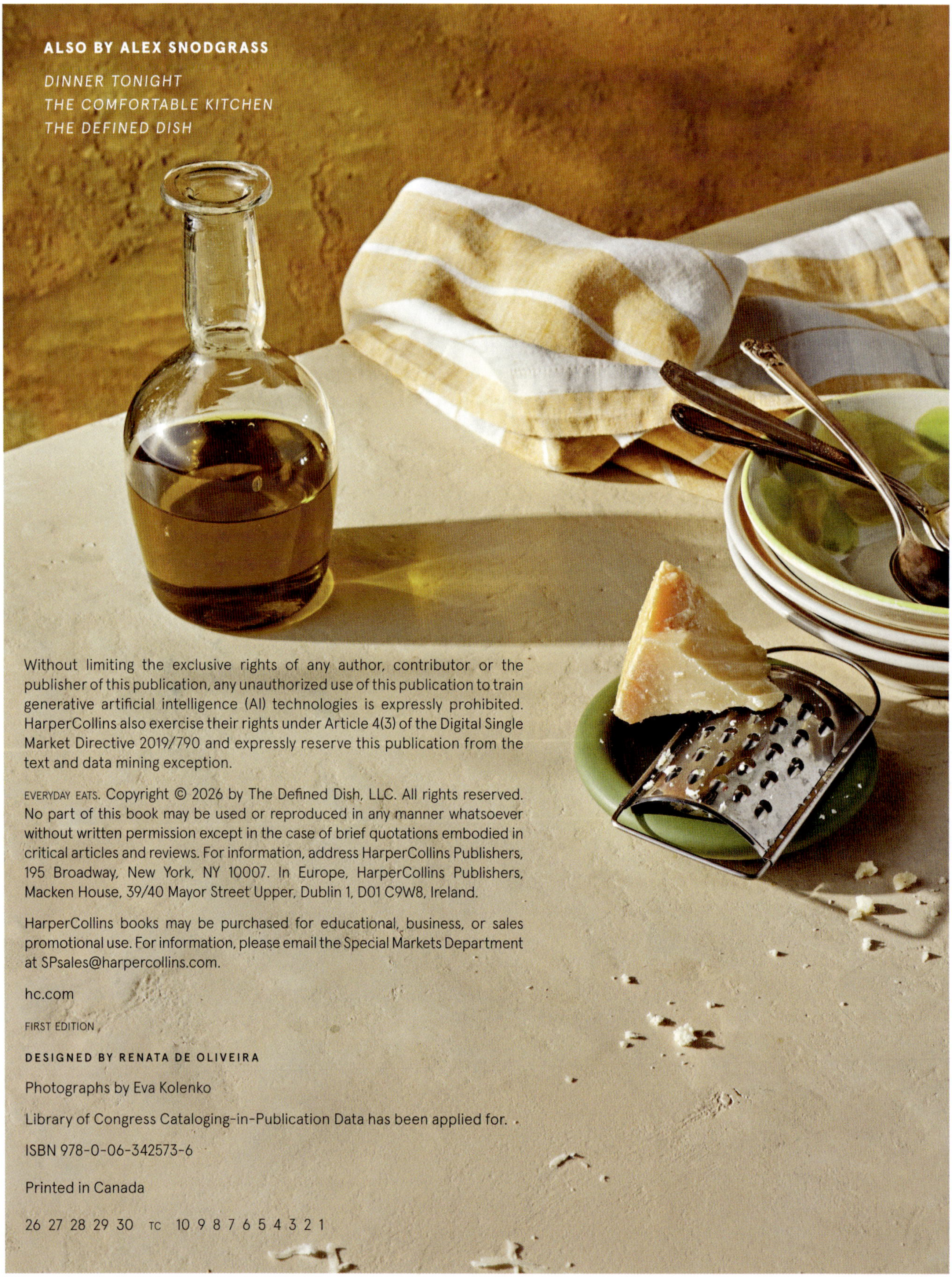

ALSO BY ALEX SNODGRASS

DINNER TONIGHT
THE COMFORTABLE KITCHEN
THE DEFINED DISH

 For information, address HarperCollins Publishers, 195 Broadway, New York, NY 10007. In Europe, HarperCollins Publishers, Macken House, 39/40 Mayor Street Upper, Dublin 1, D01 C9W8, Ireland.

HarperCollins books may be purchased for educational, business, or sales promotional use. For information, please email the Special Markets Department at SPsales@harpercollins.com.

hc.com

FIRST EDITION

DESIGNED BY RENATA DE OLIVEIRA

Photographs by Eva Kolenko

Library of Congress Cataloging-in-Publication Data has been applied for.

ISBN 978-0-06-342573-6

Printed in Canada

26 27 28 29 30 TC 10 9 8 7 6 5 4 3 2 1